How to Succeed in Psychiatry

A Guide to Training and Practice

EDITED BY

ANDREA FIORILLO MD PhD
Professor of Psychiatry
University of Naples SUN, Italy

IRIS TATJANA CALLIESS MD PhD
Department of Psychiatry, Social Psychiatry and Psychotherapy
Institute for Standardized and Applied Hospital Management
Hanover School of Medicine, Germany

HENNING SASS MD
Medical Director
Chairman of the Board, and Professor of Psychiatry
Hospital of the University of Technology
RWTH Aachen, Germany

WILEY-BLACKWELL
A John Wiley & Sons, Ltd., Publication

Library of Congress Cataloging-in-Publication Data

How to succeed in psychiatry : a guide to training and practice / edited by
Andrea Fiorillo, Iris Calliess, and Henning Sass.
         p. ; cm.
     Based on: Professione psichiatra / a cura di Andrea Fiorillo, Mariano Bassi,
Alberto Siracusano. 1. ed. 2009.
     Includes bibliographical references and index.
     ISBN 978-1-119-99866-2 (pbk)
     I. Fiorillo, Andrea.   II. Calliess, Iris Tatjana.   III. Sass, Henning.
IV. Professione psichiatra.
     [DNLM: 1. Psychiatry.   2. Professional Practice.   3. Psychiatry–education.
4. Vocational Guidance.   WM 21]
     616.89–dc23
                                              2011043614

A catalogue record for this book is available from the British Library.

Wiley also publishes its books in a variety of electronic formats. Some content that appears in print may not be available in electronic books.

Typeset in 10/12.5pt Meridien by Laserwords Private Limited, Chennai, India.
Printed and bound in Malaysia by Vivar Printing Sdn Bhd

First Impression 2012

Contents

List of contributors

Olivier Andlauer
Department of Psychiatry, University Hospital, Besançon, France

Julian Beezhold
Norfolk and Waveney Mental Health NHS Foundation Trust, United Kingdom, University of East Anglia, Norwich, UK

Joshua Blum
Department of Psychiatry, University of Massachusetts Medical School, Worcester, MA, USA

Stavroula Boukouvala
Norfolk and Waveney Mental Health Care NHS Foundation Trust, Norwich, UK

Emma Brandon
Norfolk and Waveney Mental Health NHS Foundation Trust, Norwich, UK

Otilia Butiu
Psychiatric Department, University of Medicine and Pharmacy Tg Mures, Romania

Victor Buwalda
Altrecht ggz, Utrecht/Den Dolder and Department of Psychiatry,

Free University of Amsterdam, The Netherlands

Iris Tatjana Calliess
Department of Psychiatry, Social Psychiatry and Psychotherapy, Institute for Standardized and Applied Hospital Management, Hannover School of Medicine, Germany.

Giuseppe Carrà
Department of Mental Health Sciences, University College Medical School, London, UK; Department of Neurosciences and Biomedical Technologies, University of Milano Bicocca Medical School, Monza, Italy

Massimo Clerici
Department of Neurosciences and Biomedical Technologies, University of Milano Bicocca Medical School, Monza, Italy

Stephanie Colin
AP-HP, Hôpital Avicenne, Service de psychopathologie de l'enfant, de l'adolescent, psychiatrie générale et addictions, Bobigny, France

Michael Davis
Department of Psychiatry and Biobehavioral Sciences, Semel

Institute, University of
California Los Angeles (UCLA),
Los Angeles, CA, USA

Valeria Del Vecchio
Department of Psychiatry,
University of Naples SUN,
Naples, Italy

Corrado De Rosa
Department of Psychiatry,
University of Naples SUN,
Naples, Italy

Abigail L. Donovan
Harvard University,
Massachusetts General
Hospital, Boston, MA, USA

Defne Eraslan
Department of Psychiatry,
Faculty of Medicine, Acibadem
University, Istanbul, Turkey

Silvia Ferrari
Department of Mental Health,
University of Modena and
Reggio Emilia, Policlinico di
Modena, Italy

Andrea Fiorillo
Department of Psychiatry,
University of Naples SUN,
Naples, Italy

Domenico Giacco
Department of Psychiatry,
University of Naples SUN,
Naples, Italy

Cecile Hanon
EPS Erasme, Antony, France

Sameer Jauhar
Sackler Institute of
Psychobiological Research,
Institute of Neurological
Sciences, Southern General
Hospital, Glasgow, UK

Sarah Johnson
Department of Psychiatry,
University of Louisville, KY,
USA

Nikolina Jovanović
Department of Psychiatry,
University Hospital Centre and
Zagreb School of Medicine,
Croatia

Marianne Kastrup
Centre Transcultural Psychiatry,
Psychiatric Centre
Copenhagen, Denmark

Patrick Kelly
Division of Child and Adolescent
Psychiatry, Department of
Psychiatry and Behavioral
Sciences, The Johns Hopkins
Hospital, Baltimore, MD, USA

Mario Luciano
Department of Psychiatry,
University of Naples SUN,
Naples, Italy

Gregory Lydall
Castel Hospital, La Neuve Rue,
Guernsey; University College
London, London, UK

Amit Malik
Southern Health NHS
Foundation Trust, Aerodrome
House, Gosport, UK

Kate Manley
Norfolk and Waveney Mental
 Health Care NHS Foundation
 Trust, Norwich, UK

Dominique Mathis
Institut Paul Sivadon, Hôpital de
 l'Elan Retrouvé, Paris, France

Nya Maughn
Norfolk and Waveney Mental
 Health Care NHS Foundation
 Trust, Hellesdon Hospital,
 Norwich, UK

Molly McVoy
University Hospitals of
 Cleveland/Case Western
 Reserve, Cleveland, OH, USA

Adriana Mihai
Psychiatric Department,
 University of Medicine and
 Pharmacy Tg Mures, Romania

Davor Mucic
Psychiatric Centre "Little Prince",
 Copenhagen, Denmark

Alexander Nawka
Department of Psychiatry, First
 Faculty of Medicine, Charles
 University, Prague, Czech
 Republic

Fiona Nolan
Centre for Outcomes Research
 and Effectiveness (CORE), Sub
 Department of Clinical Health
 Psychology, University College
 London, London, UK

Kajsa B. Norstrom
Psychiatric Unit Angered, Capio
 Lundby Hospital, Goteborg,
 Sweden

Clare Oakley
St Andrew's Academic Centre,
 Institute of Psychiatry, King's
 College London, London, UK

Paul J. O'Leary
Department of Psychiatry, Emory
 University, Atlanta, Georgia,
 USA

Magdalena Peckskamp
Department of Psychology,
 University of Vienna, Austria

Felipe Picon
Department of Psychiatry,
 Federal University of Rio
 Grande do Sul, Porto Alegre,
 RS, Brazil

Florian Riese
Psychiatric University Hospital
 Zurich, Switzerland

Martina Rojnic Kuzman
Department of Psychiatry, Zagreb
 University Hospital Centre and
 Zagreb School of Medicine,
 Zagreb, Croatia

Larissa Ryan
Warneford Hospital, Oxford, UK

Virginio Salvi
Mood and Anxiety Disorders
 Unit, Department of
 Psychiatry, University of Turin,
 Italy

Henning Sass
Department of Psychiatry,
    University of Technology
    RWTH, Aachen, Germany

Paola Sciarini
Department of Neurosciences and
    Biomedical Technologies,
    University of Milano Bicocca
    Medical School, Monza, Italy;
Department of Health Sciences,
    Section of Medical Statistics
    and Epidemiology, University
    of Pavia Medical School, Pavia,
    Italy

Joseph Stoklosa
Harvard Medical School, McLean
    Hospital, Boston, MA, USA

Kai C. Treichel
Medical Center Friedrichshain
    Berlin, Germany

Umberto Volpe
Department of Psychiatry,
    University of Naples SUN,
    Naples, Italy

Preface

What does it take to become a psychiatrist today? What are the training and educational needs for modern psychiatrists? What does it mean to be a psychiatrist today? What are the professional responsibilities of psychiatrists and of other mental health workers? And what will be their perspectives in the future? These are only some of the questions we have tried to address in this book, promoted by the EPA Early Career Psychiatrists Committee and the European Federation of Psychiatric Trainees, which includes 21 chapters by 50 authors from 16 different countries.

The book "How to succeed in psychiatry: a guide to training and practice" is not a source of clinical information, but rather a survival guide to help young colleagues through the first years of practice. A "survival" kit seems to be particularly needed by young psychiatrists in our days, who are very different from colleagues starting their career only a few years ago. The clinical choices of young psychiatrists today seem to be driven predominantly by the need to avoid professional errors rather than the wish to find the best and most effective therapeutic treatment. In clinical practice, young psychiatrists quite often adopt "defensive" medical styles in order to avoid complaints and litigation with patients, family members, stakeholders and also with managers. More often than in the past, young psychiatrists report not being able to bear stressful working situations and experiencing high levels of burn-out, with anxiety and depressive symptoms. Belonging to scientific and professional associations is one way to prevent these feelings and to improve young doctors' skills. Other ways to overcome these possible difficulties are reported in this book; they include setting the correct priorities for one's own life and career or choosing the "right" career among the various possibilities (e.g. private practice, community or hospital settings, academic career).

The volume is organized as an ideal path from training to employment, presenting all the relevant difficulties of being a psychiatrist today, as well as possible solutions, being represented. The book opens with an overview of psychiatric training, describing the similarities and differences among various countries. Subsequent chapters address the opportunities for research studies and for getting the results published. Chapters 4 and 5 describe training in psychotherapy and in community psychiatry, both of which are particularly relevant for young psychiatrists, as they represent two of the most frequent possible working scenarios. In chapter 7 the importance of telecommunication resources for the psychiatric profession and the risks associated with the use of new technologies are described. Chapter 8 addresses cultural factors that can influence psychiatric training. Chapter 9 deals with the problem of the shortage of psychiatrists, focusing on the transition from medical school to training in psychiatry.

Next, the book guides the reader through the transition phase into a job, discussing job opportunities in both the public and private sectors and suggesting how to choose the best career. Chapter 12 deals with job opportunities in the private sector; this is an ever-expanding sector and often represents one of the first employment opportunities after specialization. In chapter 19 the topics of mental health, work stress and burnout, to which mental health professionals seem to be particularly vulnerable, are addressed. Authors report data from the literature showing an increased risk of stress in younger colleagues and provide, at the same time, practical advice that we should all learn to follow.

The following section of the book reviews important general and legal considerations, such as ethics, professionalism, leadership and management, and how to liaise with other specialties. Professional responsibility in medicine today is a "hot" issue, and the emphasis given to this topic reflects the sensitivity of young psychiatrists to these issues. What the authors of this volume have not lost is the ethics of medical work. Chapter 17 is a useful discussion of the most significant ethical and deontological aspects of medicine in general, not only of psychiatry. In chapter 18 practical suggestions regarding compulsory hospital treatments and the use of coercive measures are offered. Again, this is a hotly-debated issue in clinical psychiatry, for which early career psychiatrists do not seem to have all the necessary information, being too often overlooked in the curricula of psychiatrists. The book closes with an account of the role of psychiatric associations and continuing professional development.

Although this book is aimed mainly at recently qualified psychiatrists or those looking to qualify soon, we believe it will be useful for all psychiatrists, including more experienced colleagues: while reading the book, they will go back in time to when they were young psychiatrists and re-experience the curious and exploratory approach to life, which is – in our opinion – the true essence of being a psychiatrist today. We hope that young psychiatrists worldwide will succeed in their aims and careers, but will never lose this attitude of "curious determination" that brought them to choose psychiatry.

We are grateful to a number of people. It is almost impossible to name all of them. Basically, we want to thank here our contributors, who have provided excellent chapters and who have enthusiastically joined this initiative; the leadership of the European Psychiatric Association, which has supported us throughout the preparation of the book; Professors Bhugra and Sartorius, for their valuable advice in selecting chapters and authors; Joan Marsh and her team at Wiley-Blackwell. We are greatly indebted and grateful to all of them.

Andrea Fiorillo, Iris Tatjana Calliess, Henning Sass

CHAPTER 1

Training in psychiatry today: European and US perspectives

Martina Rojnic Kuzman,[1] Kajsa B. Norstrom,[2] Stephanie Colin,[3] Clare Oakley[4] and Joseph Stoklosa[5]

[1]Department of Psychiatry, Zagreb University Hospital Centre and Zagreb School of Medicine, Zagreb, Croatia
[2]Psychiatric Unit Angered, Capio Lundby Hospital, Goteborg, Sweden
[3]AP-HP, Hôpital Avicenne, Service de psychopathologie de l'enfant, de l'adolescent, psychiatrie générale et addictions, Bobigny, France
[4]St Andrew's Academic Centre, Institute of Psychiatry, King's College London, UK
[5]Harvard Medical School, McLean Hospital, Boston, MA, USA

Introduction

The last few decades have brought rapid social changes, which have greatly influenced health, communication, ethics, politics and economics. Psychiatry, as a significant component of the health-care system, has also been affected by these changes. Nowadays, trainees and early career psychiatrists worldwide are facing several challenges, quite different from those faced previously. Young psychiatrists acquire the competencies requisite of a mental health professional through medical schools and postgraduate residency trainings, and this formative stage is crucial for the development of competent mental health professionals.

Psychiatric training in Europe

In Europe, training programmes in psychiatry are developed and subsequently implemented by educational policy-makers, at national levels in each European country. Accreditation policy as well as quality assurance mechanisms also fall within the remit of authorities at national levels. The need for harmonized postgraduate training in psychiatry has developed

How to Succeed in Psychiatry: A Guide to Training and Practice, First Edition.
Edited by Andrea Fiorillo, Iris Tatjana Calliess and Henning Sass.
© 2012 John Wiley & Sons, Ltd. Published 2012 by John Wiley & Sons, Ltd.

in parallel with the development of the European Union. Today, the Section and Board of Psychiatry of the Union Européenne des Médecins Spécialistes (UEMS) play an active part in shaping the future of European psychiatrists. UEMS was established in 1958 as a response to the signing of the Treaty of Rome in 1957, where harmonization and mutual recognition of diplomas was foreseen.[1] In 1990, the Section of Psychiatry was formed to deal primarily with general issues related to psychiatric practice and quality assurance of psychiatric care. In 1992 the Board of Psychiatry was formed, focusing on training issues. In 1993 the Treaty of Maastricht was signed on an EU level, which opened up the internal market and free movement of goods, persons, services and capital. Today, 27 European countries benefit from this Treaty, and in the last decade this has been reflected in an increasing migration of psychiatric trainees and psychiatrists across Europe.

Due to the observed huge variations in training standards, training programmes and training facilities in European countries, in 1993 the UEMS published the Charter of specialist training.[2] The Section and Board of Psychiatry have drafted and approved numerous reports and guidelines to enhance the speed and recognition of the harmonization process in psychiatric training. These documents concern several areas, such as training in psychotherapy, supervision, quality assurance and accreditation of training schemes in psychiatry, and in 2009 a European framework for competencies in psychiatry was published.[3] These documents are considered as guidelines and it is intended that the member countries use them in order to reform their national training programmes. UEMS has no legal authority to enforce changes in any particular country; therefore, it is important to have a continuous process of discussion and to promote a supportive attitude in order to make progress with the harmonization of psychiatric training.

Trainees' perspectives in Europe are represented by the European Federation of Psychiatric Trainees (EFPT), the first and only international organization of national psychiatric trainees' associations. EFPT has full voting rights at the European Board of Psychiatry of the UEMS, contributing significantly to the cooperation between the two organizations. The Federation has grown rapidly over the years and currently encompasses more then 30 member countries across Europe.[4]

As regards child and adolescent psychiatry (CAP) training in Europe, the UEMS CAP training logbook states that 'children are not simply small adults'. Nevertheless, the core identity of child and adolescent psychiatry has been at stake for the last few decades. Whereas in most European countries CAP has slowly grown to become an independent specialty, separated from adult psychiatry, in others it is still a subspecialty or is still strongly linked with paediatrics. Hence, there are huge discrepancies in the training programmes in CAP in Europe. Within the UEMS, CAP psychiatrists used to be represented in the Section and Board of Psychiatry, until the establishment of a separate Section and Board in 1992. The ideas behind this initiative to split within the UEMS were to promote high standards of mental health care for children across Europe, both directly and indirectly, by establishing standards and improving the quality of postgraduate CAP training, with a particularly strong emphasis on training in psychotherapy.[5]

Again, the perspective of European CAP trainees is represented by the EFPT, which now provides a valuable framework for European child and adolescent psychiatry trainees to discuss and exchange ideas. Its inner structure has recently been modified in response to the growing identity claims of CAP trainees, as a new board position for a 'CAP secretary' was created, allowing specific representation of CAP trainees in European CAP meetings, and enhanced links with international organizations, such as UEMS-CAP and the European Society for Child and Adolescent Psychiatrists (ESCAP).

Psychiatric training in the USA

The young psychiatrist training and practising in the USA today faces a different set of challenges than the psychiatrist training just a few decades ago. The structure of psychiatric training itself has shifted from a participation-based into a competency-based model, in response to pressures from government, practitioners and patients to make physicians more accountable to the public. Psychiatric training is regulated by a single governing body for all US residencies, which is a private, non-profit council called the Accreditation Council for Graduate Medical Education (ACGME). The ACGME was established in 1981 from demands in the academic medical community for an independent crediting association with the mission to 'improve health care by assessing and advancing the quality of resident physicians' education through exemplary accreditation'.[6] Comprising 28 specialty-specific Residency Review Committees (RRCs), each RRC is formed by 6–15 volunteer physicians appointed by the American Medical Association (AMA) and individual specialty boards. It is these RRCs that then determine the specific programme requirements for each specialty training programme, including psychiatry. RRCs also have direct oversight on each specific training programme institution to ensure sufficient support within each programme. Each residency training programme submits to a review by its RRC at least every 5 years. During review, each programme provides extensive information on all aspects of training, which is then verified by the site visit to solicit trainee and faculty feedback, and make direct observations on patient care, staff and facilities.[7]

In 1959, child and adolescent psychiatry was established as an official subspecialty of general psychiatry. Residents wishing to pursue this subspecialty can enter the two-year fellowship after either their third or fourth year of general psychiatry training. The core requirements of child and adolescent specialty training also fall under the purview of the psychiatry RRC.

Around this system of regulation, several unique situations in US culture have evolved that sculpt the modern psychiatry resident's experiences, including the rise of core competency-driven education, the advent of national duty hours regulations, and the US health-care system of managed care.

State of the art of psychiatric training in Europe

For the majority of European countries, curricula for psychiatric training across Europe are set by national authorities. In a significant proportion of European countries, the curricula are developed in accordance with the UEMS requirements for the specialty of psychiatry and standards, as defined in the document called the 'Charter on training of medical specialists in the EU: requirements for the specialty of psychiatry'.[2] A selection of the UEMS recommendations is given in Table 1.1.

While in most European countries the structures of training programmes are reasonably compatible with standards set by the UEMS, the duration of different placements, as well as the duration of training as a whole, varies across Europe. This is more pronounced in some parts of Europe – the shorter duration of training is seen in some parts of Eastern and southeastern European countries, but not in all countries. There are great differences in the psychiatric trainees' assessment before they become specialists: some countries have neither examinations nor other methods of assessment, while other countries employ a range of assessment methods, including different types of examination, workplace-based assessments, portfolios and supervisor's reports.[8] An overview of the structure of training programmes in Europe is given in Table 1.2.

Recently, a UEMS survey aiming to find out whether the UEMS directives had an impact on the conditions of psychiatry training across Europe was conducted.[9] The authors concluded that while there were great differences between the training centres in different countries, progress towards developing high standards had been made. The parts of the training programmes that display major variations and that show little coherence even within a country seem to be supervision (especially educational supervision) and psychotherapy training.[9] These findings are compatible with recent EFPT data, where the most important problems faced by postgraduate psychiatric trainees across countries

Table 1.1 A selection of requirements for the specialty of psychiatry according to charter on training of medical specialists in the EU released by the Union Européenne des Médecins Spécialistes (UEMS).[2]

Article	Content
CENTRAL MONITORING AUTHORITY FOR PSYCHIATRY (defines the requirements for the monitoring Authority, the recognition of teachers and training Institutions, quality assurance mechanisms and recognition of quality)	
GENERAL ASPECTS OF TRAINING IN PSYCHIATRY (in addition, it defines the selection and access to the training, the circumstances of the interruption of training, training abroad and funding)	Training duration The minimum duration of training will be 5 years in psychiatry; can take place in different institutions if they are recognized nationally as training institutions; part-time training should be possible in every EU member state Definition of common trunk Within the national training programme in psychiatry there is a common trunk of fundamental knowledge and skills that is required of all candidates. The common trunk is compulsory. This common trunk includes training in inpatient psychiatry (short, medium and long stay), outpatient psychiatry (community psychiatry, day-hospital), liaison and consultation psychiatry, and emergency psychiatry. Psychotherapy training is also part of the common trunk. Training should cover general adult psychiatry, old age psychiatry, psychiatric aspects of substance misuse, developmental psychiatry (child and adolescent psychiatry, learning difficulties and mental handicap) and forensic psychiatry. The training programme can include not more than one year of flexible training (e.g. research or other related subjects to be approved by the head of training) Practical training Practical training should evolve around routine clinical work under supervision. As training progresses there should be an increasing level of responsibility. During the period of training rotation within different sections of an institution should be compulsory. Rotation to different institutions should be facilitated

(*continued overleaf*)

Table 1.1 (Continued)

Article	Content
	Supervision
	Clinical supervision should be available on a daily basis. In addition to clinical supervision and psychotherapy supervision, individual educational supervision (dealing with such subjects as attitude, growth in the profession, etc.) is compulsory for a minimum of 1 hour per week, at least 40 weeks per year
	Implementation of training programme/training logbook
	The theoretical and practical training will follow an established programme approved by the national authorities in accordance with national rules and EU legislation as well as with the requirements and recommendations of the European Board of Psychiatry. The different stages and the activities of training and the activities of trainees should be recorded in a training logbook
	APPENDIX 1: Theoretical training
	Training should include a structured training (lectures, seminars, etc.) over 4 years, on average for 4 hours per week. The subjects to be covered are the scientific basis of psychiatry, psychopathology, examination of a psychiatric patient, diagnosis and classification, psychological tests and laboratory investigations, specific disorders and syndromes, child and adolescent psychiatry, mental handicap, psychiatric aspects of substance misuse, old age psychiatry, diversity in psychiatry, legal, ethical and human rights issues in psychiatry, psychotherapies, psychopharmacology and other biological treatments, multidimensional clinical management, community psychiatry, social psychiatric interventions, research methodology, epidemiology of mental disorders, psychiatric aspects of public health and prevention, medical informatics and telemedicine, leadership, administration, management, economics

(continued overleaf)

Table 1.1 (Continued)

Article	Content
	APPENDIX 2: Training in psychotherapy
	Psychotherapy is an integral part of training in psychiatry. The content that is considered essential for training in psychotherapy include a mandatory part of the training curriculum that takes place within working hours, practical application of psychotherapy in a defined number of cases, theory of psychotherapy over at least 120 hours, supervision provided on a regular basis for at least 100 hours, individual (at least 50 hours) but preferably also group supervision. Experience should be gained with a broad range of diagnostic categories, including assessment and evaluation of outcome. Experience in psychotherapy should be gained with individuals as well as families and groups. As a minimum, psychodynamic, cognitive behavioural therapy (CBT), and systemic theory and methods should be applied, but integrative psychotherapies are highly recommended. Personal therapeutic experience/feedback on personal style is highly recommended. Research methodology should be included
	Training should if possible take place within different parts of mental health services. Supervisors should be qualified. Training should be publicly funded
REQUIREMENTS FOR TRAINING INSTITUTIONS (defines the criteria for the recognition of training institutions, their size and the quality assurance of training institutions)	
REQUIREMENTS FOR TEACHERS (defines the qualification of the chief of training and the training programme)	
REQUIREMENTS FOR TRAINEES (defines the required experience, language skills and specialization for trainees)	

Table 1.2 Training programmes for adult psychiatry across Europe.

Country	Duration of training (years)	Structure of training programme	Assessments and examinations	Separate CAP training	Meeting UEMS recommendations
Austria	5	NA	Examinations Portfolio	Yes	Yes, in part
Belarus	1	Only covered acute psychiatric care, outpatients, substance abuse, daily programmes, CAP, rehabilitation	Examinations Portfolio	No	No
Belgium	5	Basic schema*	Examinations Portfolio	No	Yes, significantly
Bosnia	4	Three programmes, but in one followed the basic schema*, but no old age, liaison	Examinations Portfolio	No	Yes, in part
Czech Republic	5.5	Basic schema*, but fulfilled the requirements for psychotherapy, no liaison and forensics	Examinations Portfolio	No	Yes, significantly
Croatia	4	Basic schema*, no old age, liaison	Examinations Portfolio	No	Yes, in part
Denmark	5	Basic schema*, no liaison		Yes	Yes, significantly
Estonia	4	Basic schema*, no old age psychiatry, no liaison and forensics	Examinations WPBA Portfolio	No	Yes, significantly
Finland	6	Basic schema*	Examinations Portfolio	Yes	Yes, significantly
France	4	Basic schema*, no psychotherapy	None	No	Yes, significantly
Germany	5	Basic schema*, no forensics, no liaison plus neurosurgery/ neuropathology	Examinations Portfolio	Yes	Yes, in part
Greece	5	Basic schema*, no psychotherapy, no liaison	Examinations	Yes	Yes, in part
Ireland	6	Basic schema*	Examinations WPBA Portfolio	Yes	Yes, significantly
Italy	5	Basic schema*, no psychotherapy, no old age	Examinations	Yes	Yes, significantly

(continued overleaf)

Table 1.2 (Continued)

Country	Duration of training (years)	Structure of training programme	Assessments and examinations	Separate CAP training	Meeting UEMS recommendations
Latvia	4	Basic schema* plus rehabilitation	Examinations Portfolio	No	Yes, in part
Lithuania	4	Basic schema*	Examinations Portfolio	NA	Yes, in part
Malta	5	Basic schema*	Examinations Portfolio	NA	Yes, significantly
Netherlands	4,5	Basic schema*	Examinations WPBA Portfolio	Yes	Yes, significantly
Norway	5	Basic schema*	Portfolio	Yes	Yes, in part
Poland	5	Basic schema*, no old age	Examinations Portfolio	Yes	Yes, significantly
Portugal	5	Basic schema*, no old age, no psychotherapy	Examinations	Yes	Yes, significantly
Romania	5	Basic schema*	Examinations Portfolio	Yes	Yes, significantly
Russia	2	NA	NA	No	No
Serbia	4	Basic schema*, no old age and psychotherapy, liaison	Examinations Portfolio	Yes	Yes, in part
Slovakia	5	Basic schema*, no liaison	Examinations Portfolio	Yes	Yes, in part
Slovenia	5	Basic schema*, no liaison	Examinations Portfolio	Yes	Yes, significantly
Sweden	5	Basic schema*, no liaison	Portfolio	Yes	Yes, significantly
Switzerland	6	Basic schema*	Examinations WPBA Portfolio	Yes	Yes, significantly
Turkey	5	Basic schema*, no old age, liaison, no psychotherapy	Examinations Portfolio	Yes	Yes, significantly
UK	6	Basic schema*	Examinations WPBA Portfolio	Yes	Yes, significantly
Ukraine	1.5	Inpatient psychiatry, outpatient psychiatry, drug abuse	Examinations	No	No

*Basic schema = training in in-patient psychiatry (short, medium and long stay), outpatient psychiatry (community psychiatry, day-hospital), liaison and consultation psychiatry, and emergency psychiatry in general adult psychiatry, old age psychiatry, psychiatric aspects of substance misuse, developmental psychiatry, and forensic psychiatry.
*CAP, child and adolescent psychiatry; UEMS, Union Européenne des Médecins Spécialistes; WPBA, workplace-based assessments.

were implementation of postgraduate curricula, psychotherapy training and lack of supervision.[10] Problems with the implementation of training programmes are related to the implementation of newly developed programmes in some countries, while in others there is a significant gap between the conception of the training systems that are prescribed by the national educational bodies and their delivery at a local level. This issue might be related to the overall shortage of psychiatrists,[11] leaving the trainees without proper educational and clinical supervision, but also leaving the trainees to engage in the tasks of fully trained specialists, which they are not yet competent to do. It may also be due to the lack of accredited or high quality facilities in many parts of Europe (especially in eastern and southern countries) and to the heterogeneity of standards of training in different centres, even within the same country, with a consequent relative overload of trainees in some placements and thus long waiting lists for some rotations. Another reason for explaining implementation problems of training programmes might be the lack of adherence to the recommended quality assurance mechanisms at the national and international levels.

In recent years, a significant shift in the philosophy of training has occurred. As the result of the work of the UEMS and of national authorities in several European countries, a competency-based framework for training, including a competency-based curriculum and assessment programmes ranging from workplace-based assessments to exit examinations, was designed and it is now being implemented in several European countries.[12] Whilst this introduction of competency-based training represents a major shift in medical education, new challenges arise with this transition, due to the high demands on trainers to deliver this relatively intensive method of providing postgraduate training and to the new regulations for residents. Nevertheless, the benefits of the new programme are clear and, thus, it is firmly supported by both the UEMS and the EFPT.

Although European child and adolescent psychiatry has undergone impressive development over the past 50 years, there is still a huge variability in the structure of CAP training across Europe, and a long way to go for full harmonization in the programs. CAP is now an independent specialty in more then 20 countries and a subspecialty in the rest of them, but some countries still do not have any structured CAP training curriculum (Table 1.2).[13] One of the main achievements of the UEMS CAP Board was to publish a training logbook, which has been implemented at least partially in two-thirds of the countries.[14] It specifically states that the minimum duration of postgraduate training should be 5 years, of which 4 years should be pure CAP. Training differences are marked even within the EU member countries, and not only in terms of content of training programmes, but also of duration, trainee selection and graduation procedures. Moreover, a lack of detailed information regarding training curricula in several countries has also to be acknowledged. While the UEMS-CAP logbook emphasizes training in psychotherapy as being mandatory, only half of the countries have integrated structured psychotherapy training as a full component of CAP training. Interestingly, trainees in almost all countries have to pay with their personal funds for their psychotherapeutic education within CAP training. In virtually all European countries, experience in psychiatry with adults of working age is a necessary component of training in CAP. Similarly, experience in paediatrics is welcome, or required, in many countries. Training in research, however, is integrated as a structured part of the training only in one-third of the countries.

Leaving the tradition of any particular country aside, and devising an adequate yet realistic training schedule that would incorporate such experiences, the UEMS CAP Board recommended a 12-month minimum time for training in adult psychiatry. Similar rotations in paediatrics or neurology are recommended, but they are optional. The logbook has already proven to be important in helping new EU member countries to develop their own training programme in CAP.[15] However, standards set in the logbook are high and may well exceed those set by relevant authorities in each country: they should therefore be inspirational.

State of the art of psychiatric training in the USA

The Accreditation Council for Graduate Medical Education policy defines a set of specific requirements for psychiatric training programmes that are seeking accreditation. Currently, residency education in psychiatry requires 4 years of training.[16] Thus, the newly graduated doctor, having just completed medical school, must undertake an additional 4 years of training prior to practising as an independent physician. The first year of training includes 4 months in a primary care setting (internal medicine, family medicine and/or paediatrics), and 2 months in neurology. The second 6 months can comprise additional medical training or introductory psychiatry training. The second year of residency marks the true beginning of psychiatry training; this includes at least 9 months of inpatient psychiatry and 12 months of continuous outpatient psychiatry that uses both psychotherapy and biological therapies. Additional requirements exist to ensure diversity of experience within the inpatient and outpatient training, including at least 2 months of child and adolescent psychiatry, 1 month of geriatric psychiatry, 1 month of addiction psychiatry, and 2 months of consultation/liaison psychiatry. Residents must also have clinical experience in the following areas: forensic psychiatry, emergency psychiatry, community/public sector psychiatry, group, couples and family therapy, and psychological testing. Residents must participate in a didactic curriculum that includes neurobiology, psychopharmacology, major theories of psychotherapy, child development and cultural issues in psychiatry. Training must encompass a wide variety of clinical experiences with different patient populations. The ACGME is committed to achieving a balance between psychodynamic and biological psychiatry, in both education and clinical care.

Beyond the specific educational components, the ACGME also sets recommendations on the hierarchical structure of programmes and specific monitoring parameters. These various requirements include regulations for necessary programme personnel, faculty qualifications, educational resources, specific competencies, scholarly activities' participation, resident and faculty evaluations, and duty hours. In order to meet ACGME certification, these requirements must all be met during RRC review.

The ACGME previously guided psychiatric training by a set of 'minimum standards' that needed to be met by each trainee in order to complete training. These 'minimum standards' were met through completion of the required rotations and clinical experiences; thus, the model was largely participation-based.[17] Each training programme was responsible for defining and implementing its own system to assess satisfactory performance on these required rotations. However, in 2000 the ACGME dramatically changed the requirements for education assessment from merely participation-based to competency-based. The idea of measuring competence grew out of a culture in the USA that prized directly measurable outcomes. This 'outcomes movement' began in the 1980s in a variety of non-medical industries, such as aviation and business, with great success.[17] In medicine, this movement followed society's shift toward research and evidence-based outcomes and away from traditional physician judgment and intuition. This was soon embodied nationally with the establishment in 1989 of the Agency for Health Care Policy and Research. The outcomes movement reached educational programmes when the Department of Education mandated that graduate educational institutions shift to an outcomes model. In the 1990s, this model reached residency training when the ACGME endorsed its own definition of outcomes-based competence by defining a set of basic skills necessary for residents to practise medicine. In 2000, the ACGME formalized its recommendations as the 'six core competencies', which now define the specific abilities and skills that comprise residency training and drive the focus for resident education. Residents must now demonstrate competency in the following six areas: patient care (including clinical reasoning), medical knowledge, practice-based learning and improvement, interpersonal and communication skills, professionalism and system-based practice.[6] While each programme may use individual models of assessment for each competency, these universal core competencies have changed the focus and face of psychiatric training on a national level.

A second major shift in US residency training is the advent of strict duty hours limitations. The days of residents working 36-hour shifts, and up to 120 hours per week, are no more. In 2003 the ACGME passed its own work hours regulations for residents, which include: (i) weekly duty hours must be no more than 80 hours per week; (ii) no shift longer than 24 hours, with an additional 6 hours for transfer of care; (iii) at least 10 hours off between shifts; (iv) call every third night or less frequently; and (v) one day off in seven.[18] There is a debate regarding the merits of duty hour regulations. Supporting duty hours regulation, studies show that residents make more serious medical errors, medication errors and diagnostic errors after long shifts in the intensive care unit.[19] Given that psychiatric evaluation requires a high level of attentiveness to the patient and empathic responsiveness, it is felt by supporters that these regulations protect residents and patients alike from poor quality therapy, consultations or evaluations.[20] Furthermore, for the increasing numbers of physicians choosing specialties based on lifestyle, shorter work hours allow for a new kind of professionalism and life balance to emerge.

However, duty hour regulations also have a number of drawbacks. More frequent pass offs (handovers or transfer of care) may also lead to a decrease in alliance and connection with patients, which are central to effective psychiatric care. There are worries that limited duty hours are leading to less overall training per resident, less exposure to patient diversity, and less direct patient contact.[21] Given that early estimates showed 86% of all psychiatry residencies had some duty hour violations, more work must be done to understand better the harms and benefits of this new system.[22]

Another major shift in training followed the dramatic changes of the health-care system in the USA over the last several decades. In the 1990s, costs for medical care rose dramatically.[23] The government and insurance companies supported 'managed care' as a way to decrease these costs. 'Managed care' requires that medical services be approved by a patient's primary care physician or an insurance reviewer. It exists in several different forms, including health maintenance organizations, point of service, or preferred provider organizations, differing in fee structure and 'in network' versus 'out of network' coverage. The goal of this system was to reduce unnecessary medical costs in order to preserve basic care for the largest number of people. This theoretical construct has merit; however, managed care in the USA has led to challenges in providing appropriate services to psychiatric patients. Practically speaking, managed care has created challenges in both the practice of psychiatry and patients' access to care, leaving only the most ill patients admitted to hospitals and shortening the length of hospitalizations. That in turn, besides leading to reduced cost, may also represent cost shifting of those with severe mental illness to the criminal justice system.[23] The criminal justice system becomes involved because many patients who do not qualify for an inpatient level of care, or who are discharged too quickly, may end up committing crimes as a result of their largely untreated mental illness, resulting in their imprisonment. Furthermore, many medications and most long-term therapies also require prior authorization. Outpatient care has now shifted to a focus on psychopharmacology and brief therapy, as managed care considers these more cost-effective treatments and will approve payment for them more readily. Thus, briefer '15-minute' medication visits are becoming more prevalent in standard outpatient practice, with an increase in prescribing psychotropic medication and decrease in psychiatrists providing psychotherapy themselves. Because of this change, early career psychiatrists in the USA must now become skilful at short-term therapy and psychopharmacological management under strict time constraints, become familiar with which types of services are authorized by which insurers, and learn how to advocate effectively for their patients' needs with an insurance reviewer. Lastly, they must know how to accurately and effectively fill out insurance paperwork that sometimes requires hours of extra work.

In 2008, the Mental Health Parity and Addiction Equity Act (MHPAEA) was approved by the US government. This act, which went into effect in late 2009 and 2010, requires that insurance-based financial requirements (such as co-pays and deductibles) and treatment limitations (such as visit limits) applicable to mental health and substance use disorders can be no more restrictive than the predominant requirements or limitations for medical and surgical illnesses. The effects of this act on care for patients with psychiatric illness in the USA remain to be seen.

Conclusions and future perspectives

The last few decades have brought rapid and important social changes, greatly influencing health, communication, ethics, politics, economics and, consequently, psychiatry. These global changes were also reflected by the shift in requirements that trainees and early career psychiatrists worldwide must fulfil, which are very different from those required only a few decades ago. These social changes also influenced the development of educational programmes worldwide. Although there are globally shared problems for trainees and early career psychiatrists, there are still significant differences between the European and US educational systems, and thus psychiatry training programmes.

In Europe, one of the most challenging tasks for European authorities that develop and implement training programmes is still the harmonization of training programmes. This is one of the major strategies for improving scientific, working and educational activities in all European regions. This task is becoming more and more important now that the expansion of the EU has brought more countries with different historical and socio-cultural backgrounds into the Union. While efforts towards the harmonization of psychiatric training in Europe started a few decades ago, progress in this challenging task is slow, especially for the observed discrepancy between what is happening in respect of training and what occurs in actual practice. The UEMS and the EFPT, as the major players in psychiatric educational policies at the pan-European level, are working together to develop effective strategies that can enhance the full implementation of the harmonization process. The UEMS strategy and aims for the next decade include harmonization of postgraduate medical training to the highest standards, including evaluating performance and proposing changes. This will be achieved by advocating the harmonization of training based upon the published document 'European framework for competencies in psychiatry',[12] which outlines the competencies and assessments required for psychiatric trainees, and by the development of high-quality assurance mechanisms. In this perspective, developing stronger links with responsible national training authorities and bodies, and providing advice and feedback about the development of high-quality psychiatric training programmes that are nationally driven, are crucial. Moreover, proper executive power should be allocated to the national bodies that are responsible for quality control, while international bodies, such as UEMS, should provide an additional external quality control source by enhancing national clinical visits throughout Europe.

Psychiatric training in the USA needs to embody the ACGME core competencies as caring, informed, up-to-date, professional communicators able to function within the US health-care system. In the USA there are strict limits on duty hours, requiring a mastery of more frequent transfers of care. It is also essential to learn to function within a regulated system of managed care via briefer outpatient visits and shorter inpatient stays; the effect of the Mental Health Parity and Addiction Equity Act remains to be seen. For psychiatrists entering the field today, these new challenges come at a time when psychiatry is rapidly expanding its knowledge base of diagnosis and treatment. European trainees have faced similar challenges with a recent reduction in working hours to 48 hours per week as a result of the European working time directive. A shift to competency-based training is also beginning in many countries, as opposed to the participation-based model.

Despite the still significant differences between the European and US educational and health-care systems, and societal differences, globalization has contributed to the increase in global sharing of challenges among the communities of trainees and early career psychiatrists and to the formation of a 'global community of young psychiatrists'. This fact is also evident by the formation of international networks of trainees and young psychiatrists aiming to serve as a platform allowing colleagues to share and learn from each others' experiences. In light of the growth of globally shared challenges in psychiatric training, learning from international experiences is crucial to develop more effective training systems. Ultimately, to succeed as psychiatrists, trainees worldwide must remember that their responsibility to their patients is paramount, and they must learn to effectively balance the demands of the health-care industry, training bodies and society.

References

1. Maillet B. The Union of European Medical Specialists. *World Med J* 2008; **54**: 50–54.
2. UEMS Section for Psychiatry. Charter on training of medical specialists in the EU: requirements for the specialty of psychiatry. *Eur Arch Psychiatry Clin Neurosci* 1997; **247**(Suppl.): S45–47.
3. UEMS Section and Board of Psychiatry (http://www.uemspsychiatry.org).
4. European Federation of Psychiatric Trainees (http://www.efpt.eu).
5. Hill P, Rothenberger A. Can we – and should we – have a neuropsychiatry for children and adolescents? The work of the UEMS Section and Board for Child and Adolescent Psychiatry/Psychotherapy. *Eur Child Adolesc Psychiatry* 2005; **14**; 466–470.
6. Beresin E, Mellman L. Competencies in psychiatry: the new outcomes-based approach to medical training and education. *Harv Rev Psychiatry* 2002; **10**: 185–191.
7. Bhatia SK, Bhatia SC. Preparing for a successful residency review committee site visit: A guide for new training directors. *Acad Psychiatry* 2005; **29**: 249–255.
8. Oakley C, Malik A. Psychiatric training in Europe. *The Psychiatrist* 2010; **34**: 447–450.
9. Lotz-Rambaldi W, Schafer I, ten Doesschate R, Hohagen F. Specialist training in psychiatry in Europe – results of the UEMS-survey. *Eur Psychiatry* 2008; **23**: 157–168.
10. Nawka A, Rojnic Kuzman M, Giacco D, Malik A. Challenges of the postgraduate psychiatric training in Europe: a trainee perspective. *Psychiatr Serv* 2010; **61**: 862–864.
11. World Health Organization. MhGAP: Mental Health Gap Action Programme: scaling up care for mental, neurological and substance use disorders. 2008; available at: www.who.int/mental_health/mhgap_final_english.pdf.

12. UEMS Section for Psychiatry – European Board of Psychiatry. European framework for competencies in psychiatry. UEMS, 2009.
13. Karabekiroglu K, Doğangün B, Hergüner S, von Salis T, Rothenberger A. Child and adolescent psychiatry training in Europe: differences and challenges in harmonization. *Eur Child Adolesc Psychiatry* 2006; **15**: 467–475.
14. Rothenberger A. The training logbook of UEMS Section/Board on Child and Adolescent Psychiatry/Psychotherapy (CAPP) – progress concerning European harmonization. *Eur Child Adolesc Psychiatry* 2001; **10**: 211–213.
15. Costello, Jane E. Increasing awareness of child and adolescent mental health. *Am J Psychiatry* 2010; **167**: 1411.
16. Berestin EV. The administration of residency training programs. *Child Adolesc Psychiatr N Am* 2002; **11**: 67–89.
17. Swick S, Hall S, Beresin E. Assessing the ACGME Competencies in Psychiatry Training programs. *Acad Psychiatry* 2006; **30**, 330–351.
18. Sattar SP, Basith F, Madison J, Bhatia SC. New ACGME work-hour guidelines and their impact on current residency training practices. *Acad Psychiatry* 2005; **29**: 279–282.
19. Landrigan CP, Rothschild JM, Cronin JW, *et al.* Effect of reducing interns' work hours on serious medical errors in intensive care units. *N Engl J Med* 2004; **351**: 1838–1848.
20. Rasminsky S, Lomonaco A, Auchincloss E. Work hours regulations for house staff in psychiatry: bad or good for residency training? *Acad Psychiatry* 2008; **32**: 54–60.
21. Petersen LA, Brennan TA, O'Neil AC, Cook EF, Lee TH. Does house staff discontinuity of care increase the risk for preventable adverse events? *Ann Intern Med* 1994; **121**: 866–872.
22. Landrigan CP, Barger LK, Cade BE, Ayas NT, Czeisler CA. Interns' compliance with accreditation council for graduate medical education work-hour limits. *JAMA* 2006; **296**: 1063–1070.
23. Hoge MA, Jacobs SC, Belitsky R. Psychiatric residency training, managed care and contemporary clinical practice. *Psychiar Serv* 2000; **51**: 1001–1005.

CHAPTER 2

How to start a research career in psychiatry

Domenico Giacco,[1] Mario Luciano,[1] Sameer Jauhar[2]
and Andrea Fiorillo[1]
[1]Department of Psychiatry, University of Naples SUN, Naples, Italy
[2]Sackler Institute of Psychobiological Research, Institute of Neurological Sciences,
Southern General Hospital, Glasgow, UK

Introduction

Research has always been a source of great interest for young doctors starting a complex and fascinating specialty such as psychiatry, and this is particularly true in recent years.[1-3] J.A. Lieberman says that 'there has never been a better time to go into biomedical research. The science is burgeoning and better than ever. The current funding levels are generous. There are numerous training opportunities. And, finally, the field is eagerly seeking the next generation of psychiatric researchers.'[1]

Despite several difficulties and obstacles, research in psychiatry is advancing rapidly, and has a diversity that few other medical specialties can rival.[2,3] Acquiring research skills is considered by most university professors as an essential part of training.[4] In fact, all psychiatrists, even those not primarily involved in research activities, clearly benefit from an understanding of research methodology and from the ability to think critically about research findings.[5-7] The section of psychiatry of the Union Européenne des Médecins Spécialistes (UEMS) has recently produced a document called 'UEMS Framework for competencies in psychiatry', which states that psychiatrists have to 'contribute to research and to the development of new knowledge', and that they should acquire the following specific research competencies:[8]
- recognize the principles, methodology and ethics of research and scholarly inquiry;

How to Succeed in Psychiatry: A Guide to Training and Practice, First Edition.
Edited by Andrea Fiorillo, Iris Tatjana Calliess and Henning Sass.
© 2012 John Wiley & Sons, Ltd. Published 2012 by John Wiley & Sons, Ltd.

- formulate a research question and conduct a systematic search for evidence;
- select and apply appropriate methods to address the question;
- analyse, interpret and report the results;
- appropriately disseminate and utilize the findings of a study.

Furthermore, the European Federation of Psychiatric Trainees (EFPT) has also produced a statement on research training, according to which 'Psychiatric residents should be trained in basic knowledge of research theories and methodologies. They should have basic training in analyzing the quality of research. Trainees should also be encouraged to develop scientific attitudes towards their professional activities and an ability to effectively implement new research evidence into their clinical practice.'[9]

Despite the increasing emphasis on the importance of research skills for all psychiatrists, early career psychiatrists often meet several difficulties when they try to acquire the skills needed to participate in research activities and to start a research career; these fall into three large categories:[6]

- regulatory factors, such as time in training programmes dedicated to research experiences and to development of research skills;
- institutional factors, such as lack of mentors and limited technological access, knowledge and resources; and
- personal factors, such as female gender, non-Caucasian ethnic group, lack of motivation and financial difficulties.

This chapter is intended as a practical guide for early career psychiatrists wishing to work in psychiatric research. The different steps to follow to get started in research activities, the international opportunities available for improving research skills, the different phases of a research project, and the different settings and stages of a research career will be outlined. At the end of the chapter, some practical tips will be provided.

How to get started: choosing a career in research

Assessing one's own research interests

Before starting a career in research, it is essential to identify the fields of interest. Research in psychiatry is, by its very nature, interdisciplinary and involves several different approaches, which focus on the different aspects of mental disorders.[10,11] The choice should be guided by personal interests and values but, most importantly, by the personal experience of research activities during training.[1,12] It is important to avoid spending energy on too many projects that are not of interest. Nevertheless, maintaining a very narrow focus may also be a mistake. The mind of a prospective psychiatry researcher must be open to different influences and be aware of the 'big picture' of mental disorders.[12]

Reading scientific literature

The knowledge acquired from textbooks studied during training is already at least 1 year old, at best, due to the time required for the author to finish the manuscript, and for the publisher to print and circulate the book.[13] Therefore, in order to keep up to date on the continuous advances in the field, articles published in scientific peer-reviewed journals are of utmost importance throughout the whole medical career. This is particularly true for researchers: the development of valid research hypotheses requires an in-depth knowledge of the updated literature evidence.

Currently, several online databases exist; to access articles of interest, keywords – and sometimes combination of keywords – must be used. Hundreds of abstracts must be screened, among which only a few need to be identified and read in detail. When one or few articles have been identified, it is advisable to go through the methodology of the study first. If this section seems adequate, suggesting that the results can be trusted, then it is worthwhile reading the results, discussion and introduction sections.[13] This process requires experience, which can only be acquired by practice and by the guidance of senior experts. In particular, discussing with professors or senior colleagues how a study has been designed, why a given methodology has been used and, possibly, identifying methodological flaws is a very useful exercise for those wanting to learn research methods and to improve research skills. The so-called 'journal clubs' (i.e. groups of individuals who meet regularly to critically evaluate recent articles in scientific literature) help students to become more familiar with the advanced literature in their field. In addition, these journal clubs help to improve students' skills of understanding and debating current topics of active interest in their field. Research laboratories may also organize journal clubs for all researchers in the lab to help them keep up with the literature produced by others who work in the same field.[14] A continuing medical education course aimed to provide early career psychiatrists with competencies on how to critically read and review scientific literature, and to write scientific papers, is offered by the European Psychiatric Association; see www.europsy.net for further information.

Joining a research group

After the self-assessment of research preferences, the next and crucial step is to join a research group. Learning how to undertake high-quality research requires membership of a group that publishes regularly, and offers a rich learning environment. To be part of a research group, team orientation, team spirit, team management skills and the ability to handle one's own tasks are required.[15] It is important to become active in the group and to help experienced researchers as much as possible; in turn these will give guidance, mentorship and feedback to younger researchers.

Choosing a mentor

As in other walks of life, it is very important to choose a mentor who can be a guide and a teacher for young and inexperienced researchers. The role of a research mentor is to be a constant key-point for the young researcher. In particular, mentors should: (i) provide 'research directions'; (ii) involve young colleagues in writing scientific papers; (iii) introduce young colleagues to public speaking at conferences; and (iv) help them interact with members of the research community. It has been documented that having a good research mentor is one of the strongest predictive factors for embracing a successful research career.[16,17]

Participating in international scientific initiatives (congresses, fellowships, courses)

Participation in international scientific initiatives is essential for early career researchers. Attending a congress provides the opportunity to listen to inspiring lectures by prominent experts and, possibly, to meet them in person. This may be an occasion to establish contacts with them, to ask for their advice on research and receive their feedback, or to propose that they act as mentors or advisors of one's own research projects. Furthermore, there are several international fellowship programmes and courses for young psychiatrists who want to improve their research skills. These programmes give the opportunity to establish contacts with different research institutions, to work in research centres with advanced technical facilities for research,[1] and to acquire expertise in specific research fields. Box 2.1 presents some recent international initiatives aimed at improving early career psychiatrists' skills in research.

Box 2.1 International opportunities for research training

World Psychiatric Association (WPA) (www.wpanet.org)

The WPA recently established a fellowship programme in order to encourage research activities and networking between early career psychiatrists, particularly those from low- and middle-income countries. Past fellowship programmes have been held, among others, at the Institute of Psychiatry in London and at the University of Maryland School of Medicine, Baltimore, USA.

American Psychiatric Association (APA) (www.psych.org)

The APA research colloquium, offered annually, is aimed to provide guidance, mentorship and encouragement to young investigators in

(Continued)

Box 2.1 (Continued)

the early phases of their training, and feedback about their past, present and future research from mentors in a small group setting, as well as general information about career development. Furthermore, the APA website has a detailed list of more than 100 fellowships for early career psychiatrists, funded in collaboration with several US universities and international societies.

European Psychiatric Association (EPA) (www.europsy.net)

The EPA scholarship programme is aimed to support early career psychiatrists' professional development and to facilitate their networking. Scholars have the opportunity to participate actively in the congress, are exempted from payment of the Congress registration fee, have their travel and accommodation expenses covered by the EPA, and participate at the mentors' luncheon where they have the opportunity to establish mutual agreements for mentorship during the subsequent years with internationally renowned experts. Furthermore, the EPA is organizing a Summer School for psychiatric trainees and early career psychiatrists, which aims at developing clinical skills on topic of relevance for psychiatric practice.

European College of Neuropsychopharmacology (ECNP)
(http://www.ecnp.eu)

The ECNP fellowship award is presented to individuals who are engaged full-time in clinical or basic research, training or teaching activities in the field of neuropsychopharmacology and closely related disciplines. The posters presented by the Fellowship Award winners are reviewed for publication on the ECNP website, their expenses for participation in the ECNP Congress are covered and they receive a certificate.

American College of Neuropsychopharmacology (ACNP)
(http://www.acnp.org)

The ACNP annually selects distinguished young scientists in the field of neuropsychopharmacology to be a part of their travel award programme. These awards offer an opportunity to attend an outstanding scientific programme in clinical and basic research on brain–behaviour–drug interactions, become aware of the most

(Continued)

Box 2.1 (Continued)

recent, and often unpublished, advances in psychopharmacology, and meet and interact with internationally distinguished researchers and scientists.

Association for the Improvement of Mental Health Programmes (AIMHP) (http://aim-mental-health.org/)

This Association created the project 'Leadership development in psychiatry', which is primarily aimed to provide ECPs with leadership skills. However, the workshops on topics such as 'How to carry on research and find sponsors', 'How to prepare a scientific paper', 'How to make a presentation', the collaborative and informal atmosphere, and the scientific prominence of invited lecturers makes this course a relevant tool for young researchers.

Maudsley Forum (www.maudsleyforum.iop.kcl.ac.uk/)

This is a course aimed at graduate students and European young specialists in psychiatry, and includes topics ranging from epidemiology to genetics, neuroimaging to drug therapy and cognitive-behavioural psychotherapy. For those who have already attended the Maudsley Forum, or who already have basic skills, there is the possibility of joining the Advanced Maudsley Forum, with lessons to design a scientific study, to develop statistical skills necessary to analyse data, to write and publish scientific papers, and to submit results to a scientific conference.

Pittsburgh/Stanford Research Career Development Institute (www.cdipsych.org)

The Career Development Institute for Psychiatry (CDI) is a 4-day intensive institute for junior investigators interested in a research career, with continuing communication with mentors and peers. Its aims are to increase the number of new researchers, to shorten the time between their research training period and initial extramural grant support, to foster relationships among young and senior researchers, and to facilitate peer support and collaborative research among their cohort group of developing investigators.

Creating a network with peers

The establishment of a network with colleagues interested in the same research field provides the possibility of being involved in multi-centre studies or of using the existing network when developing a new research project. There is no substitute for meeting colleagues in person; however, to maintain regular contacts with colleagues from other countries a number of web tools are available, such as mailing-list groups (e.g. Google groups, Yahoo! groups), Skype or Dropbox.

The participation of young psychiatrists in international meetings and associations is also a very useful way of meeting other persons interested in the same research fields. In this respect, the European Federation of Psychiatric Trainees (EFPT) in 2008 started a research group with the aim to facilitate trainee-led collaborative studies focused on activities relevant for European psychiatric trainees. The EFPT research group has contributed three major projects, presented work at international meetings, and published in major peer-reviewed journals. The group is run through a web-group format, and has representatives from most European countries. Further details are at www.efpt.eu.

How to conduct a research project: the phases

The Early Career Psychiatrists' Committee (ECPC) of the European Psychiatric Association (EPA) recently carried out a survey on research experiences during training in psychiatry, which showed that early career psychiatrists are mostly involved in data collection (87 %) and review of the literature (67 %) (Figure 2.1). Some other activities, such as statistical analyses and study design, are often performed by senior colleagues only, resulting in a lack of research experience for early career researchers.

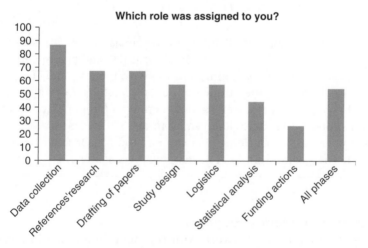

Figure 2.1 Participation of European early career psychiatrists in the different phases of a research project.

Research projects can be ideally subdivided into the following phases, which will be described in detail in the following paragraphs: (i) development of the study concept; (ii) preparation of the study protocol; (iii) search for funding; (iv) development of study plans and procedures; (v) submission of the study protocol to the Ethics Committee; (vi) implementation and data collection; (vii) data analysis and interpretation of findings.[18-20]

Development of the study concept

Study design is probably the most important stage of a research project. In fact, 'a bad research idea will produce bad results, no matter how good the methods used are'.[20] A good study design should be based on: (i) an extensive review of the literature; (ii) relevance of the topic and expected impact of results (including both positive and negative findings) on clinical practice and public opinion; and (iii) discussion with and feedback from the other members of the research group. Hypotheses in scientific research are usually null hypotheses[19] (i.e. predicting negative results). If a null hypothesis is disproved, then it is reasonable to entertain the opposite (positive results) until this is tested again. The study hypotheses should be prepared with adequate care and be precise and well defined, not vague statements[19] (i.e. not 'do rehabilitative interventions have any effect on outcome of bipolar patients?' but 'does a 20-session psychoeducational family intervention improve social functioning of bipolar patients compared with a waiting-list control group?').

Preparation of a 'study protocol'

The 'study protocol' should clearly describe the plan for conducting the study, the purpose and function of the study, and how to carry out the study. More specifically, the study protocol should include the rationale of the study, the number of participants, eligibility and exclusion criteria, details of the experimental intervention (and of the control intervention), data collection and data analysis, and ethical considerations. The structure of the protocol is broadly similar across most disciplines, though there are some variations among the different research fields. An example of the headings is given in Box 2.2.

Producing a protocol is a fairly disciplined process. It is important to adhere to the structure of a protocol given by the local ethical committee, funding body or academic department. At this stage, during protocol development and study design, it would be worthwhile to consult a statistician (or a statistically minded colleague) about the study methodology, the data analyses, and whether the proposed design is adequate to answer study aims and research questions.

Box 2.2 Outline of a study protocol

Title
Background
Hypothesis to be tested
Aims
Design
Population and sample
Inclusion criteria
Exclusion criteria
Sample size
Effects on clinical practice
Ethical considerations
Statistical analysis
References

Search for funding

Whilst a lot of meaningful research can be achieved with minimal funding, to undertake major collaborative projects, and to utilize advanced techniques, such as genetics or neuroimaging, funding is required. Different agencies, such as national ministries for scientific research or health, the European Commission, non-profit organizations, pharmaceutical industries, etc., may offer grants for research activities. In some cases, especially for large or long-term studies, funding may come from more than one source. In any case, researchers must follow a specific process comprising a number of steps, including planning, writing and submitting an application, and going through the peer-review process. Also here, proper guidance will be provided by a research mentor and senior colleagues. However, it is important that researchers participate and gain experience in establishing networks and contacts with colleagues, public and private institutions, etc., and develop fundraising skills, which will be useful throughout their entire research career. Examples of grants dedicated to young researchers are provided in Box 2.3.

Development of study plans and procedures

Before participants are recruited, the study procedures, training and documentation must have been finalized. Good research teams usually develop a 'Manual of Operations' (also known as 'Standard Operating Procedures Document'), which provides detailed steps on study recruitment, enrolment, administration of informed consent, use of study forms

Box 2.3 Research grants dedicated to early career researchers

European Research Council (ERC) – Starting Independent Researcher Grant	ERC Starting Independent Researcher Grant has been designed to support the establishment of excellent new research teams. Topics of the research proposal are pioneering frontier research in any field of science, engineering and scholarship; the principal investigators can be of any nationality, and must have obtained their PhD, or equivalent degree, more than 2 years but less than 10 years prior to the opening date of the relevant call for proposals. More information available at: http://erc.europa.eu/index. cfm?fuseaction=home.FILMDownload&fileId=9
Burroughs Wellcome Fund Career Awards for Medical Scientists (CAMS)	The CAMS programme is designed to address the ongoing problem of increasing the number of physician scientists and keeping them in research. The programme offers $700 000 over 5 years to bridge postdoc/fellowship training and the early years of faculty service. The ideal candidate will be 2 years from becoming an independent investigator, have at least 2 years or more of research experience, and have a significant publication record. Research proposals must be in the area of basic biomedical, disease oriented, translational, or molecular, genetic or pharmacological epidemiology research. More information available at: http://www.bwfund.org/ page.php?mode=privateview&pageID=188
The European College of Neuropsychopharma- cology (ECNP) Research Grant for Young Scientists	The ECNP Research Grant for Young Scientists aims to provide European young researchers who work in the field of neuropsychopharmacology and related disciplines with the opportunity to expand their knowledge and skills by working on scientific projects in different countries, thereby also creating new international networks. Each year a maximum of three European young scientists are awarded a research grant, which consists of a maximum of 50 000 euros. Further information can be found at www.ecnp.eu.

(Continued)

Box 2.3 (Continued)

European Psychiatric Association (EPA) Early Career Psychiatrists research prize	The EPA provides a special research prize awarded to ECPs, to support their involvement in research activities. The candidates have to meet the following criteria: (i) work as a psychiatrist, or work in research in psychiatry, or be a resident in psychiatry in a European country; (ii) be younger than 40 years of age; (iii) be the first author of a scientific paper published in that year in a journal indexed in the Current Contexts. More information available at: http://www.europsy.net.
APA Early Career Award	This award recognizes the best nominated paper published during the year by an early career psychiatrist. It is designed to promote health services research, support young investigators in their research efforts, and recognize significant contributions to the field. More information available at: http://www.psych.org.

and documentation of data. Study forms may be case report forms, questionnaires, or other data-collection or data-tracking instruments. In this phase it is extremely useful to start a research diary reporting the most important timepoints of the study and with personal annotations, motivations for excluding/including particular subjects and even interesting anecdotes. This will facilitate the analysis of data and the writing up of papers.[20]

Submission of the study protocol to the Ethics Committee
The Ethics Committee (EC) is responsible for ensuring that the study design meets the ethical requirements so that the research may be carried out without risks for participants, ensuring respect of their privacy. The ethical principles to which all researchers should adhere are outlined in the Declaration of Helsinki, developed by the World Medical Association (WMA).[21] The EC also approves participants' consent forms and information sheets, where information is provided on procedures, study rationale and possible risks and benefits of participating in the protocol. The process of submitting to an EC can be time consuming; unless all the necessary steps are in order, resubmissions may be requested.

Study implementation and data collection

Study implementation involves recruiting participants, screening them to ensure they meet eligibility criteria, obtaining participants' informed consent, enrolling, registering and, if appropriate, randomizing participants into the relevant study group. One of the main tasks is to recruit an adequate number of participants in the study to respect the study protocol. Retrospective studies, based on case notes or clinical reports, are not affected by these problems, but the generalizability of their findings is limited.[20] In prospective studies, Lasagna's law predicts that the recruitment rate will fall by at least half at the moment the study starts.[20] The best way is to incorporate this variability in the study methodology, and to arrange the study so that the estimated number is doubled, widening the survey area or increasing the time for recruitment. There are different approaches to increase the recruitment of subjects: (i) prepare flyers to advertise the study; (ii) establish dedicated services (i.e. assessment or treatment programmes) dedicated to patients who are eligible to be recruited; (iii) offer financial incentives. In all cases, it must be considered that the adoption of these strategies will have an impact on the characteristics of the final recruited sample.[17]

Data analysis and interpretation of findings

The analyses proceed according to the plan outlined in the study protocol. Generally, study aims and research questions should guide the selection of the type of analyses. In addition to the primary analyses, which should have been defined in advance, exploratory or secondary analyses can be performed after the study is completed. Primary analyses are used to reach conclusions, while exploratory analyses are used to generate new ideas or hypotheses for planning future studies. Statistics can be intimidating to anyone, though in the modern era (and with internet aids and new software) all one requires are the broad principles of medical statistics (which can be gleaned from any introductory statistics book). It is worth spending some time acquainting oneself with software programs for analysing data.

Working in research: settings and stages

Research activities may be performed in different settings and institutions, such as universities, governmental agencies, community services, non-profit organizations, pharmaceutical industries or private research facilities.[22–24] The choice of work setting has to be made according to one's own priorities, qualifications and even personality.[25] In a survey carried out in 2000 on the preferences of scientists regarding working in industry or in academia, the main reasons for preferring working in industry were income, availability of advanced technological equipment, career development and advancement. On the other hand, scientists stated that working in universities meant more creative freedom, a stronger learning environment and greater job security.[26]

In most cases, the mobility of researchers between academia and other settings (especially industries) is limited and predominantly in one direction, with university-trained doctors finding work positions in industry or other research organizations.[26] This could be due to the different evaluation of the research activities. In university settings, the academic 'merits', represented by original scientific papers and by experience in teaching and mentoring students, are essential for progression into an academic career, whereas in other settings the desired outcomes of research are more related to patenting key discoveries for commercial or other (social, political, etc.) interests.[23] Even if variability exists among countries, centres and work-settings, a career in research may be schematically conceptualized as a progression through four different stages.[23]

Stage I. Doctoral training

A PhD degree represents the highest level, internationally recognized, of academic education. When a medical doctor has completed it, he/she is awarded with the title of PhD (i.e., *Philosophiae Doctor*). Entry to a funded PhD programme, usually autonomously managed by individual universities, is quite competitive. However, self-funding for a PhD is also possible, though it can be expensive (up to 10 000 euros per year). During a PhD, the researcher has to complete a specific research project. The duration of PhD programmes is 3 to 4 years of full-time work.[27] However, in many countries the requirement for a doctoral thesis are expressed as a minimum recommended number of original publications. Therefore, more than 4 years may be needed in some cases, in particular when PhD students experience difficulties related to poorly structured training, insufficient supervision and huge workload from other duties (clinical work, teaching responsibilities, part-time working elsewhere, etc.).

Stage 2. Postdoctoral training

There is a great variability in job positions for researchers in this stage. In some countries eligibility for a postdoctoral position does not extend beyond 5–8 years after completion of doctoral training, whereas in other countries postdoctoral researchers may also be doctors in the later stages of their career. Researchers in postdoctoral training may receive specific funding from national funding schemes or from international programmes (e.g. the Marie Curie individual fellowship scheme, or the Human Frontiers science programme), work in different types of teaching position or research project, or receive personal grants or salaries obtained through highly competitive examinations. This stage represents a true 'bottleneck' for establishing a research career, since the number of postdoctoral positions and the opportunities for funding in this stage are very few, thus leading to high competitiveness among early career researchers.

Stage 3. Independent researchers

Universities and other research organizations have a limited number of highly competitive positions in this category, funded by both national and international programmes. Most scientists at this stage receive salaries. Initially, independent researchers work under fixed-term contracts, with low job security, but there are possibilities for tenure, which may range from the assistant/associate professorship in the university to a long-lasting work position in industries and other research agencies. Researchers who succeed in face of the strong competition for funding are usually highly advantaged in achieving academic positions or other research jobs due to the high scientific productivity that they must have shown during this period of their career.

Stage 4. Established scientist stage

This is the final stage of a research career. In the academic institutions it corresponds to the full or associate professor stage. Job titles are quite different in industries, governmental organizations and other research agencies, but nearly all scientists at this stage receive high salaries; however, some of them work under fixed-term contracts. This applies in particular to researchers who work outside academic institutions, and to academics who have not reached high-ranking permanent positions. On the other hand, high demands in teaching and administrative responsibilities faced by full and associate professors are often the main obstacles for remaining competitive in research.

Recommendations for early career psychiatrists interested in research

Some practical advice on what early career psychiatrists should do and know about a career in research is given below. These ten suggestions reflect the authors' personal experiences and are derived from the available literature.[11,12,13,21,22]

1. *Start early with the help of an experienced mentor:* It is advisable that aspiring researchers become active in their local research groups, and attempt to collaborate early with more experienced researchers. Learning how to complete high-quality studies requires membership of a group that publishes regularly, and offers a rich learning environment.

2. *Learn how to read scientific literature:* It is important to first read the abstract, in order to understand the major points of the work, and then attempt to understand the study methodology. One of the best ways to learn how to read scientific literature is by joining a research group.

3. *Keep abreast with international scientific literature:* Improvement of research skills does not finish when early career psychiatrists complete their training, but it is a life-long learning activity. Researchers have to devote a considerable part of their time to continuously updating their knowledge of scientific literature.

4. *Create a network:* Creating (or joining) a network is essential for many reasons, including the possibility of being involved in multi-centre studies or of using an existing network when trying to develop a project. There is no substitute for a face-to-face meeting, though regular web-based contact can be very useful.

5. *Develop innovative strategies for funding:* A major problem faced by young researchers is the scarcity of resources. In turn, this stimulates innovative strategies to obtain adequate financing, such as sponsorship from private institutions without specific interests (e.g., large local firms, foundations, industry associations).

6. *Learn how to work fairly in collaboration with pharmaceutical companies:* The pharmaceutical industry provides a large amount of funding to prospective researchers, and working with them can have some benefits. However, it is important for ECPs to establish and follow some specific rules and ethical principles to govern their relationship with industry and/or ask for advice from more experienced researchers.

7. *Don't spend too much energy on too many projects:* Early career psychiatrists who want to start a research career usually tend to work on every opportunity offered. Acquiring as much experience as possible is fundamental; nevertheless, it is advisable to focus on a specific field.

8. *Do not choose an ultra-specialized research topic too early:* On the other hand, a very narrow focus may be a mistake for young psychiatrists. It is important to keep in mind the 'big picture' of the complexity of mental disorders.

9. *Keep a close link with clinical experience:* As for any other medical specialty (and probably more so), in psychiatric research it is always important to draw new ideas for research from clinical experience. This can give critical perspectives on data that at times conflict with the literature.

10. *Cultivate personal qualities:* The real secret of good research is the people involved. Good researchers have qualities such as humility, curiosity, a spirit of cooperation and perseverance.

Conclusions

Despite many difficulties experienced by early career psychiatrists in starting a research career,[6] the significant attention paid by the public and private agencies to the development of a new generation of researchers in psychiatry, and the increased opportunities for research training and funding, make this decade one of the best times ever to undertake a career in research.[1] The role of modern research in psychiatry is clear: it is to produce evidence that will help improving mental health care and, hence, the lives of many people with mental health problems.[28] The new possibilities offered by recent advances in psychiatry and neuroscience[29] bring hope that in the coming years research in the mental health field will significantly improve. The genomic revolution will probably soon enable us to track the pathogenic processes in many psychiatric disorders to their roots in molecular abnormalities and allow better pharmacological treatments. At the same time, the evidence-based support for psychotherapeutic and other psychosocial interventions is constantly increasing, and technologies for epidemiological, cognitive and social science research have also advanced markedly.[1-3] These advances, particularly if they are achieved in collaboration with other medical professionals (geneticists, psychologists, etc.), will require a vision and an understanding of the complexity of the mental functioning and illnesses that only psychiatrists have.[13] Therefore, this will constitute one of the major challenges for the new generation of psychiatrists.

References

1. Lieberman JA. Starting a career in psychiatric research: the lessons of experience. *Acad Psychiatr* 2001; **25**: 28–30.
2. Gaebel W, Zielasek J, Cleveland HR. Psychiatry as a medical specialty: challenges and opportunities. *World Psychiatry* 2010; **9**: 36–38.
3. Heninger GR. Psychiatric research in the 21st century: opportunities and limitations. *Mol Psychiatry* 1999; **4**: 429–436.
4. DeHaven MJ, Wilson GR, O'Connor-Kettlestrings P. Creating a research culture: what we can learn from residencies that are successful in research. *Fam Med* 1998; **30**: 501–507.
5. McGuire MT, Fairbanks LA. Research training. In: Yager J (ed.) *Teaching Psychiatry and Behavioural Science*. New York: Grune & Stratton, 1982; pp. 243–251.
6. Board on Neuroscience and Behavioral Health (NBH) of Institute of Medicine (IOM) (eds Abrams MT, Patchan KM, Boat TF). *Research Training in Psychiatry Residency: Strategies for Reform*. Washington, DC: National Academies Press, 2003.
7. Pato MT. Generating and implementing research ideas. In: Kay J, Silberman EK, Pessar L. (eds) *Psychiatric Education and Faculty Development*. Washington, DC: American Psychiatric Press Inc., 1999; pp. 181–193.

8. Union Européenne des Médecins Spécialistes (UEMS) – Section and Board of Psychiatry (www.uemspsychiatry.org).
9. European Federation of Psychiatric Trainees (www.efpt.eu).
10. Insel TR, Wang PS. Rethinking mental illness. *JAMA* 2010; **303**: 1970–1971.
11. Patil T, Giordano J. On the ontological assumptions of the medical model of psychiatry: philosophical considerations and pragmatic tasks. *Philos Ethics Humanit Med* 2010; **5**: 3.
12. Ferrari S, Caraci F, Salvi V. Percorsi di ricerca in psichiatria in Italia [Pathways to psychiatric research in Italy]. In: Fiorillo A, Bassi M, Siracusano A. (eds) *Professione Psichiatra: Guida Pratica alla Formazione, all'Inserimento Lavorativo e all'Aggiornamento* [*Psychiatry as a Profession: a Practical Guide for Training, Job Placement and Continuing Professional Development*]. Rome: Il Pensiero Scientifico Editore, 2009.
13. Munk-Jorgensen P. La responsabilità accademica di essere uno psichiatra [The academic responsibility of being a psychiatrist]. In: Fiorillo A. (ed.) *Lezioni di Psichiatria per il Nuovo Millennio* [*Psychiatry Lessons for the New Millennium*]. RomeL Il Pensiero Scientifico Editore, 2010.
14. Swift G. How to make journal clubs interesting. *Adv Psychiatr Treat* 2004; **10**: 67–72.
15. Ursin J. *Characteristics of Finnish Medical and Engineering Research Group Work*. Jyväskylä, Finland: Jyväskylä University Printing House, 2004.
16. Fahy TA, Beats B. Psychiatric training at the Maudsley Hospital: a survey of junior psychiatrists' experiences. *Psychiatr Bull* 1990; **14**: 289–292.
17. Castle DJ, Refault S, Murray RM. Research during psychiatric training as a predictor of future academic research career: the Maudsley experience. *Eur Psychiatry* 1991; **6**: 115–118.
18. Chow SC, Liu JP. *Design and Analysis of Clinical Trials: Concepts and Methodologies*. New York: John Wiley and Sons, 2004.
19. Pocock SJ. *Clinical Trials: a Practical Approach*. Chichester: John Wiley and Sons, 1983.
20. Freeman C, Tryer P. *Research Methods in Psychiatry*, 3rd edn. London: Royal College of Psychiatrists, 2006.
21. World Medical Association. WMA Declaration of Helsinki. Ethical principles for medical research involving human subjects. Available at: http://www.wma.net/en/30publications/10policies/b3.
22. Kelley WN, Randolph MA. *Careers in Clinical Research: Obstacles and Opportunities*. Washington, DC: National Academy Press, 1994.
23. European Science Foundation Member Organisation Forum on Research Careers. Research careers in Europe: landscape and horizons. 2009. Available at: http://www.esf.org/fileadmin/links/CEO/ResearchCareers_60 p%20A4_13Jan.pdf.
24. Searls DB. Ten simple rules for choosing between industry and academia. *PLoS Comput Biol* 2009; **5**: e1000388.
25. Grimwalde A. Working in academia and industry: The Scientist surveys researchers about the two distinct work environments. *The Scientist* 2001; **15**: 28.

26. European Commission. Communication from the Commission to the Council and the European Parliament. Better careers and more mobility: a European partnership for researchers. EC, 2008.

27. European University Association. Glasgow declaration: strong universities for a strong Europe. EUA, 2005. Available at: http://www.eua.be/eua/jsp/en/upload/Glasgow_Declaration.1114612714258.pdf.

28. Slade M, Priebe S. *Choosing Methods in Mental Health Research: Mental Health Research from Theory to Practice.* Hove, UK: Routledge, Taylor & Francis Group, 2006.

29. Spitzer M. Decade of mind. *Philos Ethics Humanit Med* 2008; **3**: 7.

CHAPTER 3

Publications in psychiatry: how to do and what to do

Amit Malik[1] and Gregory Lydall[2]
[1]Southern Health NHS Foundation Trust, Aerodrome House, Gosport, UK
[2]Castel Hospital, La Neuve Rue, Guernsey; University College London, London, UK

Introduction

Getting published as a postgraduate trainee in psychiatry is an important and valuable achievement, whether a career in academia or as a clinician or a manager is intended. Adding one's own research or opinions to the scientific literature is satisfying, but can be daunting. A number of benefits and barriers exist to getting published, as reported in Table 3.1.

Requirements for research and publication in psychiatric training vary by country. In general some experience of research is a requirement in order to complete specialist training. Several countries require a full thesis, dissertation or publication. Others require proof of research skills or competencies, while others have no absolute research requirements.

Despite the barriers, psychiatric trainees do produce publications. A study carried out in the UK noted that psychiatric trainees contributed 16–32 % of published articles in 12 top English-language journals. However, very few trainees were first authors.[1]

In the present chapter we will suggest a procedure for planning, writing and editing a paper and guide the reader in choosing a suitable journal and subject, and discuss the role of the editor and peer reviewers in a refereed journal. It is assumed that data collection and analysis have already been completed before attempting publication (see chapter 2).

How to Succeed in Psychiatry: A Guide to Training and Practice, First Edition.
Edited by Andrea Fiorillo, Iris Tatjana Calliess and Henning Sass.

Table 3.1 Benefits and barriers to publication as a trainee.

Benefits	Barriers
Advancing science	Time limitations (examinations, night shifts)
Improved patient care	Lack of confidence with scholarly writing
Professional, personal and institutional recognition and reward	Lack of confidence with scientific method or statistics
Improved curriculum vitae and career prospects	Failure to recognize expertise or collaborate
Professional obligation	Difficulty handling editorial rejection
Spread good practice	Reluctance to subject work to scrutiny
Learn new skills, competencies	Methodological limitations of study
Learn to handle rejection	Difficulty with the language of the journal
Financial reward	

Planning a paper

The ingredients of good science are obvious: novelty of research topic, comprehensive coverage of the relevant literature, good data, good analysis including strong statistical support, and a thought-provoking discussion. The ingredients of good science reporting are obvious: good organization, an appropriate use of tables and figures, the right length and writing to the intended audience.[2]

If these principles are followed, the chances of getting a paper published are greatly increased. The process of research, from raw data to publication, is illustrated in Figure 3.1.

Essential decisions, such as what kind of article to write and for which target journal, must be agreed upon by all authors before starting to write. In Box 3.1 some decisions, as well as a number of helpful strategies to start writing a paper, are reported.

Box 3.1 Decisions and strategies to get started

Essential decisions
- What kind of article?
- Which journal?
- Who will take responsibility for which sections of the paper (including abstract, images, etc.)?
- Who will take overall responsibility (the guarantor)?
- Who will be coauthors, and in which order?

(Continued)

Box 3.1 (Continued)

- Time frames (first draft, final draft, submission)
  Strategies to get started
- Plan ahead: allocate appropriate responsibilities to coauthors
- Set yourself achievable goals and deadlines
- Start writing as the research (or the literature search) starts
- Select a topic of interest
- 'Brainstorm' ideas for the article onto a single page
- Write a quick first draft and then enrich it
- Attend a journal club to learn critical appraisal and see examples of publishable quality
- Write with a mentor or group
- Find a coauthor who speaks the language of the journal
- Become a reviewer: help the journal and understand how others get published

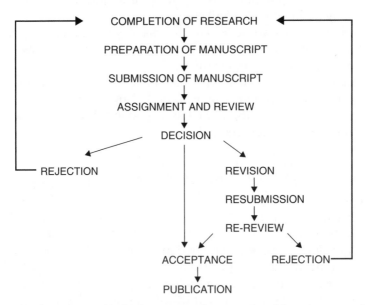

Figure 3.1 The process of publishing research. Reproduced from Benos *et al.* (2005),[12] with permission.

Table 3.2 Types of articles (requirements vary by journal).

Letter	Correspondence, often in response to an article or with an important finding
Short communication	Shorter article, typically fewer than 1200 words with fewer than 10 references
Full-length article	Full length article, typically 3000–5000 words
Filler	Usually brief and interesting, up to 200 words
Case study	Clinical case presentation. Signed patient consent required
Review article	A coherent summary of the current state of research on a topic
Rapid communication	Quickly disseminate 'hot' or important public health findings, usually in a brief communication format

Article type

Knowing what type of article is important in order to adopt the correct structure and word limit. To help decide on the type of article, some options are given in Table 3.2. Table 3.3 itemizes selected psychiatric journals, their impact factors and websites.

Author selection

It is important to decide on the authors, and their order, as early as possible. Authors should include only those who have made a substantive

Table 3.3 Psychiatric journals and impact factors.

Journal name	Impact Factor* (2010)	Website
Archives of General Psychiatry	10.78	http://archpsyc.ama-assn.org
Molecular Psychiatry	15.47	http://www.nature.com/mp/index.html
American Journal of Psychiatry	12.76	http://intl-ajp.psychiatryonline.org/
Biological Psychiatry	8.86	http://journals.elsevierhealth.com/ periodicals/bps/home
Neuropsychopharmacology	6.69	http://www.nature.com/npp/index.html
The British Journal of Psychiatry	5.95	http://intl-bjp.rcpsych.org/
Schizophrenia Bulletin	8.27	http://schizophreniabulletin.oxford journals.org/
World Psychiatry	5.562	http://wpanet.org

*The impact factor is a measure of citation rate per article, and is calculated by dividing a year's worth of citations to a journal's articles published in the previous two years by the number of major articles published by that journal in the same period. Source: *2010 Journal Citation Report* (Thomson Reuters, 2010).

intellectual contribution to the project reported, and can defend the data and conclusions publicly. According to the Vancouver Protocol, which is internationally recognized as the standard for determining authorship on publications, 'in order to be credited as an author, each and every author on a publication needs to have been involved in all three of these criteria: a) having generated at least part of the intellectual content (i.e., conception or design of the work; data analysis and interpretation); b) having drafted, critically reviewed or revised the intellectual content; c) having approved the final version of the manuscript to be submitted.'

Journal selection

Careful journal selection is essential to successful publication. This will define the form and level of detail and assumed novelty of the work. Many scientific journals have a pre-submission enquiry system that should be used. Even before the paper is written, it is possible to obtain a sense of the novelty of the work by reading and discussing widely with colleagues, and whether a specific journal may be interested. It is helpful to reflect with mentors and supervisors on how important the work really is, and which types of editors and readers would be most interested. When choosing journals, the following factors should be considered: (i) general psychiatric, medical or specialist journal (e.g. *British Journal of Psychiatry, New England Journal of Medicine, Addiction Biology*); (ii) impact factor (i.e. the 'strength' of the journal based on the frequency of citations); (iii) readership (the public, or general medical, psychiatric or specialist audience); (iv) themed future issues (which are advertised in the journal); (v) language (English language journals are often considered to have higher impacts and wider readership).

Publication in journals that have high impact factors means it is more likely that a paper is cited and has a higher impact. However, lower impact factor journals are perhaps less selective about the articles they accept, and more likely to publish work by inexperienced authors. It is said that every paper can be published, somewhere. This may be useful for trainees aiming to get a quick publication. But if we are striving for quality in science, then aiming for a good quality journal is the ideal.

Another opportunity is to make an initial enquiry with the journal editor. This person's name can be found in the author guidelines, which are often published in the journal, online at the journal's website, or in the masthead located in the front of the journal. The masthead includes the names of journal staff and editorial board members and the address for correspondence.

Sending an enquiry letter offers several advantages. First, it avoids wasting your time writing an article only to learn that the editor is not interested or has already accepted a manuscript on the same subject.

Table 3.4 Literature search and other web tools.

Literature sources	Web reference
PUBMED	www.ncbi.nlm.nih.gov/pubmed
PsycLIT	www.apa.org/pubs/databases/training/index.aspx
Google Scholar	www.scholar.google.com
Psychiatric Journal Impact Factors	http://workinfo.com/products tools/analytical/jcr/
Gunning Fog Index (readability scale)	http://gunning-fog-index.com/

Second, the editor can give a feedback on the idea, which will help craft the article to best meet readers' needs. Finally, if the editor expresses an interest in the paper, there is a higher possibility of successful publication – but even editorial interest does not guarantee publication.[3]

Reference management

An extensive and comprehensive quality search of the scientific literature is an essential first step to producing a good quality publication. Reading through the current state of knowledge in the area will ensure that the writer builds on good quality existing research. MEDLINE is the US National Library of Medicine's bibliographic database covering the fields of medicine, and beyond. It is possible to search scientific literature via a number of sources (Table 3.4), including the PubMed database. A tutorial is provided on the home page at http://www.ncbi.nlm.nih.gov/entrez/.

The most efficient way of managing literature is by adding the references to a software program called a reference, or bibliography, manager. A reference manager creates a database of bibliographic details (author, journal, abstract, etc.), and some may store or download the papers for easy referencing. A good reference manager integrates with word processing software. The ability to cite a reference while writing, and then automatically create a reference list in the correct journal style, is an important feature. Commercial options include EndNote, RefWorks, Papers and Mendeley. Open source options include Zotero, Wikindx and BibTeX. Word processors like Microsoft Word typically include some reference manager capabilities. References should be in exactly the format required by the journal. A common style is the Vancouver style, which is displayed as: Snowdon J. (2002) Severe depression in old age. *Medicine Today*. **3**, 40–47.

Title and abstract

The title and abstract are arguably more important than the completed paper. This is because editorial teams and referees can often make a judgment about the paper from the impact of the headline and quality of the abstract. After the title, the abstract is usually the first part read by the audience. A good title catches the eye, is brief, yet conveys the 'headline message'.

A good abstract will: (i) keep within the word limit; (ii) explain why the topic is important; (iii) convey the important findings; (iv) be accurate; (v) use simple, clear language; and (vi) use standard headings (Introduction, Method, Results, Discussion).

The main article

Each journal has its own requirements. It is essential to read and follow the relevant instructions to authors carefully. For example, those of the *British Journal of Psychiatry* are available at: http://bjp.rcpsych.org/site/misc/resourcesforauthors.xhtml.

Scientific articles typically use a number of standard headings to provide a logical structure and format to the paper. The Introduction, Methods, Research and Discussion (IMRAD) style is a common format used for academic research papers (Box 3.2) and is used by the American Psychological Association.

Box 3.2 Standard publication headings (IMRAD style)

Introduction/background (Why did you look at it?)
- Formulate your research question
- Why is it important?
- Will I and others find it interesting?
- Will it add to the body of scientific evidence?

Method (What did you do?)
- Sampling
- Population
- Measuring instruments
- Statistical methods

Results (What did you find?)
- Give significant results only

Discussion (What did it mean?)
- Validity
- Generalizability
- Methodological strengths and limitations
- Refer to previous literature

Conclusions (Sum it all up)

Statistics

Journals increasingly require good quality statistical methodology and descriptions. The *British Journal of Psychiatry* requires that 'methods of statistical analysis should be described in language that is comprehensible to the numerate psychiatrist as well as the medical statistician'. The statistical analyses should be planned before data are collected. Involving a medical statistician before starting research increases the chances of being selected for review and possibly publication.[4] Quality journals usually require justification for the statistical procedures used, how the tests were interpreted, and whether they were appropriate for the hypotheses tested. Journals usually request justification for analyses carried out post hoc.

Authors are encouraged to include estimates of statistical power (a power calculation) where appropriate. To report a difference as being 'statistically significant' is generally considered insufficient. Both the magnitude and direction of change and confidence intervals, if appropriate, should be reported. A brief and useful introduction to the place of confidence intervals is given by Gardner and Altman.[5]

Many editors discourage the use of percentages to report results from small sample sizes. The value of statistical tests and their significance levels should be given so that their origins can be understood. Standard deviations and errors should be specified and referred to in parentheses. The number of decimal places to which numbers are given should reflect the accuracy of the original data measures.

Examples of incorrect practices that persist despite published warnings include: (i) using correlations to compare two methods of measurement; (ii) using significance tests to compare baseline characteristics in randomized trials; (iii) conducting multiple tests of data recorded at multiple times; and (iv) ignoring clustering in the design and analysis of cluster randomized trials.[6]

For the interested reader, an elegant guide and some recommendations on the use of statistics for psychiatric journals was published by Haque and George.[7]

A question of style

A simple formula states that the extent of effective communication depends on the ratio of expectation of reward to effort required.[8] Ideally, for the editor and reader, the expectation of reward is high and the effort required is low. The task as a writer is to increase the level of reward while decreasing the effort readers must exert to understand the material. Reward can be increased by choosing topics of interest, and the effort can be decreased by writing in a way that is easy to understand. Of course being familiar with the journal 'house style' is the first step. An

> **Box 3.3** The 4 Cs of editing. Adapted from Saver (2006)[3]
>
> Clear
> - Consistent and appropriate tone
> - Sentences written in the active voice
> - Transitions used between paragraphs
>
> Concise
> - Focus on 'need-to-know' (not 'nice-to-know') information
> - Logical organization
> - Extraneous words removed
>
> Correct
> - Grammar and spelling checked
> - Appropriate use of references, each with complete citation
>
> Compelling
> - Easy to read
> - Fulfils your intended purpose
> - Contains enough information to fully address the topic
> - All questions answered, and no gaps in logic

example of a journal house style guide is available on the Royal College of Psychiatrists website.[9]

When writing, consider the 'four Cs' of effective communication as described by Saver:[3] *clear, concise, correct and compelling* (Box 3.3). If an author is not confident in the language of the journal, he/she should consider employing or collaborating with a fluent speaker of that language, ideally someone who has published in that field.

Here we discuss briefly some common potential errors of style.
- Abbreviations should be spelt out on first usage and only widely recognized abbreviations are recommended.
- The generic names of drugs should be used. Drug dosages should be double checked.
- Generally, Système Internationale (SI) units should be used; where they are not, the SI equivalent should be included in parentheses. Units should not use indices: i.e. report g/mL, not $g\ mL^{-1}$.
- Tables should be numbered and have an appropriate heading. The tables should be mentioned in the text, and should be self-explanatory, but must not duplicate information in the text.
- Figures should be clearly numbered and mentioned in the text and include an explanatory legend. The desired position of the figure in the manuscript should be indicated.

- For figures and tables, authors must obtain permission from the original publisher if they intend to use figures or tables from other sources, and due acknowledgement should be made in the legend.

Ethical issues

It is vital to ensure that a published article complies with the generally accepted ethical rules as follows.

- Ensure that local ethical permissions as appropriate have been given before starting the project. As a guide, a *clinical audit* or *service evaluation* does not usually need ethical approval; every other study does. Supervisors, local hospital staff or ethical committee will have more information.
- If the study includes original data, at least one author must confirm that he or she had full access to all the data in the study, and takes responsibility for the integrity of the data and the accuracy of the data analysis.
- Many journals recommend that clinical trials are registered in a public trials registry. Further details of criteria for acceptable registries and of the information to be registered are available on the website of the International Committee of Medical Journal Editors (http://www.icmje.org/index.html#clin_trials). For reports supported by pharmaceutical industry funding, registration is usually a requirement for the paper to be considered for publication in many journals.
- In a case report, the patient's consent must usually be obtained and submitted with the manuscript. The patient should read the report before submission. Where the individual is not able to give informed consent, it should be obtained from a legal representative or other authorized person. A sample patient consent form can be downloaded at: http://www.rcpsych.ac.uk/pdf/BJPconsentForm.pdf.
- Most journals require that the authors assign copyright to the journal. The authors usually, however, retain the right to use the article in certain ways (e.g. for teaching), as long as the journal is acknowledged, and the authors do not sell the article, which would conflict with a journal's business interests.
- Never submit a given article to more than one journal concurrently.
- A study must not mislead; otherwise it could adversely affect clinical practice and future research.

Revisions

Usual practice is for one author to draft the paper, which is then distributed to the coauthors for amendments. Using a word processor that tracks and highlights changes allows all authors make their own alterations or comments and also to spot those of others.

Authors should put all their energy into improving the quality of the manuscript *before* submission. They should revise it and then ask coauthors for their comments. Once it is ready, they could leave it for a few days to reflect on it and then review it. Then they could ask a colleague or expert in the field, but one not associated with the paper (if they can be trusted), to read it and comment. In particular the author might ask the external colleague to appraise readability and flow, clearness of language and scientific method.

Usually journal reviewers assess the following points:
- originality;
- readability;
- topicality;
- validity;
- likely appeal;
- generalizability;
- whether it matches the editorial interests of the submitted journal;
- references (relevant, up-to-date and correctly cited).

Paragraphs must be easily readable. The Gunning Fog Index (Table 3.4) is a test designed to measure the readability of a sample of English writing. The resulting number is a rough estimate of the number of years of formal education that a person requires in order to understand the text on a first reading. Texts that are designed for a wide audience generally require a Fog index of less than 12; however, scientific articles may score higher and still be readable for a specialist audience. Useful readability principles are: keep words small and sentences short.

Lastly, keep a note of the contact details and affiliations of each author. When ready for final submission, a signed declaration of authorship or financial interests is often required from each author. Many journals accept electronic signatures but some require facsimiles or even originals.

Online submission

Most journals now require an online manuscript submission. This allows them to automate the process, and it allows authors to keep track of progress. Register with the relevant website, usually using a personal email address. The submission process will require all the contact details of the authors. Typically the process will require uploading of: a covering letter; an abstract; the main paper; tables; figures; declarations of interest; and declarations of authorship.

Helping the journal editor understand why the submitted work is important and relevant is the key to achieving acceptance for publication. The covering letter to the editor, like the abstract, can make or break publication chances. A polite letter addressed to the editor should briefly explain why the author thinks the topic is important, and convey the headline findings. No more than one A4 page should be used. This covering letter should not replicate the abstract. It may be useful to conclude with a paragraph similar to: 'We look forward to your comments, and those of the reviewers. We would be very grateful if you will consider this work for publication in your journal.'

Handling rejection

Before long a letter from the editor will be sent to the corresponding author with one of the following outcomes: the paper has been accepted; rejected; or rejected as is, but it may be resubmitted with some changes. *Very few* papers are accepted on the first attempt. It is important not to lose hope, and to learn from the experience. After all, even experienced professors get their papers rejected! Peer review is an important process to maintain standards in the published literature. Reviewers' comments are often valuable and may usefully be incorporated into a revised version. When resubmitting the paper, the editor and reviewers should be thanked for their comments. Each point in the reviews must be addressed in a new covering letter sent to the editor. Changes must be visible in the revised manuscript, if required.

Engaging the next generation: junior trainees and students

Encouraging early involvement in research and publication increases the chances of future publication.[10] Senior trainees may wish to mentor junior trainees into the rewarding world of science. Lambert and Garver[11] described a step-wise process of mentoring trainees from start to finish of the research cycle, in which key training elements are identified. These include: identifying the key research question and reframing as a hypothesis (training elements: engage the trainee, encourage curiosity); designing a study; data collection; data analysis and forming conclusions; manuscript preparation; and managing the publications process (training elements: journal selection, managing and interpreting criticism and reviewers' comments). The same authors present a number of case studies as useful examples.

Conclusions

Publishing one's work as a trainee is important and can be extremely rewarding and helpful for the psychiatric trainee's career, resumé, job prospects and overall satisfaction. Publications enrich the scientific litera-ture and may contribute towards any aspect of psychiatry and psychiatric education. Common obstacles to achieving successful publication include lack of time, confidence and knowledge of scientific method and statistics.

Planning a winning paper requires good organization, an appropriate use of tables and figures, aiming for the right length, and writing to the intended audience. Before starting to write, all authors must agree on what kind of article to write and for which target journal; and on authorship inclusion and order. Intelligent management of references using free or commercial software can save a lot of time and energy. Common errors of style include poor grammar and punctuation, mixed tenses, not spelling out abbreviations, and incorrect table/figure labelling and referencing. Where figures or tables have been quoted, their source should be given, and permissions acquired where needed.

Particular attention should be paid to clear descriptions of study designs and objectives, and evidence that the statistical procedures used are both appropriate for the hypotheses tested and correctly interpreted. When writing the text, consider the four Cs of effective communication: *clear, concise, correct* and *compelling*. Ethical issues include ensuring appropriate approvals have been given, ethical rules adhered to, and not submitting to more than one journal at once. Electronic submission and revision are now the norm. Reviewers are typically asked to assess an article's originality, readability, validity and likely appeal, as well as style. Authors are encouraged to guide the next generation in getting their research published. The mentoring process includes identifying the key research question; study design, data collection and analysis and forming conclusions; manuscript preparation; and managing the publication process. When the trainee (or perhaps professor) is long gone, their scientific legacy is largely the literature left behind, the impact it represents, and the skills passed on to the next generation.

It is sincerely hoped that this chapter has enabled psychiatric trainees to feel more competent and confident in adding their valued research to the body of published scientific literature, and also in training others in these essential skills. If these principles are followed, the chances of getting a paper published successfully are greatly increased.

References

1. Junaid O, Daly R. An audit of research activity among trainee psychiatrists. *Psychiatr Bull* 1991; **15**: 353–354.
2. Bourne PE. Ten simple rules for getting published. *PLoS Comput Biol* 2005; **1**: e57.
3. Saver C. Writing for publication series. *AORN Journal* 2006; **84**: 373–376.
4. Altman DG, Goodman SN, Schroter S. How statistical expertise is used in medical research. *JAMA* 2002; **287**: 2817–2820.
5. Gardner MJ, Altman DG. Confidence – and clinical importance – in research findings. *Br J Psychiat* 1990; **156**: 472–474.

6. Altman DG. Poor-quality medical research: what can journals do? *JAMA* 2002; **287**: 2765–2767.

7. Haque MS, George S. Use of statistics in the Psychiatric Bulletin: author guidelines. *Psychiatr Bull* 2007; **31**: 265–267.

8. Schramm WL. How communication works. In: Schramm WL (ed.) *The Process and Effects of Mass Communication*. Urbana, IL: University of Illinois Press, 1961; pp. 5–6, 24.

9. Royal College of Psychiatrists. *House Style. A Guide for Editors and Writers*. London: RCP, 2009. Available at: http://www.rcpsych.ac.uk/PDF/RCPsych %20house%20style%20guide%20Nov09.pdf.

10. Chusid MJ, Havens PL, Coleman CN. Alpha Omega Alpha election and medical school thesis publication: relationship to subsequent publication rate over a twenty-year period. *Yale J Biol Med* 1993; **66**: 67–73.

11. Lambert MT, Garver DL. Mentoring psychiatric trainees' first paper for publication. *Acad Psychiatry* 1998; **22**: 47–55.

12. Benos DJ, Fabres J, Farmer J et al. Ethics and scientific publication. *Adv Physiol Educ* 2005; **29**: 59–74.

CHAPTER 4

Training in psychotherapy: where are we now?

Clare Oakley,[1] Larissa Ryan[2] and Molly McVoy[3]
[1]St Andrew's Academic Centre, Institute of Psychiatry, King's College London, UK
[2]Warneford Hospital, Oxford, UK
[3]University Hospitals of Cleveland/Case Western Reserve, Cleveland, OH, USA

Introduction

Psychotherapy has traditionally been a core component of postgraduate training in psychiatry, although the methods and models of training have varied over time and between places. More than a decade ago the European Board of Psychiatry, a committee of the Union Européenne des Médecins Spécialistes (UEMS), set standards for the provision of psychotherapy training in Europe, which are: psychotherapy training should be compulsory with one theoretical course a week; psychotherapeutic theory should include at least psychodynamic and cognitive behavioural approaches; personal therapy is highly recommended but not mandatory; and a minimum of 100 hours of psychotherapy supervision should offer the trainee experience in different therapeutic approaches.[1] However, these guidelines remain aspirational for many psychiatric trainees in Europe.

In the USA, no hourly requirements are in place for psychiatry trainees.[2] However, the Accreditation Council for Graduate Medical Education (ACGME) requires that all trainees demonstrate competency in applying psychodynamic, supportive and cognitive behaviour therapy.[2] The ACGME also requires that each psychiatry residency facilitates further training for those psychiatrists with more interest in practising psychotherapy.[2] However, the application of these requirements remains quite varied across training programmes in the USA.[3]

How to Succeed in Psychiatry: A Guide to Training and Practice, First Edition.
Edited by Andrea Fiorillo, Iris Tatjana Calliess and Henning Sass.
© 2012 John Wiley & Sons, Ltd. Published 2012 by John Wiley & Sons, Ltd.

In this chapter we will consider the current state of training in psychotherapy for psychiatrists in Europe and the USA, as well as the obstacles and possible solutions to improving this training.

Psychotherapeutic models

Central to the modern practice of psychiatry is the biopsychosocial approach, of which psychotherapy has been described as an essential component.[4] The development of psychological therapies has led to the creation of many different therapeutic models, from psychodynamic therapy and cognitive behavioural therapy (CBT), on to the more recent cognitive analytic therapy (CAT) and dialectical behavioural therapy (DBT). Most models have been able to accumulate a body of evidence to support their treatment effectiveness, with some models now accepted as at least as effective as medications for certain conditions. The most common psychotherapeutic models are briefly summarized below.

Supportive psychotherapy
This form of psychotherapy is widely used and has various definitions. The term is commonly used to describe the psychological support given to patients with chronic and disabling mental illnesses. The objectives of supportive psychotherapy include optimizing the patient's psychological and social functioning, helping them to cope with the effects of their illness, increasing self-esteem and self-confidence, education about their illness and the prevention of relapse.

Cognitive behavioural therapy
Cognitive behavioural therapy (CBT) is structured, time limited, and problem- and goal-orientated. CBT has been evaluated in randomized controlled trials and been shown to be effective in the treatment of depression (it is as effective as medication in mild to moderate depressive illness), eating disorders, anxiety disorders, obsessive compulsive disorder, post-traumatic stress disorder and chronic psychotic symptoms.

Interpersonal psychotherapy
Interpersonal psychotherapy (IPT) was originally developed to treat major depression, and this is the disorder for which there is the strongest evidence base, although there is a growing literature relating to eating disorders. In IPT the biopsychosocial signs of depression are understood in the context of current social and interpersonal stressors, defined in terms of role transitions, role disputes, grief and interpersonal sensitivities. In therapy, the patient learns to understand the interactions between symptoms and interpersonal difficulties and is helped to break this pattern

to achieve a reduction in depressive symptoms and an improvement in interpersonal functioning.[5]

Cognitive analytic therapy

Cognitive analytic therapy (CAT) is a brief, focal therapy informed by cognitive therapy and psychodynamic psychotherapy. CAT was developed for treating neurotic conditions but evolved to treat patients with borderline personality disorder. After initial sessions with the patient, the therapist will write a reformulation letter that outlines the main problems and the repetitive maladaptive procedures or reciprocal roles that underlie them; the patient is encouraged to amend this letter in negotiation with the therapist so that it can become the basis for the therapy.[6] Similarly there is a goodbye letter summarizing achievements at the end of the therapy.

Dialectical behaviour therapy

Dialectical behaviour therapy (DBT) is a special adaptation of behavioural therapy. It is a manualized therapy that includes functional analysis of behaviour, cognitive techniques and support.[7] It was originally used for a group of female patients with borderline personality disorder who had made suicide attempts. DBT aims to reduce self-harm and then to promote change in the emotional dysregulation at the core of the disorder. Whilst effective at reducing self-harm, there are concerns that the long-term effectiveness of DBT as a treatment for the personality itself is unproven.[7]

Systemic therapy

Family therapy is also referred to as systemic therapy as it involves seeing and treating people in context. There is considerable diversity of systemic therapy models, and different phases of therapy require different techniques. There is evidence for the effectiveness of systemic therapy in eating disorders in adolescents, drug and alcohol misuse, conduct problems in children, marital distress, mood disorders and psychotic disorders.[8]

Psychodynamic psychotherapy

Psychodynamic theories stress that early childhood experiences are crucial in shaping the personality. In psychodynamic psychotherapy unconscious conflicts are explored and the insight gained aims to change patients' maladaptive behaviour. The main goals of psychotherapy are symptom relief and personality modification through exploration of the unconscious. The relationship between the therapist and patient is crucially important. Therapies can be offered on an individual, couple, group and therapeutic residential community basis. Psychodynamic psychotherapy has been shown to be a highly efficacious treatment in a range of psychological disorders but patient selection for therapy is important, with consideration of psychological mindedness and a concern with the antecedents as well as the relational contexts of the presenting problem being key.[9]

Current perspectives

Why is psychotherapy training important?

For trainees in psychiatry, an understanding of psychological therapies is important for many reasons. Early exposure to psychotherapy is important for trainees to decide whether they want to specialize in this field. For psychiatrists who do not go on to specialize in psychotherapy, experience of this area also represents an essential part of their training. For all psychiatrists there is likely to be a psychological component to the presentations of most patients seen in mental health services, and for some there will be significant transference and counter-transference reactions. To care for these patients, doctors will need to be able to understand and deal with these factors appropriately. Psychodynamic factors are also important in many interactions within mental health teams, both community- and ward-based. Doctors who can perceive these, and adapt to them, will make better leaders within these teams.

Another relevant factor relates to appropriate referrals for psychological therapies. One model of psychological therapy does not fit every problem, or every patient. Patients must also understand the process of therapy, including what they will need to contribute to it. Considerable resources could be wasted by attempting to carry out psychological treatments on unsuitable patients, or on patients who discontinue therapy because they were not prepared for what would be involved. Psychiatrists will frequently be responsible for assessing and diagnosing a patient, and deciding on a course of treatment, which may be biological, psychological or both. To assess and refer appropriately the treating psychiatrist must understand the indications for a particular therapy, and be able to have an idea of its likely success in a particular patient.

For many trainees, the successful completion of training depends on acquiring psychotherapy competencies, whether this relies on a knowledge base tested as part of written examinations, a skill base tested in practical examinations, or on completion of seeing cases for therapy.

Opinions on psychotherapy

Surveys have generally found that trainees in psychiatry rate psychotherapy highly in terms of its importance in their training.[10,11] The majority of trainees report that the prospect of learning and practising psychotherapy was an important factor in their decision to specialize in psychiatry, and more than four out of five trainees expected to practise psychotherapy in some form throughout their careers.[10]

However, it has also been noted that attempting to conduct a psychodynamic therapy before a trainee psychiatrist is fully ready for this, is likely to result in the trainee feeling high levels of anxiety, and being discouraged from pursuing further cases.[12] This is supported by surveys of trainees, in which more than 1 out of 10 trainees felt that some of their psychotherapy experiences had a negative impact on their lives.[10] These negative experiences were described as problems with inadequate supervision, and feelings of stress and insecurity. A mix of good preparation and clear supervision arrangements is required to reduce some of these anxieties. It has been found that satisfaction with psychotherapy training, or the lack of this, is associated with trainees choosing whether or not to practise psychotherapy in their ongoing careers.[10]

In a UK survey, trainee psychiatrists reported that psychoanalytical thinking was aloof, and not always relevant to psychiatry.[13] Another in-depth study, which interviewed 21 participants in Balint groups, found that the groups were anxiety provoking, and at times experienced as persecutory.[14] In this study a particular problem was noted to be the shift away from a medical model of thinking, with participants finding it hard to relate their own feelings to the clinical material. However, this study also found that Balint groups helped participants to learn new skills, and have an increased awareness of their emotions.

How can trainees be taught psychotherapy?

Education and training in psychotherapy can be divided into two areas. The first is theoretical knowledge – both about how different therapeutic modalities work, as well as a historical perspective on the development of psychotherapy. The second area is the acquisition of skills, obtained through practice in psychotherapy, where trainee psychiatrists can deliver therapy under supervision.

Formal teaching

As with other areas of medical education, lecture-based learning is a frequently used option for the teaching of theoretical knowledge in psychotherapy. This format has the advantage of being relatively easy to arrange and low in use of resources, as one educator may teach several trainees at once. However, this format does not allow trainee psychiatrists to have practical experience of psychotherapy, and therefore does not permit them to achieve competence in using the techniques described.

Balint groups

Balint groups have become established as a widespread part of training in psychotherapy, often covering both the theoretical knowledge base, and starting to look at dynamics within patient-doctor relationships. They were started by Michael Balint, a psychoanalyst who led case discussion groups first in Budapest, and from the 1950s, in the Tavistock Clinic in London. The main aim of the Balint group is to 'examine the relationship between the doctor and the patient, to look at the feelings generated in the doctor as possibly being part of the patient's world and then use this to help the patient'.[15] Often Balint groups are used as an introduction to thinking in a psychotherapeutic way, although for many trainee psychiatrists they may continue throughout their training and beyond. A typical format for a Balint group would be all trainee psychiatrists working in a hospital meeting on a regular basis, usually weekly and usually with consistent timing and location. The group is often facilitated by a senior clinician, usually a psychotherapist. During the group one trainee psychiatrist might present a patient that they have seen, and the group will discuss the psychological factors that may be relevant. Balint groups can be a useful bridge between didactic teaching and the actual practice of psychotherapy, as it provides an environment where trainees can start to explore psychodynamic components in a clinical relationship, without requiring the trainee to conduct any therapeutic interventions. Participation in a weekly Balint group over the course of a year was shown to significantly improve trainee psychiatrists' performance in a written response to a clinical case vignette.[13]

Clinical cases

For most trainees, their training in psychotherapy will include seeing at least one patient for a course of therapy. This could be in a variety of modalities, and most trainees will be expected to attempt more than one case in total. Requirements regarding numbers of therapy cases for trainees are not in place in all European countries, and where present these requirements vary between countries (discussed later in this chapter). In the USA there are no requirements for the number of psychotherapy cases.[2] However, the ACGME does require evaluation and treatment of ongoing individual psychotherapy patients, some of whom should be seen weekly under supervision.[2] Of course, trainees with an interest in psychotherapy may choose to see more patients than the minimum required.

Supervision

As discussed above, conducting psychotherapy can be an anxiety-inducing process for trainees, who may feel they are entering a very unfamiliar area where they lack any personal experience to guide them. The process of supervision should help to support trainees through this anxiety. For trainee psychiatrists, supervision is an important element of their training in psychotherapy. It is likely to be provided by a senior psychotherapist, who may or may not have a medical training. Supervisors are likely to be involved in identifying suitable patients for trainee psychiatrists. The supervisor will then meet regularly with the trainee to discuss each therapy session, guiding the trainee psychiatrist in his or her understanding of the therapy process, and helping to plan for upcoming sessions. Supervision may be on a one-to-one basis, or one supervisor may see a group of trainees together. As well as being more efficient in terms of the supervisor's time, group supervision allows trainees to follow the progress of each other's cases, and hence expand their learning opportunities.

The quality of supervision is key to the success of clinical training in psychotherapy; however, it is a subjective process, which may vary between locations and between supervisors. A recent survey asked trainee psychiatrists whether they knew what they were supposed to be learning in their psychotherapy supervision. Half of respondents said they did not, and the majority had not actually discussed this with their supervisor. In addition, the majority did not know how they were being assessed, or how to improve their performance.[16]

Personal therapy

Trainee psychiatrists may or may not undertake personal therapy as part of their psychotherapeutic development. This obviously has financial and time implications, but may be felt to be beneficial for training. A recent survey of trainee psychiatrists in London found that 16 % had had personal therapy, and 73 % would consider it in the future.[17] Most of the respondents in this survey gave their psychiatry training as a reason for having therapy. Another survey in Canada found that 67 % of trainees thought that personal therapy was important, and 25 % had entered personal psychotherapy.[10]

New developments in teaching methods

A recent literature review of psychotherapy training in psychiatry looked at three steps to improve psychotherapeutic skills, which were described as modelling, rehearsal and feedback.[3] Modelling involves the demonstration of skills by an expert, following which learners can practise these skills by the process of rehearsal, or repetition. Finally feedback is the process by which experts comment on the learner's performance, to promote new learning. The review identified that feedback using recordings of therapy sessions was particularly useful, and many innovative developments in psychotherapy training use modern technology to facilitate this.

An interesting study from Brazil combined modelling with theoretical teaching. It described a course of teaching sessions where trainee psychiatrists selected one of their own patients, whom they had been treating in their clinic with a primarily pharmacological focus. The patient came to a teaching session, where he or she was interviewed by the supervisor, and following this all the trainee psychiatrists discussed the case in a psychodynamic framework.[18] A specific aim of this method was to address the mind-body split and promote a unified approach to treating patients. As part of this study trainee psychiatrists were assessed by means of a written test at the start and end of the course, which demonstrated a significant improvement in knowledge and understanding.

Another area generating interest is the idea of allowing trainees to learn basic psychotherapeutic skills by the use of role play. This method has the advantage of removing the unpredictability of real patients, including eliminating the possibility of the patient discontinuing therapy. It also may be a helpful option if there is a shortage of suitable patients for training cases. Attempts have been made to formally assess the value of such standardized, or scripted, patients. One study involved trainee psychiatrists seeing scripted patients on a weekly basis for 18 weeks.[19] This paper assessed performance, and found that it varied widely between the doctors, but that overall it did not improve after the therapy. Another model suggests that the role plays set up a series of escalating difficulties to desensitize trainees to their fears and learn appropriate therapeutic responses to patients.[20] Use of simulated patients should not be a replacement for direct patient interaction, but it may be a useful environment in which to begin to learn key skills, and a systematic review on the topic of simulated patients in psychiatry was broadly supportive of their use in psychotherapy training.[21]

Assessment of psychotherapeutic competencies

For any educational training, consideration must be given to how learners will be assessed on their attainment of the objectives of that training. This presents particular challenges for psychotherapy, which can be very subjective in terms of both the patient and the therapist. Theoretical knowledge can be tested in written examinations, as for any other discipline. Assessment of clinical performance is more difficult, and this is particularly relevant in psychotherapy, where a clinical interaction is likely to take place over months or years, and a good outcome is not always easy to define. However, methods have been established for assessing competence. Trainees will usually keep a logbook, recording their attendance at Balint groups and sessions of therapy conducted. This logbook can be used as a basic measure of progress, together with reports from tutors and supervisors. Some trainees are required to write an essay describing the process of therapy for one of their cases, which then can be marked by a local or external assessor.

The review mentioned above also looked for all published papers relating to assessing competence in psychotherapy,[3] and concluded that there had been a general shift towards more objective methods of assessing competence, such as video or audio recordings of therapy sessions. It identified nine empirically validated assessment scales that can be used to assess therapists' psychotherapeutic skills, and suggested that these could be used to assess recordings in weekly supervision. Another approach has been the development of a written examination that aims to assess psychodynamic technique and applied theory.[22] This examination presents a small number of detailed clinical vignettes, with multiple choice questions relating to these. The questions consider the areas of therapeutic alliance, transference and counter-transference, resistance, defensive organization, therapeutic change and interventions. The examination was validated by an external group of experts, and when taken by trainees it was found that higher scores were positively associated with the number of hours of therapy conducted by the student, and the number of hours of supervision. For more senior trainees, the score of the test was found to significantly correlate with their overall evaluations by the programme director. Written examinations of this sort may be a useful additional objective tool, although they are unlikely to be sufficient as a sole measure of competence in psychotherapy.

In order to assess the attainment of objectives, it must also be clear what those objectives are. In the UK, the Royal College of Psychiatrists has a curriculum that requires all trainee psychiatrists to undertake at least two therapy cases, one in a longer modality and one in a shorter modality.[23] There is a further set of competencies for doctors who wish to specialize in psychotherapy.[24] The European Board of Psychiatry, in collaboration with the European Federation of Psychiatric Trainees, has also produced a framework of competencies in psychiatry, which includes the following standards in psychotherapy: 'The psychiatrist is able to understand the theories that underpin standard accepted models of individual, group and family psychotherapies available for treatment of mental disorders, [and] practise psychotherapy safely and effectively on the basis of values and the best evidence available'.[25]

The Accreditation Council on Graduation Medical Education (ACGME) in the USA requires that all psychiatry residents 'develop competence in applying supportive, psychodynamic, and cognitive behavior psychotherapies to both brief and long-term individual practice, as well as to assuring exposure to family, couples, group, and other individual evidence-based psychotherapies'.[2,3]

What are the challenges in training in psychotherapy?

Training in psychotherapy is likely to be more consuming of resources than other areas of postgraduate study in psychiatry. For example, an area such as psychopharmacology can be learnt in a more self-directed way, relying mainly on written information, whereas the main activity of psychotherapy training is seeing patients, and being supervised in their treatment. This requires the trainee to have time available to see their patient and for supervision, time that may take them away from their regular clinical work. Facilities must be available for the therapy to take place, such as a designated room, and ideally administrative support. Both of these may not be readily accessible in all services.

The availability of supervision may also be a difficulty, as many trainees may work in areas where there is no provision of psychological therapies and hence no senior clinician to supervise them. If there are senior clinicians working locally, they may not be able or willing to supervise trainee psychiatrists. In particular non-medical psychotherapists may have their own trainees from other disciplines, and may feel less confident in supervising trainee psychiatrists. All senior psychotherapists are likely to have many competing demands on their time, and they may struggle to accommodate supervision time for one or several trainees. One solution to a lack of designated psychotherapy services is to optimize the training opportunities in other psychiatric settings. For example, it has been suggested that trainees can undertake psychotherapeutic interventions such as ward groups in inpatient settings, behavioural interventions in learning disability placements, motivational interviewing in addiction clinics, and family work in child psychiatry.[20] However, appropriate supervision for this work would again be key, and the same problems are likely to arise in obtaining this.

For busy doctors, finding time for psychotherapy training is likely to be a major issue to address. Some doctors may not have protected training time, and will need to fit their psychotherapy sessions around full-time jobs. For those doctors who do have specified time set aside to acquire these skills, this might be a regular weekly session, or perhaps a 6-month or year-long stint working full-time in a psychotherapy service. A paper estimating the amount of training provided by these approaches suggested that a half-day session over 3 years would give around 400 hours total training time, compared to around 500 hours for a 6-month post in psychotherapy.[26]

The availability of psychotherapy for patients also varies between different countries and areas, with a resultant variability in how accessible training is for doctors. With the financial challenges of recent times, mental health services as a whole are likely to be asked to make significant cuts to services. Psychotherapy, particularly longer models, may be a target for reduced services, leading to a further restriction in the availability of training.

There is no shortage of studies showing that trainee psychiatrists feel they struggle to access psychotherapy training,[27–30] and some that also show that doctors are often unclear as to what the objectives of that training should be.[31] Desirable changes suggested by trainee psychiatrists in these surveys commonly related to increased availability of cases and supervision. Particular problems included lack of seniors specializing in psychotherapy, and lack of a local psychotherapy department to coordinate training.

Another survey by UEMS attempted to assess the extent to which their guidelines (outlined in the introduction to this chapter) had influenced the development of psychotherapy training in Europe.[32] The survey found that on the whole psychotherapy was a mandatory part of the psychiatry training programme, but that there were still great differences in the extent of theoretical teaching and practical supervision of psychotherapy, with some countries falling considerably short of the UEMS standards. Personal therapy was mandatory in 53 % of the training centres surveyed. The level of trainees' personal financial contribution to their psychotherapy training varied from nothing to more than 10 000 euros.

A more recent survey of the 22 member countries of the European Federation of Psychiatric Trainees (EFPT) found that, in contrast to the UEMS survey, only half of trainees reported that psychotherapy training was mandatory in their country.[33] In 10 of the countries it was possible to work as a specialist in psychotherapy after completing training. Trainees had access to training in psychodynamic psychotherapy and cognitive behavioural therapy in nearly all countries, with family therapy in 17 countries, systemic therapy in 16 countries, interpersonal therapy in 12 countries and dialectical behavioural therapy available in 7 of the 22 countries. There was a wide range of requirements for the psychotherapy training, with some countries having no specifications for types or lengths of therapy undertaken or number of patients seen. Austria and Switzerland expected trainees to see more than 10 patients for therapy but Sweden, Ireland and the UK expected three or less. The expected duration of therapy varied between 3 and 24 months. In 10 countries trainees had to pay for their own supervision of the psychotherapy they administer, even though in three of these countries (Estonia, Germany and Italy) it is a compulsory part of their training. In four countries it is compulsory to have personal therapy. In 19 countries trainees have to pay for personal therapy, and in three of these countries (Austria, Switzerland and Germany) it is a compulsory part of their training.[33] Similar results have been found in a more recent study carried out by the Early Career Psychiatrists Council of the World Psychiatric Association.[34]

Future directions

The provision of appropriate psychotherapy training to psychiatric trainees continues to be a priority for both trainers and trainees. This has been reflected in the recent surveys described here that were undertaken by the UEMS and the EFPT. It is clear that improvements have been made, but there is still further work to be done. In order to achieve this it will be crucial for scientific associations and political or organizational bodies to continue to work together and for representatives to engage the relevant training bodies in their own countries in improving psychotherapy training.

The EFPT statement on training in psychotherapy provides a useful outline of what needs to be achieved:[35]

> 'A working knowledge of psychotherapy is an integral part of being a psychiatrist and this must be reflected in training in psychiatry. All trainees should gain the knowledge, skills and attitudes to be competent in psychotherapy. Competence should be gained in at least one recognized form of psychotherapy (of the trainee's choice) and basic knowledge should be gained in the other forms of psychotherapy to allow the trainee to evaluate suitability for referral to a specialist psychotherapist.'
>
> Training in psychotherapy must include supervision by qualified therapists. A personal psychotherapeutic experience is seen as a valuable component of training. It is crucial that trainees have access to relevant psychotherapy experience to cater to the needs of the appropriate patient group that the trainee is dealing with or is expected to deal with in the future. Relevant training authorities should guarantee that time, resources and funding are available to all trainees to meet the above mentioned psychotherapy training needs.

Conclusions

Psychotherapy training is accepted as being a core component of postgraduate training in psychiatry. There is an established need for psychiatrists to understand psychological techniques, and psychodynamic factors in a relationship, such that they can use these skills in their day-to-day work. They must also be able to refer patients appropriately for such therapies, and inform patients knowledgeably about what to expect from the referral. The growing body of evidence for the effectiveness of psychological therapies suggests that, rather than becoming of less importance with the advances in biological psychiatry, psychological therapies will continue to be an essential part of psychiatric treatments and practice.

There are many challenges for trainees in obtaining good quality training in psychotherapy, both in terms of finding time and resources, and dealing with the emotional stress that may result from seeing a patient for therapy. Supportive and well-resourced supervisors, innovative teaching methods, and above all the efforts made by trainees themselves, will help to ensure that psychotherapy training of an excellent standard is clearly defined and readily available for trainee psychiatrists.

References

1. Hohagen F. Training in psychiatry in Europe – recommendations of the European Board of Psychiatry. *Eur Psychiatry* 1996; **11**: s4, 248s.
2. ACGME Program Requirements for Graduate Medical Education in Psychiatry. Available at: http://www.acgme.org/acwebsite/rrc_400/400_prindex. asp.
3. Weerasekera P, Manring J, Lynn DJ. Psychotherapy training for residents: reconciling requirements with evidence-based, competency-focused practice. *Acad Psychiatry* 2010; **34**: 5–12.
4. Denman C. A modernised psychotherapy curriculum for a modernised profession. *The Psychiatrist* 2010; **34**: 110–113.
5. Law R. Interpersonal psychotherapy for depression. *Adv Psychiatr Treat* 2011; **17**: 23–31.
6. Denman C. Cognitive-analytic therapy. *Adv Psychiatr Treat* 2001; **7**: 243–256.
7. Bateman AW, Tyrer P. Psychological treatment for personality disorders. *Adv Psychiatr Treat* 2004; **10**: 378–388.
8. Asen E. Outcome research in family therapy. *Adv Psychiatr Treat* 2002; **8**: 230–238.
9. Fonagy P. Psychotherapy research: do we know what works for whom? *Br J Psychiatry* 2010; **197**: 83–85.
10. Hadjipavlou G, Ogrodniczuk JS. A national survey of Canadian psychiatry residents' perceptions of psychotherapy training. *Can J Psychiatry* 2007; **52**: 710–717.
11. Hwang KS, Drummond LM. Psychotherapy training and experience of successful candidates in the MRCPsych examinations. *Psychiatr Bull* 1996; **20**: 604–606.
12. Wilson J. Starting out in psychodynamic psychotherapy. *Psychiatr Bull* 2001; **25**: 72–74.
13. Fitzgerald G, Hunter MD. Organising and evaluating a Balint group for trainees in psychiatry. *Psychiatr Bull* 2003; **27**: 434–436.
14. Graham S, Gask L, Swift G, Evans M. Balint-style case discussion groups in psychiatric training: an evaluation. *Acad Psychiatry* 2009; **33**: 198–203.
15. Balint M. *The Doctor, his Patient and the Illness*. London: Pitman, 1964.
16. Rojas A, Arbuckle M, Cabaniss D. Don't leave teaching to chance: Learning objectives for psychodynamic psychotherapy supervision. *Acad Psychiatry* 2010; **34**: 46–49.
17. Dover D, Beveridge E, Leavey G, King M. Personal psychotherapy in psychiatric training: study of four London training schemes. *Psychiatr Bull* 2009; **33**: 433–436.
18. Zoppe EHCC, Schoueri P, Castro M, Neto FL. Teaching psychodynamics to psychiatric residents through psychiatric outpatient interviews. *Acad Psychiatry* 2009; **33**: 51–55.

19. McGowen KR, Miller MN, Floyd M, Miller B, Coyle B. Insights about psychotherapy training and curricular sequencing: Portal of discovery. *Acad Psychiatry* 2009; **33**: 67–70.
20. Margison F. Psychotherapy: advances in training methods. *Adv Psychiatr Treat* 1999; **5**: 329–337.
21. McNaughton N, Ravitz P, Wadell A, Hodges BD. Psychiatric education and simulation: A review of the literature. *Can J Psychiatry* 2008; **53**: 85–93.
22. Mullen LS, Rieder RO, Glick RA, Luber B, Rosen P. Testing psychodynamic psychotherapy skills among psychiatric residents: the psychodynamic psychotherapy competency test. *Am J Psychiatry* 2004; **161**: 1658–1664.
23. Royal College of Psychiatrists. A competency-based curriculum for specialist training in psychiatry: core module. London: RCPsych, 2009. Available at: www.rcpsych.ac.uk/training/curriculum2010.
24. Royal College of Psychiatrists. A competency-based curriculum for specialist training in psychiatry: specialist module in psychotherapy. London: RCPsych, 2009. Available at: www.rcpsych.ac.uk/training/curriculum2010.
25. Union Européenne des Médecins Spécialistes. European Framework for Competencies in Psychiatry. UEMS, 2009. Available at: www.uemspsychiatry.org/board/reports/2009-Oct-EFCP.pdf.
26. Wildgoose J, McCrindle D, Tillett R. The Exeter half-day release psychotherapy training scheme – a model for others? *Psychiatr Bull* 2002; **26**: 31–33.
27. McCrindle D, Wildgoose J, Tillett R. Survey of psychotherapy training for psychiatric trainees in South-West England. *Psychiatr Bull* 2001; **25**: 140–143.
28. Pretorius W, Goldbeck R. Survey of psychotherapy experience and interest among psychiatric specialist registrars. *Psychiatr Bull* 2006; **30**: 223–225.
29. Rooney S, Kelly G. Psychotherapy experience in Ireland. *Psychiatr Bull* 1999; **23**: 89–94.
30. Kuzman MR, Jovanović N, Vidović D et al. Problems in the current psychiatry residency program in Croatia: residents' perspective. *Collegium Antropol* 2009; **33**: 217–223.
31. Agarwal S, Singh Y, Palanisamy V, Basker R, van der Speck R. Psychotherapy requirements as recommended by the College: awareness and achievement by senior house officers. *Psychiatr Bull* 2007; **31**: 394–396.
32. Lotz-Rambaldi W, Schäfer I, ten Doesschate R, Hohagen F. Specialist training in psychiatry in Europe – results of the UEMS survey. *Eur Psychiatry* 2008; **23**: 157–168.
33. Oakley C, Malik A. Psychiatric training in Europe. *The Psychiatrist* 2010; **34**: 447–450.
34. Fiorillo A, Luciano M, Giacco D et al. Training and practice of psychotherapy in Europe: results of a survey. World Psychiatry 2011; 10:238.
35. European Federation of Psychiatric Trainees. Psychotherapy statement. EFPT, 2009. Available at: www.efpt.eu/staticpages/index.php?page=statements.

CHAPTER 5

Training in community psychiatry

Giuseppe Carrà,[1,2] Paola Sciarini,[2,3] Fiona Nolan[4] and Massimo Clerici[2]

[1]Department of Mental Health Sciences, University College Medical School, London, UK
[2]Department of Neurosciences and Biomedical Technologies, University of Milano Bicocca Medical School, Monza, Italy
[3]Department of Health Sciences, Section of Medical Statistics and Epidemiology, University of Pavia Medical School, Pavia, Italy
[4]Centre for Outcomes Research and Effectiveness (CORE), Sub Department of Clinical Health Psychology, University College London, London, UK

The community psychiatrist must be a dreamer as well as a pragmatist

Leonard I. Stein

Introduction

Academia and community psychiatry have experienced a long and varied history of relationships, and a mutual understanding of the partners' differing missions is critical. Involvement of medical schools' departments of psychiatry with public sector programmes is diverse but needs to be increased because of challenges posed by new clinical populations such as court-remanded patients, assertive outreach services' clients, and persons with comorbid drug and alcohol disorders.[1] Major changes in community psychiatry over the last 40 years have significantly influenced training programmes in psychiatry worldwide. New and emerging training needs, which include services planning, relevant tasks and roles, characteristics and core components of community psychiatry programmes, must be satisfied for early career psychiatrists. There is also a need for uniform curricula, through the identification of common theoretical and field placement core elements in the implementation of community psychiatry

How to Succeed in Psychiatry: A Guide to Training and Practice, First Edition.
Edited by Andrea Fiorillo, Iris Tatjana Calliess and Henning Sass.
© 2012 John Wiley & Sons, Ltd. Published 2012 by John Wiley & Sons, Ltd.

training programmes. The obstacles faced by early career staff in community psychiatry, the lessons learned and possible solutions are described in this chapter, giving practical guidance on organizational solutions to overcoming relevant barriers.

What is community psychiatry?

The practice of mental health care in the second half of the twentieth century changed fundamentally. Such changes were largely influenced by principles of the human rights movement and led to an impressive decline in the number of beds in mental hospitals, preventing inappropriate admissions and discharging long-term institutional patients into the community.[2] The closure of the large asylums, with a progressive shift from a mainly hospital-based care to a community-care system, was the final milestone of such a process, known as deinstitutionalization.[3]

The definitions of community psychiatry proposed over the years have constantly been reframed to accommodate changing practice on the ground.[4,5] However, there remains a gap between 'values-based' and 'operational' definitions. The best available example of the former is arguably provided by Thornicroft and Szmukler,[5] who regard community psychiatry as comprising the principles and practices needed to provide mental health services for a local population by: 'a) establishing population-based needs for treatment and care; b) providing a service system linking a wide range of resources of adequate capacity, operating in accessible locations; and c) delivering evidence-based treatments to people with mental disorders'. On the other hand, a relatively up-to-date operational definition from an authoritative European body describes community psychiatry as a series of practices, covering all aspects of mental health care, which encompass all or any of the following settings: day hospitals, day centres, hospital settings and, of course, community mental health teams (including tertiary level ones, such as crisis resolution, assertive outreach and early intervention teams). Such services build up a network whose aims are the delivery of continuous treatment, employment and social support programmes to help mentally ill people to maintain or reach a satisfactory social role.[6] A definitive choice between the two kinds of definitions is almost impossible as any structure of community psychiatry must be placed within the restrictions of a social and historical context. Although there may be similarities in different cultural and social contexts, there will always be differences.[4]

Further issues contribute to the characterization of community psychiatry. First, it is strictly influenced and guided by the results of social psychiatry research,[6] which is concerned with the effects of the social environment on the mental health of the individual, and with the effects of the mentally ill person on his/her social environment.[7] Second, community psychiatric care is provided by a wide range of mental health professionals, including psychiatrists, community psychiatric nurses, psychologists, psychiatric social workers, occupational therapists and community psychiatric workers, all of which are found in community-based multidisciplinary teams.[3] Such teams are challenged by the transition from a hospital-based to a community-based system of care, with its inherent major changes and an emphasis on integration between mental health and primary care services and a multidisciplinary approach to clients. Indeed, that approach is consistent with the theoretical framework of social psychiatry – dealing with the social, environmental and cultural factors in the aetiology and outcomes of psychiatric disorders – and provides a link with other disciplines in the field of mental health, such as social anthropology, cultural psychiatry and sociology, while being equally influenced by them.[8] Similarly, community mental health care has to establish close collaborations with services addressing different but interlinked areas (e.g. health, welfare, employment, justice and educational agencies), which are often challenging for mentally ill people to negotiate.[3]

Planning community mental health services delivery: the first step for education and training

These major changes described above have important implications for the role of mental health staff. Key issues involve restructuring staff from inpatient settings to community facilities; developing recovery-oriented competencies; extending the range of workers in need of appropriate training; and implementing evidence-based training models.[3]

Any training programme for community mental health care has to be framed within consistent human resources planning,[9] which includes an analysis of the existing services, in terms of number and type of staff members and service utilization. Analysis and planning of staffing requirements for community mental health services with regard to the care needs of the population must take into account the prevalence and incidence of the most common mental disorders in the local area. Staff management and training will ultimately be guided by the identified priorities.[3]

The multidisciplinary nature of services, responsibility for mentally ill people living in a defined area and emphasis on external (e.g. domiciliary) interactions with patients are the principal domains of community psychiatry.[6] Prime targets are the promotion of rehabilitation programmes and the improvement of quality of life scores, by means of controlling and minimizing risk factors for relapses and impairment. Good mental health community practice should be characterized by harmonization and integration of care delivered by community mental health teams and inpatient services, constituting a balanced care approach. This is, of course, also relevant for appropriate training. The balanced model of care delivery focuses on providing community services that are close to home and easy to access for service users, facilitating hospital admission efficiently and quickly when needed, and minimizing the duration of inpatient treatment.[10]

Tasks and roles in community psychiatry

The main tasks of community psychiatry include the provision of integrated community and hospital-based mental health care for mentally ill people and their families, as well as supporting the mental health, resilience and well-being of whole communities in conjunction with other experts and agencies. In brief, community psychiatry should take a public health approach to mental health in terms of prevention, early detection and interventions. Community psychiatrists' skills should therefore cover both direct clinical inputs and the well-being of relevant communities.[11]

Working within large multidisciplinary teams makes the role of the community psychiatrist perhaps unique among medical disciplines. The best trained psychiatrist cannot meet all of the many potential treatment needs of severe mental health disorders. Other mental health professionals will share significant proportions of the overall responsibility for treatment programmes, providing coordinated interventions. There is a definite need for clarity in community psychiatry in differentiating medical expertise in assessing, diagnosing and prescribing, as well as medico-legal signatory and reporting functions, from other clinical roles and related responsibilities.[12] Working with other professionals in performing joint assessments and planning care, and cultivating an open attitude towards a continued, mutual exchange of knowledge in clinical and research activities, are examples of skills not traditionally covered in psychiatric training, but which are essential in community psychiatry. On the other hand, in vivo experiential apprenticeship[13] seems the only possible framework for training community mental health professionals, including psychiatrists, in activities such as formal and regular interdisciplinary debriefing of clients' health and social care needs (Care Programme Approach Review for National Health Service in England and Wales), which ensure that all team members are aware of each others' work. As a whole, multidisciplinary community mental health teams must both maintain specific professional roles and increase joint core tasks, with robust transformational leadership and management[14] provided by the most skilled team member, regardless of his/her professional background.[11]

Core skills in community psychiatry

Critics may imply that psychiatrists possessing in-depth training in community mental health care have clinical competencies that are weaker than those of colleagues trained and working in traditional hospital settings. Indeed, good psychiatrists must be competent and skilled clinicians regardless of whether their training and practice are community or hospital based. However, there is a case for all community mental health professionals, including psychiatrists, needing a firmer grounding in public health competencies.[15]

According to Rosen,[11] the more traditional clinical skills of community mental health care professionals should focus on the following aspects:

1. Providing a more streamlined service between outpatient and inpatient care.[16]
2. Tailoring the way in which assessments and reviews are conducted in non-traditional settings, including those aimed at negotiating an admission, arranging a compulsory treatment, and evaluating a risk of violence. This is particularly needed in the delivery of modern mental health services, such as assertive community treatment (ACT), crisis resolution teams (CRTs) and other models based on research evidence.[17]
3. Comprehensively updating professional grounding in both biological and psychosocial domains, through a critical use of best available guidelines (see, e.g., ref. 18).
4. Working as part of a multidisciplinary team, which efficiently complements the programmes of other similar teams (e.g. drug and alcohol and vocational rehabilitation services).
5. Implementing both clinical and operational transformational leadership and management.[15]
6. Using screening instruments to detect the main mental disorders, and employing other evaluation tests to communicate with clients and teams, and to monitor outcomes.[11]
7. Working closely with service users, family carers, primary care professionals, and any other medical and welfare agencies, regardless of their statutory or charitable status.[19]

However, a public approach, incorporating skills in epidemiology, community-oriented scholarship, leadership and advocacy, requires community mental health professionals to address several additional domains and develop related skills by:

1. Capitalizing on methods and findings in social science research, particularly when dealing with special populations.[20]

2. Assessing met and unmet needs of the catchment area in question, in terms of preventive and treatment programmes,[21] including those for comorbidities and physical risk factors.[22]
3. Supporting initiatives aimed at improving resilience, mental health and well-being in the community by changing knowledge, attitudes and behaviour relating to mental health.[23]
4. Challenging stigmatization and discrimination of mentally ill people.[24]
5. Advocating the improvement of mental health facilities and addressing policy-makers and the general public about mental health issues.[25]

Characteristics of community psychiatry training programmes

John Talbott in 1991[26] speculated, 'Does the university have a role or responsibility in training psychiatrists for community work, in operating community services, and/or in performing research in or about community psychiatry settings?' He stated that, though some US-specific training programmes in psychiatry were deeply involved in the community in the 1950s and 60s through services delivery, research and/or training, many of the key aspects of these programmes, such as continuity of care and home treatment, have currently become pillars of 'good psychiatry', not just of 'community psychiatry'. However, it has to be acknowledged that a similar gap between universities and national health services remains a major issue in most Western countries, as regards transfer of knowledge into practice.[27]

Community psychiatry training programmes should be developed to provide supervision and mentoring to trainees while they are engaged in full-time community practice, as well as opportunities to participate in relevant didactic activities. Training courses in leadership, management, appraisal techniques, team building and negotiation skills should be given equal importance to courses in clinical skills. The main characteristics of community psychiatry training programmes, in terms of knowledge, skills, attitudes and activities, are shown in Table 5.1.

Recovery-oriented training
Mental health staff who are to be trained to work in community psychiatry settings must review their professional approach as identifying recovery as the main aim. This implies authentic cooperation with service users, carers, other agencies and allied disciplines, as well as with any relevant external stakeholders.[28] Nevertheless, defining the components of recovery-oriented training presents a challenge. The extent to which staff can be trained in elements such as therapeutic optimism and

Table 5.1 Community psychiatry training programmes: main characteristics.[28]

Knowledge of	Skills (i.e. to be able to...)	Attitudes	Activities
• Prevention and public health approaches to community mental health • Professional ethics and advocacy	• Navigate system policies and mediate with other agencies through joint approach	• Openness to considering opinions of service users, families and community as a whole	• Advocacy programmes
• Historical basics of community mental health • Social psychiatry and psychiatric epidemiology	• Act as team members as well as team leaders according to circumstances • Integrate all staff contributions in the care programme	• Develop partnerships with service users, families and significant others	• Primary field placement
• Effective leadership practices and consultation methods	• Develop appropriate treatment plans within a multidisciplinary team • Practise case management activities • Provide supervision, mentoring and teaching	• Integrate multiple contributions into problem-solving outputs • Respect multi-disciplinary mental health team members	• Both academic and field placement weekly supervisions
• Integrated care (mental health, substance use, physical health and developmental disabilities) for co-occurring disorders • Group and family treatments	• Assess and address substance use, developmental and physical health issues • Use medication in collaboration with non-medical team members as regards compliance and informed consent • Integrate non-pharmacological interventions	• Respect, compassion, integrity and honesty	• Implementation of active community agencies' networks • Teaching, presenting and supervising learning formats

(*continued overleaf*)

Table 5.1 (Continued)

Knowledge of	Skills (i.e. to be able to…)	Attitudes	Activities
• Engagement practices and recovery-focused care and approaches to maintaining healthy communities • Motivational techniques • Risk assessment and benefit analysis	• Support people in self-management and recovery • Determine areas of need in treatment planning process • Assess readiness for and commitment to change	• Use engagement strategies, plain language and assess non-verbal communication • Cope with emotional and stressful situations	• Recovery-oriented opportunities such as collaborative service planning, service development, housing, medication management
• Services for special populations	• Provide culturally and spiritually sensitive care	• Be aware of the differences of the diverse populations also in terms of gender, age, ethnicity and sexual orientation	• Programmes focused on special populations
• Quality improvement, use of documentation and guidelines, implementation of evidence-based practices	• Critically appraise health-care literature	• Openness to critical review by peers	• Research and/or quality improvement projects opportunities
• Primary care, homelessness and housing policies • Difference between intervention and prevention	• Design and implement health delivery services • Plan community-based research	• Use professional networks to solve problems	• Trust management secondment

ability to infuse hope[29] is questionable, as these can be seen as personal rather than professional characteristics. Perhaps the exposure, within an experiential and role modelling framework, to highly regarded and valued local staff, may itself contribute to these ends. Possession of a social conscience and an egalitarian attitude is also related to personal values and cultural influences. Concepts that may be more easily learned concern prioritizing service users' goals – valuing their self-determination and control over the recovery process – as well as interweaving treatment and rehabilitation.[11]

Knowledge and skills

The knowledge and skills required for community-oriented psychiatry are wide ranging. The key training requirement is the development of appropriate attitudes to allow better cooperation between inpatient and community teams. Staff should be given time to accompany other members of the community team for adequately supervised joint assessments.[30] In contrast to the traditional paternalistic medical approach, it is essential that psychiatrists, community psychiatric nurses, social workers, occupational therapists, psychologists and support workers have an in-depth, working knowledge of each others' roles in relation to community treatment. A simple means of achieving this is by sharing working activities, as well as participating in interdisciplinary learning opportunities. Furthermore, a genuine interest in exploring the whole range of views from all staff and carers – not to mention service users – is needed. However, for the benefit of current and future community mental professionals, skills in planning weekly activities and, more importantly, efficient case-load management skills, must be developed. Competencies in facilitating continuity of care can be honed by appropriate planning in terms of duration of treatment within teams. Generally, capacity for community follow-up of small caseloads is a minimum of 2 years.[31]

Competencies

Staff working in community mental health settings need additional competencies in designing, implementing and providing community- and home-based treatment programmes, and in working within specific populations. They must have a good working knowledge of local legislation pertinent to mental health as well as that concerning other relevant issues, such as benefit entitlements, employment, housing and education. They should advocate the rights of mentally ill people both as individuals and as a group – people whose interests need negotiation within a competitive environment. Administrative and managerial competencies are also needed.[3]

Core elements of community psychiatry training programmes

The definition of training objectives, within a programme for community mental health staff, needs to be stated in behavioural terms (e.g. 'The professional should be able to...'). A good example is provided in the UK by the Capable Practitioner Framework,[32] which covers five areas: ethical practice, knowledge of mental health and mental health services, the process of care (including effective communication and partnerships), evidence-based interventions, and their application to specific service settings. However, community psychiatry is a discipline in continuing transformation, and cultural, social and health policy issues significantly influence related implementation across countries, with evident training implications.[33] In order to deal with the resulting educational gap, training targets and curricula should be updated in relation to current best clinical practice and available evidence. Three core principles should be followed: (i) assessing the current training provision; (ii) assessing the future needs for which training is carried out; and (iii) setting targets for adapting current training towards future needs.[3] There is also a need for integration between theoretical lectures and more participative techniques.[3] In terms of format, the European Union of Medical Specialists (UEMS)[6] recommends that training in community psychiatry should last at least 6 months, should comprise supervised activities, modelled by an appropriate staff member of a multidisciplinary team, and should entail a significant amount of joint work with a range of agencies for mentally ill people. It should also include consultations with patients outside hospital settings (e.g. home assessment, day care), and furnish the knowledge to evaluate health, services and the implementation of new programmes.

Community psychiatry training programmes have been proposed by several international organizations,[3,33–35] and professional associations.[28,36] These are intended to be used by professional and regulatory bodies to map competency-based profiles for each of the staff disciplines, as well as to guide education and training organizations. A series of core elements, which should be included in any community mental health care training programme, have been identified and described in terms of competencies, which should be achieved in the following seven domains.

1. *Clinical field*. Community psychiatry staff should acquire comprehensive clinical expertise, in terms of appropriate theoretical knowledge and practical ability for the evaluation and diagnosis of a wide range of mental disorders.[28,35] Reliable risk assessment, particularly in the area of self-harm,[36] should be a fundamental component of a comprehensive investigation plan, which considers biological, psychological and socio-cultural needs.[36] Professionals should also acquire the knowledge and clinical expertise needed to deliver appropriate interventions

to patients and their families (e.g. pharmacological and non-pharmacological interventions, psychotherapy, individual, group and family interventions)[35] and to special populations (e.g. homeless persons, criminal offenders, gay/lesbian/bisexual/transgender, addicted, child and family, rural, geriatric, institutionalized), providing integrated care for co-occurring physical, developmental or substance abuse disorders.[28]

2. *Leadership and multidisciplinarity*. Community psychiatry professionals should acquire a comprehensive knowledge of leadership practices and consultation methods,[28] and be able to work with colleagues – within multiprofessional health care teams and from different health and social care services[35] – both as team members and as team leaders.[28] They should also show successful attainment of skills in leadership and supervision, including coordination of teams, setting learning outcomes, planning, motivating, delegating, organizing, negotiating and monitoring performance. Furthermore, expertise is needed to plan and realize programmes for change and optimization of services, to use the professional background of other team members, and to recognize, mediate and facilitate recovery from conflicts within teams and with other services (e.g. other psychiatric teams, medical teams, primary care services).[36]

3. *Clinical governance*. Knowledge and abilities are required to implement evidence-based practices and guidelines, to recognize and solve problems within systems through the application of principles aimed at ameliorating quality, and to ease the accomplishment of clinical goals. In addition, appropriate management of relationship and integration problems between care system components, and appraisal and navigation of system policies and politics is needed.[28] Finally, there is the need to monitor the safety of services and to reduce the risk for patients, carers, staff members and the community.[36]

4. *Education*. Community psychiatry staff should be trained to teach particular groups (e.g. students of medicine and allied disciplines, other professionals, service users, carers and the community as a whole),[35,36] through different and appropriate educational assessment and appraisal methods.[36] They should also cooperate in the organization of continuing medical education activities and programmes.[35]

5. *Interpersonal communication*. Community psychiatrists should build authentic relationships with service users, show evidence of cultural understanding, and be able to use engaging approaches in a wide range of situations, evaluating non-verbal communication and conveying information in a straightforward and understandable manner.[28]

6. *Culture*. Community psychiatry professionals should be respectful, sympathetic, principled and honest; they should be able to adapt their

behaviour depending on situations, showing genuine sensitivity about the distinctive characteristics of patients in terms of gender, age, culture, ethnicity, religious beliefs, personal impairments and sexual orientation.[28] Furthermore, they should respect confidentiality when sharing information with both health-care and non-health-care professionals.[36]

7. *Research and literature appraisal.* Basic research methodology as well as the ability to write research protocols and carry out research projects, critically evaluating existing literature and implementing relevant evidence-based results into clinical practice, should all be fundamental components of community staff training.[36]

Hopefully, any training programmes in community psychiatry will take advantage of previous experiences of the implementation of community mental health services,[37] and lessons learned will provide guidance on steps to take, and obstacles and mistakes to avoid.[2] The most common obstacles encountered by early career staff in community psychiatry, as well as related lessons learned and possible solutions, are summarized in Table 5.2.

A practical working model: the Public Psychiatry Fellowship of New York State Psychiatric Institute at the Columbia University Medical Center

The Public Psychiatry Fellowship (PPF) of New York State Psychiatric Institute at the Columbia University Medical Center is the oldest and largest programme in the USA for training psychiatrists to become public-sector leaders. Established in 1981, it is a one-year programme that trains 10 fellows per year.[38] It identifies rehabilitation and recovery as central components of training, which constitutes an inclusive strategy to manage severely mentally ill people. Learning is achieved through active involvement rather than simply observation: theoretical principles learned during academic sessions are implemented in field placement. The fellowship is characterized by seven core elements (described in Table 5.3), which are recognized as examples of best practice and constitute the basis for the development of the guidelines of the American Association of Community Psychiatrists (AACP).[28]

Conclusions

Social psychiatry may well be 'alive and kicking',[8] but still there is the need to balance the dominant biomedical model, renegotiating the profession of psychiatry and completing a social re-engineering of community psychiatry in terms of scientific grounds, moral relevance and social influence.[24]

Table 5.2 Obstacles facing early career staff in community psychiatry, lessons learned and possible solutions.[2]

Professional obstacles and challenges	Lessons learned and solutions
Need for leadership	Psychiatrists and other mental health professionals need to be involved as experts in planning, education and research
Difficulty sustaining in-service training/adequate supervision	Training of the trainers by external staff
	Shifting of some traditional psychiatric functions to trained and willing staff
	Make this a service priority
High staff turnover and burnout, or low staff morale	Recovery-oriented services providing relevant examples
	Involving staff leaders in oversight and decision-making committees
	Avoid individual solutions, such as removing a burnt out worker from the job, as situational and organizational factors play a greater role in burnout. Intervention should be aimed at the areas of reward and fairness
Poor quality of care/concern about staff skills	Emphasize career-long continuing training programmes, including out-of-area professional meetings
	Disseminate and implement guidelines
	Cultivate staff clinical skills
	External audit procedures
	Encourage and reward quality by structured initiatives
Professional resistance, e.g. to community-oriented care and service user involvement	Governmental and professional bodies promoting and campaigning about community-care and users' involvement
	Management groups supporting psychiatrists to use their abilities more broadly and work with a range of stakeholders including consumers and carers/families
	Develop training in recovery-oriented psychosocial rehabilitation
Lack of research on community mental health services cost-effectiveness and evaluation	Prioritizing research, qualitative and quantitative, about successfully implemented examples of community mental health services

Table 5.3 Core elements of community psychiatry training.[28]

Element 1: the academic curriculum covers the essential topics in public psychiatry	The curriculum is organized in 12 sections addressing mental health care needs of both adults with a severe mental illness and of other populations, such as those of people suffering from substance use disorders, post-traumatic stress disorder (PTSD) and the homeless. The structure of public mental health, fiscal management topics and elements for public mental health advocacy, are basic components of the curriculum.
Element 2: trainees apply concepts learned in the academic curriculum in their field placements	Through seven oral presentations, trainees describe to other trainees and faculty what they are doing at their field placement sites. Such presentations give the trainee the chance both to become skilled at organizing meetings and to share comments with their field-placement site supervisors.
Element 3: weekly presentations by guest speakers illustrate topics covered in the academic curriculum	
Element 4: trainees complete a practicum in mental health administration	Six didactic sessions and six case presentations on management problems are alternated. The aim is to try to solve pragmatic problems described in the case presentations and, in the following didactic session, to examine and appraise how theoretical notions of management are put into practice in the case presentations. This element is important also in maintaining a link and creating a supportive relationship between faculty, current trainees and alumni (medical directors in public mental health organizations), with trainees being informed of the careers of the alumni.
Element 5: field placement in a public mental health organization in order to obtain comprehensive clinical and management experience	Trainees work 3 days a week in a field placement with a leadership role.

(continued overleaf)

Table 5.3 (Continued)

Element 6: weekly meetings with a faculty preceptor supporting individuals in academic and field-placement experiences	Each trainee is assigned a faculty preceptor, whose tasks include helping the trainee with her/his presentations and examining her/his experience in the field placement, in order to facilitate the integration of theoretical and practical experiences. Clinical and administrative supervision is provided by a field-placement supervisor, where possible a former trainee. The preceptor acts as a link between the faculty and the supervisor.
Element 7: faculty provides mentorship and ongoing support beyond the fellowship year	The link between the faculty members and alumni goes beyond the fellowship year: this is achieved through mentorship and supervision, as well as meetings, and different kind of contacts via the internet.

Likewise, community psychiatry training needs to be weighted equally towards science as towards encompassing diverse professional practices. We need committed, responsive and engaged practitioners, who are aware of the multifactorial nature of severe mental illness, willing to employ a genuine bio-psycho-social paradigm, culturally sensitive and focused on the service users' empowerment. Such practitioners may represent the minority at present, but it is a legitimate aspiration for the future, which may be fostered by more appropriate selection, training, role modelling and systems of reward.[11] Sound curricula and training programmes should ensure that the 'end product' community mental health worker will have acquired the knowledge, skills and attitudes to meet the newly identified responsibilities. A channel of communication is needed with educational agencies in terms of different professional groups working together in their respective roles in providing mental health care (e.g. primary care nurses and community mental health nurses, psychiatrists and psychologists, social workers and occupational therapists).[3] As community psychiatric training appears to differ across countries,[33] it is necessary to strive for more uniform curricula, through the identification of common theoretical and field placement core elements. Studies aimed at the evaluation of trainees after completion of training are limited and should be implemented in order to appraise the quality of training itself.

However, as Stein[39] stated, although 'not everyone can or should be a community psychiatrist', nonetheless 'those who possess some of the qualities' needed 'will find rich rewards in the field of community

---

Box 5.1 Web resources for training curricula in community psychiatry

- Centre for Mental Health (formerly The Sainsbury Centre for Mental Health) – UK; http://www.centreformentalhealth.org.uk/
- International Mental Health Leadership Program (iMHLP) – Australia; http://www.cimh.unimelb.edu.au/pdp/imhlp
- Mental Health Foundation – UK; http://www.mentalhealth.org.uk/
- Mental Health in Higher Education – UK; http://www.mhhe.heacademy.ac.uk/
- Center for Psychiatric Rehabilitation, Boston, MA – USA; http://www.bu.edu/cpr/training/index.html •
- Fellowship in Community Psychiatry/Public Health, within the Department of Psychiatry and Behavioral Sciences at the Emory University School of Medicine, Atlanta, GA – USA; http://www.psychiatry.emory.edu/Community_Psychiatry.cfm
- Public Psychiatry Fellowship of New York State Psychiatric Institute at Columbia University Medical Center, New York – USA; http://ppf.hs.columbia.edu/

---

psychiatry'. They deserve the best available training in terms of knowledge, skills and activities to match their innate attitudes.

References

1. Talbott JA. The evolution and current status of public–academic partnerships in psychiatry. *Psychiatr Serv* 2008; **59**: 15–16.
2. Thornicroft T, Alem A, Dos Santos RA *et al.* WPA guidance on steps, obstacles and mistakes to avoid in the implementation of community mental health care. *World Psychiatry* 2010; **9**: 67–77.
3. World Health Organization. *Mental Health Policy and Service Guidance Package. Human Resources and Training in Mental Health*. Geneva: WHO, 2005.
4. Bebbington P. Textbook of community psychiatry. *Br J Psychiatry* 2002; **180**: 383–384.
5. Thornicroft G, Szmukler G. What is community psychiatry? In: Thornicroft G, Szmukler G (eds) *Textbook of Community Psychiatry*. Oxford: Oxford University Press, 2001; pp. 1–12.
6. European Union of Medical Specialists. Report of the UEMS Section for Psychiatry. Recommendations on social and community psychiatry. UEMS, 2006. Available at: www.uemspsychiatry.org/section/reports/socCom2006.pdf [accessed 10 August 2011].

7. Leff JP. The historical development of social psychiatry. In: Bughra D, Morgan C (eds) *Principles of Social Psychiatry*, 2nd edn. Chichester: John Wiley & Sons, Ltd, 2010; pp. 3–11.

8. Bughra D, Morgan C. Social psychiatry: alive and kicking. In: Bughra D, Morgan C (eds) *Principles of Social Psychiatry*, 2nd edn. Chichester: John Wiley & Sons, 2010; pp. XV–XVI.

9. Egger D, Lipson D, Adams O. Achieving the right balance: the role of policymaking processes in managing human resources for health problems. Human resources for health, discussion paper no. 2. Geneva: WHO, 2000.

10. Thornicroft G, Tansella M. What are the arguments for community-based mental health care? Health Evidence Network report. Copenhagen: WHO Regional Office for Europe, 2003. Available at: www.euro.who.int/document/E82976.pdf [accessed 26 August 2011].

11. Rosen A. The community psychiatrist of the future. *Curr Opin Psychiatry* 2006; **19**: 380–388.

12. Diamond R, Susser E, Stein LI. Essential and nonessential roles for psychiatrists in community mental health centres. *Hosp Community Psychiatry* 1992; **42**: 187–189.

13. Cox J. Psychiatric training and professional conduct. *Curr Opin Psychiatry* 1996; **9**: 372–376.

14. Callaly T, Minas H. Reflections on clinician leadership and management. *Aust Psychiatry* 2005; **13**: 27–32.

15. Kitchener BA, Jorm AF. Mental health first aid training: review of evaluation studies. *Aust NZ J Psychiatry* 2006; **40**: 6–8.

16. Thornicroft G, Tansella M. Components of a modern mental health service: a pragmatic balance of community and hospital care: overview of systematic evidence. *Br J Psychiatry* 2004; **185**: 283–290.

17. Killaspy H, Johnson S, King M *et al.* Developing mental health services in response to research evidence. *Epidemiol Psichiat Soc* 2008; **17**: 47–56.

18. National Collaborating Centre for Mental Health. *Core Interventions in the Treatment and Management of Schizophrenia in Adults in Primary and Secondary Care (updated edition)*. Leicester: The British Psychological Society; London: The Royal College of Psychiatrists, 2010.

19. Gask L, Lester H, Kendrick T *et al. Primary Care Mental Health*. London: The Royal College of Psychiatrists, 2009.

20. Whitley R, McKenzie K. Social capital and psychiatry: review of the literature. *Harvard Rev Psychiatry* 2005; **13**: 71–84.

21. Mojtabai R, Fochtmann L, Chang SW *et al.* Unmet need for mental health care in schizophrenia: an overview of literature and new data from a first-admission study. *Schizophrenia Bull* 2009; **35**: 679–695.

22. Osborn DP, Wright CA, Levy G *et al.* Relative risk of diabetes, dyslipidaemia, hypertension and the metabolic syndrome in people with severe mental illnesses: systematic review and metaanalysis. *BMC Psychiatry* 2008; **8**: 84.

23. Kelly CM, Jorm AF, Kitchener BA. Development of mental health first aid guidelines on how a member of the public can support a person affected by a traumatic event: a Delphi study. *BMC Psychiatry* 2010; **10**: 49.

24. Pilgrim D, Roger AE. Psychiatrists as social engineers: a study of an antistigma campaign. *Soc Sci Med* 2005; **61**: 2546–2556.
25. Maj M. Are psychiatrists an endangered species? *World Psychiatry* 2010; **9**: 1–2.
26. Talbott JA. Has academic psychiatry abandoned the community? *Acad Psychiatry* 1991; **15**: 106–114.
27. Gournay K. Training for competence. In: Thornicroft G, Szmukler G (eds) *Textbook of Community Psychiatry*. Oxford: Oxford University Press, 2001; pp. 243–252.
28. American Association of Community Psychiatrists. American Association of Community Psychiatrists' Guidelines for Developing and Evaluating Public and Community Psychiatry Training Fellowships. AACP, 2008. Available at: www.communitypsychiatry.org/publications/clinical_and_administrative _tools_guidelines/AACPPublicPsychiatryFellow-V1.pdf [accessed 10 August 2011].
29. Torrey WC, Green RL, Drake RE. Psychiatrists and psychiatric rehabilitation. *J Psychiatr Pract* 2005; **11**: 155–158.
30. Royal College of Psychiatrists. Statement on approval of training schemes for basic specialist training for the MRCPsych (BSTC/01). London: Royal College of Psychiatrists, 1998.
31. Linsley K, Slinn R, Nathan R *et al.* Training implications of community-oriented psychiatry. *Adv Psychiatr Treat* 2001; **7**: 208–215.
32. The Sainsbury Centre for Mental Health. The capable practitioner: a framework and list of the practitioner capabilities required to implement the National Service Framework for Mental Health. London: Sainsbury Centre for Mental Health, 2001.
33. World Health Organization. *Atlas: Psychiatric Education and Training Across the World*. Geneva: WHO, 2005.
34. World Psychiatric Association. World Psychiatric Association institutional program on the core training curriculum for psychiatry. Yokohama: WPA, 2002. Available at: http://www.wpanet.org/uploads/Education/Educational _Programs/Core_Curriculum/curriculum-psych-ENG.pdf [accessed 16 August 2011].
35. European Union of Medical Specialists. Consensus statement – Psychiatric services focussed on a community: challenges for the training of future psychiatrists. UEMS, 2004. Available at: www.uemspsychiatry.org/section/reports/ ConsensusStatement-2004.pdf [accessed 10 August 2011].
36. Royal College of Psychiatrists. A competency based curriculum for specialist training in psychiatry. Specialist module in adult (general and community) psychiatry. RC Psych, 2009. Available at: http://www.rcpsych.ac.uk/pdf/ General Psychiatry submission October 2010 (Aug 11 Update).pdf [accessed 16 August 2011].
37. Maj M. Mistakes to avoid in the implementation of community mental health care. *World Psychiatry* 2010; **9**: 65–66.
38. Ranz JM, Deakins SM, LeMelle SM *et al.* Core elements of a public psychiatry fellowship. *Psychiatr Serv* 2008; **59**: 718–720.
39. Stein LI. The community psychiatrist: skills and personal characteristics. *Community Ment Hlt J* 1998; **34**: 437–445.

CHAPTER 6

Why, what and how should early career psychiatrists learn about phenomenological psychopathology?

Umberto Volpe[1] and Henning Sass[2]
[1]Department of Psychiatry, University of Naples SUN, Naples, Italy
[2]Department of Psychiatry, University of Technology RWTH, Aachen, Germany

We don't see things as they are, we see things as we are

Anaïs Nin, 1969

Introduction

Until a few decades ago, it was rather implicit for most trainees in psychiatry to read Jaspers' General Psychopathology or other classical books about psychopathology by Minkowski or Binswanger, since they represented the main conceptual framework from which to observe and understand mental illnesses. Today, this is no longer true. With few exceptions, psychiatric trainees usually base their initial conceptual approach to mental illnesses on a familiarization with the standardized operational criteria of major diagnostic manuals. However, a recent survey conducted among early career psychiatrists on their opinions of the quality of training during residency, clearly showed that young psychiatrists still perceive training in psychopathology as a core aspect of their education, and that educational programmes dealing with phenomenological approaches are still greatly needed within residency training in psychiatry.[1] Unfortunately, this does not seem to always happen. Actually, the gradual abandonment of classical psychopathology is not the trainees' fault, nor that of their tutors and teachers. These days, the attention of psychiatry in general

How to Succeed in Psychiatry: A Guide to Training and Practice, First Edition.
Edited by Andrea Fiorillo, Iris Tatjana Calliess and Henning Sass.
© 2012 John Wiley & Sons, Ltd. Published 2012 by John Wiley & Sons, Ltd.

is more at a strictly clinical level, to the biological basis of psychiatric disorders, or to the organization of health-care services for the mentally ill, rather than to phenomenological psychopathology. This is not even a fault of the discipline itself, but rather a consequence of its historical evolution.

Objective or subjective psychiatry?

Psychiatry has probably followed – although with some delay – a more general trend in medicine. Medicine has traditionally been considered a 'soft science', in which scientific knowledge has always been translated into the art of practising by medical doctors. However, during the 1950s, medicine began to transform itself 'from a practising art into a scientific discipline based on molecular biology'.[2] Due to the constantly growing scientific and technical knowledge and to the greater availability of diagnostic and therapeutic tools, doctors tended to assume a privileged perspective towards the patient. In most cases, they are inclined to think they know more than their patients and that they have to provide them with the 'scientific' and objective truth about their subjective symptoms (usually disregarded as unreliable and potentially false). However, this is probably not true. The so-called 'hard sciences' have long abandoned this stance and admit that, as stated by the Austrian physicist Erwin Schrödinger,[3] 'the object is affected by our observation', and therefore they do not assume anymore that a truly objective observer exists. This, in turn, implies that a scientific observation should always be confronted with the intrinsic limits of scientific methods and with the need to explore subjective limitations of observations and analytical processes. For 'soft sciences', such considerations should probably have even more relevance. Instead, surprisingly, a presumed 'objective approach' to diseases still represents the dominant model in medical schools, and the patient is rather conceptualized as an 'object' from which the doctor is supposed to extract 'hard' data, by means of a series of objective/subjective measurements. However, since the last decade general medicine has started to rethink its attitude towards patients, by estimating the risk of oversimplifying the doctor-patient relationship and of reducing it to a dehumanizing approach.[4] Saunders[5] clearly pointed out that the practice of medicine should indeed be conceived both as an 'art' and a 'science' and that evidence-based models, although correct in principle, might show significant limits in clinical practice.

Ironically, the medical discipline that – probably more than the others – should pay specific attention to human relationships still seems to be out of step and tends to favour a bioscientific 'hard' model of practice. During the second half of the twentieth century, psychiatry (probably due to parallel progress in psychopharmacology and neuropsychology, which provided new perspectives both in psychiatric research as well as in clinical psychiatry) completely adopted Griesinger's famous motto of 'mental diseases being diseases of the brain'[6] and somehow forced itself back into the mainstream of objective medicine. So, it is not surprising that the current models of psychiatric practice are still based on the objective/descriptive one, mostly derived from Kraepelin's work and oriented more to produce reliable diagnosis rather than to truly understand the characteristics of the subject's feelings.[7] Laing[8] has elegantly condensed this inner paradoxical contradiction, stating that 'psychiatry tries to be as scientific, impersonal and objective as possible towards what is most personal and subjective'. This attitude has probably represented for the psychiatrists of the last century a sort of 'natural evolution' of the discipline, given the need to standardize a discipline that had evolved towards subjectivity, given the considerable amount of biological evidence produced in the second half of the twentieth century, and given the general shift of psychiatry into neurobiology and neuroscience. However, the psychiatrists of the twentieth century were properly trained in psychopathology and had time enough to gradually adapt to such changes. However, for the psychiatrists of the twenty-first century, such an evolution may imply significant risks.

The risks of neglecting psychopathology for psychiatric training

Psychiatry is a medical discipline that traditionally has strong links to the humanities (such as, at least, philosophy, social sciences and psychology). Psychiatry's epistemological foundations should by definition be broad since its 'object' (i.e. the human mind) is complex by nature. A complex discipline should thus have a proper 'philosophical system' behind the method of clinical practice, in order to allow a true multidimensional approach to a multidimensional entity. Especially for the training of young psychiatrists, it is important to open up the broad scope of perspectives of psychiatry[9] (see Table 6.1), although it may take a special effort to bring conceptual and methodological order to the heterogeneous phenomena of psychiatry. However, today, psychiatric residents are usually well trained to use structured psychometric scales, but only seldom do they try to understand the patient's inner world. The attempt to standardize psychiatric interviews may eliminate the 'background noise' represented by subjectivity: but does this represent only a possible source of bias that should be eliminated? If a trainee is not prepared to fill the 'empty space' of what is not measurable or quantifiable with proper psychopathological knowledge of phenomenology, the answer would probably be yes; but, if phenomenological psychopathology is among the core skills of a

Table 6.1 The 'four perspectives' of psychiatry. According to McHugh and Slavney,[11] the classical integrated 'bio-psycho-social' model is rather reductionist since mental events and mental health problems should be viewed from, at least, four different perspectives (illustrated here).

Perspective	Definition	Example(s)
Disease	Impairment in brain structure and/or function	Often used to explain depression, schizophrenia, dementia
Dimension	The way in which an individual's character or trait may cause trouble to that individual	Stable/unstable, extroversion/introversion, high IQ/low IQ
Behaviour	Actions persist because they have been reinforced, or are driven by biological means	Addiction, obesity, paraphilias
Life stories	What has happened to a person that leads him/her to experience life as he/she does?	Grief

psychiatrist, that space would probably be filled with shared thoughts and feelings, and such empathic processes would greatly enhance the understanding of patients' problems and needs, as well as the quality of doctor-patient relationships and that of psychiatric care itself. The ability to enter into someone's inner world should represent the true identity of a psychiatrist. The major risk of a psychiatry in which psychopathology is just disregarded is the risk of losing its own identity. Among the major potential risks of the objectification of psychiatry is the fact that psychiatrists trained only to assess symptoms by rating scales, mainly directed to observable behaviours, might be just focused on the most obvious aspects of psychiatric daily practice. This may lead psychiatry to clinical oversimplification and the constitution of broad (and probably less meaningful) diagnostic categories. A diagnosis constructed on mere lists of clear-cut and replicable symptoms may just fail to catch substantial details and end up with a general outline of the patient's true psychopathology, a sort of 'draft diagnosis', rather than a really meaningful one. The risk of such a process has been conceptualized by Van Praag[10] as follows: 'a painting by Vermeer in which the blues have been left out may be Vermeer-like, but it is not a Vermeer.'

The risks of neglecting psychopathology for psychiatry as a whole

Beyond the clear implications for clinical practice, there is also a more subtle risk for the entire discipline: a diagnosis rising only from symptoms might be easily detached from aetiology, especially from psychological determinants of mental illnesses. Where would such a 'restricted psychiatry' end? What would be the meaning of psychiatric research if it is not led by meaningful models? Even the best designed and most technically sophisticated neuroimaging study would fail to catch the neurobiological basis of a mental illness if no satisfying model of that illness lies at its fundament. The recent trend of favouring a neurobiological approach to mental illnesses may be, of course, agreeable (if not necessary), but it has to be balanced by the awareness that the mind cannot be simply reduced to an epiphenomenon of the brain. The issue concerning the impact of the meaning of brain research on the idea of a human, on the treatment of patients with mental disorders and on the assessment of offenders is not new.[12] While some psychiatrists conceptualized feelings, thoughts and decisions as determined by causal laws of neuronal processes, others thought that they were more related to subjectivity and freedom of will; such a controversy persisted for centuries. Griesinger,[6] who held the first chair of psychiatry at the Charité in Berlin, wrote in his famous textbook: 'Even if we knew all the things going on in the brain, all chemical electrical processes in detail – what would it be good for? All oscillations and vibrations, everything electrical and mechanical is still no mental state, no visualization. How it can become like that – this riddle will remain unsolved till the end of time, and I believe if an angel would be coming down from heaven and would explain everything to us, our intellect would not be able to comprehend.' The brain-mind dilemma is not only a philosophical issue of scholarly interest, but it directly affects psychiatric teaching as well as clinical theory and practice.

What training in psychopathology?

Psychiatry training needs psychopathology. But then, what do we talk about? Stanghellini[13] characterized phenomenological-descriptive psychopathology as sorting out, defining, differentiating and describing specific psychic phenomena, which are thereby actualized and are regularly described in specific terms. Phenomenology can be conceptualized as a particular style and method of information gathering, one that groups related phenomena clearly differentiable by a patient's self-descriptions, excluding any preconceived notion or theory and focusing on the modes in which the experience comes to expression. This approach gives a special emphasis to introspection via an interactive and empathic process between the clinician and the patient, aimed at clarifying mental phenomena 'from inside'. Such descriptions are based on the work of Karl Jaspers (1883–1969), the founder of psychopathology as a methodologically reflected science. Jaspers defined objective and subjective symptoms and was the first to explicitly realize the psychiatric significance and implications of the dichotomy between (causal) *explanation* and *understanding*.[14] He stated that there can be no choice between explanation and understanding, since patients are both agents *and* organisms; they have both mind *and* brain. Because of the junction between mind and brain, the phenomenal world must be viewed from several different perspectives if it is to be fully appreciated.[15] According to Jaspers,[14,16,17] good clinicians should try to abandon their preconceived ideas about their patient, to enter into his/her inner world by means of an attitude of neutral empathy and to accept the only possible truth of the individual's subjective experience. Jaspers[14] also affirmed the relevance of this part of phenomenological description by the differentiation between *objective* and *subjective symptoms*. The latter are emotions, inner processes and sensory manifestations like fear, grief or cheerfulness. They cannot be received by sensory organs but only by putting ourselves into another's soul, by empathy. They can be easily differentiated from the *objective symptoms*, which are all the processes that can be perceived with the senses: reflexes, visible movements, the photographable face, motor agitation, speech utterances, written products, actions, lifestyle, etc. They can only be understood by thinking rationally. Jaspers remarked in his philosophical autobiography that anyone speaking about the mind must know 'what one knows, how one knows it, and what one does not know'.[16] There is no single 'optimal method' for the study of mind and brain, and the empirical method of enquiry is maintained solely by the fact of the patient's communications.[14,16,17] The crucial methodological question for Jaspersian phenomenology thus becomes the following: by what scientific method can the psychiatrist achieve valid knowledge of the subjective experiences of another person, namely, the experiences of his or her patient? This method of one person experiencing another person's experiences will require some form of empathy,[18] and we regard empathy as an indispensable tool for human relationships, of which the patient-doctor relationship is a special one.

Why psychopathology is still relevant for psychiatric training

The fascination and risks in psychiatric thinking lie in the complex nature of psychiatric disorders, which is characterized by an intricate interplay of somatic functions, learning processes, attitudes acquired during biography and situation-specific influences.[19] Mental disorders mostly occur in the 'inner perspective' of the patients. They suffer from changes due to disorder in their self-experience, in feelings, emotions, intentions, hopes, expectations, plans, in self-estimation and in estimation of other persons; thus they suffer from modification of subjectivity. These correlate indeed with brain processes, but they also have an autonomy that goes beyond and is nevertheless natural.[12] However, Jaspers showed that the subjective and objective symptoms cannot be separated when dealing with mental disorders. Understanding why patients act like they do using the phenomenological method of understanding, and in addition explaining what can be explained with the help of natural sciences, are both fundamental for a scientific analysis of the connections between mind and brain.

There is no doubt that the method of understanding a patient's inner perspective still represents the *via regia* for establishing a close relationship between patient and physician, and it is crucial for a personalized psychiatry. Understanding the subjective experience of the patient and the relationship between patient and physician cannot be fully replaced by concentrating only on observational behaviours and data from neuroscience or biological psychiatry. All techniques together can support each other and be connected in an integrated approach to find a diagnostic formulation and design a multimodal treatment strategy using psychotherapeutic, psychopharmacological and psychosocial methodology.

The phenomenological-anthropological approach in psychopathology, as we describe it here, has a special tradition in Germany, the Latin countries and Japan.[20] However, the main question for discussion is whether the phenomenological approach in psychopathology is still of worldwide relevance in psychiatric teaching, training, patient care and research; it can be formulated as follows: 'How important is the "inner perspective" of the patient's experience?'[12]

Some clinical examples

The question of whether phenomenological psychopathology is still a basic skill of psychiatrists is connected with the impact of modern classification systems on education and training, as well as on strategies for patient care. The fact that modern systems of classification have made a fundamental contribution to the ability to compare findings in therapy, research, administration and quality control is without doubt very positive.[20] Contemporary diagnostic systems are in fact derived from earlier research diagnostic criteria (RDC),[21] whose explicitly admitted purpose was to allow diagnoses to be consistent in psychiatric research. Current operational diagnostic criteria perfectly serve to improve the reliability of clinical studies of mental disorder, since that was their original aim. However, the aim of the average clinician is not to enhance the reliability of his or her assessment, but rather to comprehensively describe the complex inner reality of the patient sitting in front of him or her. In the latter case, operational criteria probably should not be regarded as a crucial reference. A paradigmatic example of that is the concept of schizophrenia and its current formulation within the *Diagnostic and Statistical Manual IV* (DSM-IV): analysing in detail its symptomatological, chronological and functional criteria, it appears evident that the current diagnosis holds only few residua of the Kraepelinian, Bleulerian and Schneiderian concepts, while diagnosis is made mainly by exclusion of other medical and mental diseases.[22] More recently, a debate published in the journal *World Psychiatry*, focusing on the pathophysiology of schizophrenia and the available biological markers for this disease,[23] clearly highlighted both the lack of reliable and useful biological tests and the need to define further subtypes of schizophrenia in order to achieve more effective models of treatment for such disease.[24] Strik,[25] within the same volume, also concluded that the clinical handling and the understanding of schizophrenia should be based on both pathophysiological findings and proper theoretical models, even if the clinician is not a scientist or a philosopher. Unfortunately, such objective biological tests and integrative phenomenological models are not available yet for schizophrenia.[26]

If one of the most important psychiatric diagnoses is currently lacking a proper paradigm, it is not surprising either that in the *International Classification of Diseases 10* (ICD-10) and DSM-IV, crucial elements of the conceptual history of psychopathology have been completely abandoned. Even basic psychiatric symptoms seem to have been 'emptied out' within modern diagnostic approaches: for example, anguish is presented, within the diagnostic glossary of DSM, as a sort of homogeneous concept, whereas it may express very different meanings (e.g. fear of failure, fear for external threats, or anxiety); similarly, aggression may be aroused by humiliation, external threats, or the need to defend one's own territory or ideas. In most cases the qualitative heterogeneity of such symptoms is simply missed in contemporary diagnostic manuals.

Another example of how modern psychiatric classification systems may fail truly to catch the essence of relevant psychopathological phenomena is probably represented by sub-threshold symptoms, which lie at the 'interface' between the objective and subjective, being 'quasi-subjective' in nature: German psychiatrists traditionally identify a specific predelusional state, called *Wahnstimmung*, a condition in which a patient's experiences might become delusional but are not yet clearly of that nature, as they are still modifiable and correctable. Would a purely objective evaluator really be able to grasp the patient's anguish and inner turmoil, if such a condition is not readily observable or easily verbalized, and falls outside the listed criteria needed to establish a standardized diagnosis? Probably asking a few standardized questions in a limited amount of time would not represent the ideal strategy to get access to and understand the patient's suffering.

Would any psychometric rating scale really be able to catch the subtle psychopathological nuances of what Jaspers defined *depressio sine depressione*, referring to the early stages of the so-called 'vital depression'?[27] Again, this psychopathological entity would likely just be missed in an excessively standardized setting. Should a patient with no marked sadness but covertly feeling spiritless, downhearted or irritable, and with persistent bodily 'hangover-like' sensations be helped by a psychiatrist? Probably yes, if only the psychiatrist could recognize such an affective state in the person sitting in front of him/her.

The relevance of 'subjective psychiatry' is not only a scholarly issue, but it has clear implications for both pharmacological and psychological treatments. For example, the presence of a Freudian 'character neurosis' has been demonstrated to exert influence over the response to psychotropic drugs, although being a non-standardized condition;[10] similarly, a psychiatrist who would just ignore 'subjective feelings' since, again, they might not be easily standardizable, is simply more prone to miss subtle changes in symptomatology and probably worsen the final outcome of any pharmacological treatment. This issue is relevant also for non-pharmacological treatments: panic attacks are described, within the DSM-IV, as the rise of anxiety symptoms 'developed abruptly' (i.e. without any apparent or demonstrable cause); most psychotherapists would not agree with the absence of a connection between life events and panic attacks (although non-immediate and probably covert), and their work would indeed concentrate on such subjective experiences and on the hidden relationships with the symptoms.

Where is psychiatry going without psychopathology?

One consequence of the recently diminished attention paid to the psychopathological tradition in psychiatry is that younger generations of psychiatrists will deal with reductive disease conceptualizations that are simply unrealistic, and whose descriptions are dangerously elusive and shallow. Another possible consequence is that the knowledge of important psychopathological concepts in which generations of young psychiatrists have been trained will tend to fade. Overall, the requirement for reliability forces one to concentrate on observable behaviours during the diagnostic process, whereas the inner experiences of the patient get less attention. Standardized questionnaires may generate subjective estimates (and not real objective measures), since they are implicitly affected by two relevant potential sources of bias. First, a severity score on a rating scale still represents the interviewer's 'translation' of a patient's subjective symptom into a presumed objective statement: this process might imply a significant bias due to the rater's ability to understand what the individual is communicating. Second, another unavoidable source of bias for 'objective assessments' lies in the subjective variations of patients' ability and/or will to recognize and correctly verbalize their own inner experiences.

In addition, the classification systems are affected by consensus procedures, political influences and even by a certain imperialism in science. Psychodynamic and psychostructural factors are set aside. There is a strong tendency to think in terms of objective criteria and disregard aspects of subjective experience and biography. There is also a trend towards horizontalization, instead of verticalization, via the comorbidity principle, which leads to sometimes curious results (e.g. when diagnosing a multitude of personality disorders for the same individual). Finally, there is the basic reservation that modern classification manuals represent a means by which one fundamental element of psychiatry, psychopathology, is used only as a technical aid for distinctions in biological psychiatry, with the consequent loss of the notion of a 'pure psychopathology', i.e. methodologically reflected thinking about structural and functional connections of the normal and abnormal inner life, and especially the mental experiences.[19,28-30] Such a reductionist approach should not be considered a satisfying endpoint for a scientific discipline, definitely implying a substantial impoverishment of our discipline, against which younger psychiatrists should make a stand.

A new era for psychopathology in psychiatric training

Of course, today's training in psychiatry is very complex and trainees face many challenges, probably unknown to their predecessors – we only have to think of the strict rules of managed care models, combined with the recent shift of psychiatric care towards integrated models of practice in which neurobiology, psychopharmacology, cognitive behavioural models, and community-oriented approaches are included.[31] Furthermore, training in phenomenological psychopathology is probably more complex and time consuming compared to other clinical approaches. So, how could training in psychopathology for psychiatry residents be improved? This question can be answered on two different levels at least.

First, some requirements for future operational classification systems have to be kept in mind. The goal of new diagnostic manuals should be to find a clinical formulation and to design a multimodal treatment strategy using psychopharmacological, psychotherapeutic and psychosocial methods. Psychosocial contexts should be emphasized more and functional psychopathology must be developed.[10] Basing diagnoses on biological markers, combining 'categorical and dimensional approaches', diagnosing *ex juvantibus*, thinking dimensional instead of atheoretical are important to a return to an integrated perspective. This is not only important for diagnosis and treatment. In addition, a differentiated approach – including phenomenological psychopathology – would allow for the evaluation of differences, details and variations in patients' experiences, which could serve as clues and indicators for the selection of patients for investigation as well as for actual research into causes.[18] The recent developments in compiling DSM-5 show some efforts to achieve harmonization with ICD-10. Axes I, II and III of DSM-IV might be collapsed into one axis containing all psychiatric and general medical diagnoses. This brings DSM-5 into greater harmony with the single-axis approach of ICD. Axis IV of DSM-5 will contain psychosocial and environmental problems; the working group on this axis is examining codes that are comparable to ICD-10. Axis V will allow clinicians to rate a patient's level of functioning so that disability and distress should be better assessed in DSM-5 and follow more closely the outlines of the World Health Organization (WHO). Of special interest for such a perspective are the tendencies in the discussion process for ICD-11 to reach a more 'personalized' approach. Laín-Entralgo[32] pointed out that 'diagnosis is more than identifying a disorder or distinguishing one disorder from another; diagnosis is really understanding what is going on in the mind and body of the person who presents for care'. Developing a person-centred integrative diagnosis as a theoretical model as well as a practical guide, and designing the best possible classification of mental disorders, has been the goal of the WHO/World Psychiatric Association (WPA) (ICD-11) and the American Psychiatric Association (APA; DSM-5), and of other national and regional psychiatric associations in recent years.[33] Hopefully, it will not be abandoned during the ongoing finalization of these diagnostic psychiatric manuals.

Second, there is the need to develop new instruments to access the patient's inner world. Subjective psychopathology is usually conceived as impossible to measure by definition, but it is probably just not well measured by currently available rating and diagnostic tools. Although psychopathologically informed empirical studies are paying more attention to subjective experiences (especially for psychotic disorders; see ref. 34), a special effort should be devoted in future to developing new evaluation and rating instruments, which may integrate objective and subjective approaches to psychiatric diagnosis. The use of oriented but yet 'free' (rather than structured) interviews or (already available) projective psychological tests might represent a valuable add-on to standardized rating scales, in order to achieve an acceptable degree of reliability without losing subjective information.

For at least a decade, new clinical models have been proposed that are considered complementary to the currently prevailing evidence-based approach: the so-called 'narrative-based medicine'[35] focuses more on the 'story behind the disease' and integrates classical medical history with the subject's personal and life history. Such models point out the limitations of traditional disease models (classically conceived as a collection of signs and symptoms) and broaden the doctors' perspective towards the person, allowing physicians to reach a deeper understanding of the pathological condition of their patients. It is highly advisable that psychiatry follows this trend of general medicine, trying to reconcile its natural predisposition for the humanities with its needs for evidence-based and scientifically grounded approaches, overcoming false dichotomies and achieving a more 'balanced' clinical approach.

However, one should avoid the risk of presenting phenomenological psychopathology as the only method capable of bringing systematic order to the complexity of empirical reality,[36] and as supposedly a basic science, independent of the natural and medical sciences.[28] In this sense, the most practical solution probably lies in an open and holistic attitude of psychiatry, which should consider phenomenological psychopathology as a conceptual foundation of the discipline itself, although it should always be able to constantly adapt current nosological systems to the growing body of clinical and research knowledge.

Conclusions

Phenomenologically oriented psychopathology is, in most cases, neglected in contemporary training in psychiatry, due to the prevalence of objective models of clinical practice and to the great relevance of neuroscience and neuropharmacology to psychiatric research on pathophysiology and therapy. The implicit assumption of contemporary psychiatry is that the latter approaches are alternatives to the empathic and subjective approaches to psychiatric patients.[37] However, as Damasio[38] correctly pointed out in referring to it as Descartes' error, such a dichotomy is probably an artificial divide. It is simply not true that greater attention to existential factors and the first-person perspective will lead to neglect of bioscientific knowledge. In turn, the integration of different ideas and clinical schemes is necessary for the growth of the discipline, whereas favouring just one or the other of the above mentioned two approaches would probably result in psychiatry's impoverishment. Eisenberg,[39] more than 10 years ago, already urged the need of a more balanced attitude in psychiatry to avoid the risk of making our discipline either 'brainless' or 'mindless'. And Fulford[40] argued that psychiatrists need to operate both in the 'world of facts' (represented by science) but also in the world of values (represented by the humanities). Psychiatric practice truly lies at that peculiar interface between biological, psychological and social factors, which are currently thought to represent the true determinants of mental illnesses. Of course, such an integration is not easily achievable, but probably represents the only way out from the possible danger of a scientific and clinical stagnation of our discipline. Kandel,[41] while attempting to define a 'new intellectual framework for psychiatry' at the dawn of the new millennium, already foresaw that psychiatry in the future should have a sort of 'double role', both asking questions on its own level (i.e. how to diagnose and treat mental disorders, including the patient's perspective) and posing questions regarding human behaviour and higher mental processes (to answer which, biology is definitely needed).

The European Psychiatric Association (EPA), in the last decades, has constantly attempted to promote such an attitude in psychiatry. On the one hand, the EPA has promoted the harmonization of standards for education and training in the different countries of Europe but, on the other hand, it has carefully preserved the broad tradition of European psychiatry, which has a long history and a unique richness in its psychopathological heritage. At the 2010 EPA Congress held in Munich, the role of the traditional phenomenological psychopathology in the era of neuroscience and biological psychiatry was specifically addressed in a 'pro-con debate' (entitled "Traditional phenomenological-descriptive psychopathology is no longer relevant in the new era of biological psychiatry"). During this debate, some experts argued in favour of such a provocative statement, but during the discussion there was a growing acceptance for the opposite position, defending the impact of phenomenology in psychopathology for the whole field of psychiatry and advocating a more balanced attitude in clinical practice.

In conclusion, it must be emphasized that understanding the inner perspective of a patient with a mental disorder is essential not only for establishing a close relationship with the patient as a basis for treatment, but also for meaningful research (and this is probably even more true in the era of neuroscientific psychiatry). Mundt and Spitzer[20] clearly stated that 'reliability does not guarantee validity, but limits it'. Thus, if we are still interested in carefully listening to our patients, in building up a relationship via empathy and in developing a common understanding of the inner experiences together with the patient, we need more than just rating scales or collecting inclusion/exclusion criteria. That is why phenomenological-descriptive psychopathology remains a fundamental element in educating and training young psychiatrists, and should be implemented with innovative instruments and approaches within psychiatric training curricula.

References

1. Giacco D, Luciano M, Volpe U, Fiorillo A. Opinions of Italian residents in psychiatry on their training course. *Eur Psychiatry* 2010; **25**(S1): P03–170.
2. Pauling L, Itano HA, Singer SJ *et al*. Sickle cell anemia: a molecular disease. *Science* 1949; **110**: 543–548.
3. Schrödinger E. The present situation in quantum mechanics. In: Wheeler JA, Zurek WH (eds) *Quantum Theory and Measurement*. New Jersey: Princeton University Press, 1983; p. 152.
4. Lown B. *The Lost Art of Healing*. Boston: Houghton Mifflin, 1997.
5. Saunders J. The practice of clinical medicine as an art and as a science. *Med Humanities* 2000; **26**: 18–22.
6. Griesinger W. *Die Pathologie und Therapie der psychischen Krankheiten*. Stuttgart, 1845.
7. Havens L. *Approaches to the Mind*. Boston: Little & Brown, 1973.
8. Laing RD. *Wisdom, Madness and Folly*. London: Macmillan, 1985.
9. McHugh PR, Slavney PR. *The Perspectives of Psychiatry*. Baltimore/London: Johns Hopkins University Press, 1983.
10. Van Praag H. Reconquest of the subjective. Against the waning of psychiatric diagnosing. *Br J Psychiatry* 1992; **160**: 266–271.
11. McHugh PR, Slavney PR. *The Perspectives of Psychiatry*, 2nd edn. Baltimore: Johns Hopkins University Press, 1998.
12. Maier W, Helmchen H, Sass H. Hirnforschung und Menschenbild in 21 Jahrhundert. *Nervenarzt* 2005; **76**: 543–545.
13. Stanghellini G. The meanings of psychopathology. *Curr Opin Psychiatry* 2009; **22**: 559–564.
14. Jaspers K. *Allgemeine Psychopathologie. Ein Leitfaden für Studierende, Ärzte und Psychologen*. Berlin: Springer, 1913/1946.
15. Slavney PR, McHugh PR. The life-story method in psychotherapy and psychiatric education: the development of confidence. *Am J Psychother* 1985; **39**: 57–67.
16. Jaspers K. *The Philosophy of Karl Jaspers* (Schilpp PA, ed.). New York: Tudor, 1957.
17. Jaspers K. *General Psychopathology*. Chicago: University Press, 1963; p. 55.
18. Wiggins OP, Schwartz MA, Spitzer MA. Phenomenological/descriptive psychiatry: The methods of Edmund Husserl and Karl Jaspers. In: Spitzer MA,

Uehlein FA, Schwartz MA, Mundt C (eds) *Phenomenological Language and Schizophrenia*. New York: Springer, 1992; pp. 48, 58, 67.

19. Sass H. (2001) Personality disorders. In: Henn F, Sartorius N, Helmchen H, Lauter H (eds) *Contemporary Psychiatry*. Berlin: Springer, pp. 161–193.

20. Mundt C, Spitzer M. Psychopathology today. In: Henn FG, Sartorius N, Helmchen H, Lauter H (eds) *Contemporary Psychiatry*, Vol 3, Part 1. Berlin: Springer, 2000; pp. 161–193.

21. Spitzer RL, Robins E. Research diagnostic criteria: rationale and reliability. *Arch Gen Psychiatry* 1978; **35**: 773–782.

22. Maj M. Critique of the DSM-IV operational diagnostic criteria for schizophrenia. *Br J Psychiatry* 1998; **172**: 458–460.

23. Lawrie SM, Olabi B, Hall J *et al.* Do we have any solid evidence of clinical utility about the pathophysiology of schizophrenia? *World Psychiatry* 2011; **10**: 19–31.

24. Kapur S. Looking for a "biological test" to diagnose "schizophrenia": are we chasing red herrings? *World Psychiatry* 2011; **10**: 32.

25. Strik W. Clinical handling and understanding of schizophrenia should be based on pathophysiological findings and theories. *World Psychiatry* 2011; **10**: 37–38.

26. Cannon TD. Objective tests for schizophrenia: window to the future. *World Psychiatry* 2011; **10**: 36–37.

27. Borgna E. Psychopathology and clinical aspects of depressio sine depressione. *Riv Sper Freniatr Med Leg Alien Ment* 1969; **93**: 1276–1290.

28. Janzarik W. Die Krise der Psychopathologie. *Nervenarzt* 1976; **47**: 73–80.

29. Janzarik W. *Die strukturdynamischen Grundlagen der Psychiatrie*. Stuttgart: Enke, 1988.

30. Sass H. Die Krise der psychiatrischen Diagnostik. *Fortschr Neurol Psychiatr* 1987; **55**: 355–360.

31. Panzarino PJ Jr. Psychiatric training and practice under managed care. *Adm Policy Ment Health* 2000; **28**: 51–59.

32. Laín-Entralgo P. *El Diagnóstico Médico: Historia y Teoría*. Barcelona: Salvat, 1982.

33. Mezzich JE, Salloum IM. Towards innovative international classification and diagnostic systems: ICD-11 and person-centered integrative diagnosis. *Acta Psychiatr Scand* 2007; **116**: 1–5.

34. Parnas J. Clinical detection of schizophrenia-prone individuals: critical appraisal. *Br J Psychiatry* 2005; **48**: s111–112.

35. Greenhalg T, Hurwitz B. *Narrative Based Medicine*. London: BMJ Publishing Group, 1998.

36. Weber M. *Wirtschaft und Gesellschaft – Grundriß der verstehenden Soziologie*. Tübingen: Mohr, 1922/1976; p. 179.

37. Beveridge A. Time to abandon the subjective-objective divide? *The Psychiatrist* 2002; **26**: 101–103.

38. Damasio A. *Descartes' Error*. New York: Avon Books, 1994.

39. Eisenberg L. Is psychiatry more mindful or brainer than it was a decade ago? *Br J Psychiatry* 2000; **176**: 1–5.

Learning about phenomenological psychopathology **97**

40. Fulford W. Analytic philosophy, brain science, and the concept of disorder. In: Bloch S, Chodoff P, Green S (eds) *Psychiatric Ethics*. Oxford: Oxford University Press, 1999; pp. 161–192.
41. Kandel E. A new intellectual framework for psychiatry. *Am J Psychiatry* 1998; **155**: 457–469.

CHAPTER 7

The psychiatrist in the digital era: new opportunities and new challenges for early career psychiatrists

Umberto Volpe,[1] Michael Davis[2] and Davor Mucic[3]
[1]Department of Psychiatry, University of Naples SUN, Naples, Italy
[2]Department of Psychiatry and Biobehavioral Sciences, Semel Institute, University of California Los Angeles (UCLA), Los Angeles, CA, USA
[3]Psychiatric Centre "Little Prince", Copenhagen, Denmark

A day in the life of the digital psychiatrist

I swipe my ID badge at the door; the light flashes green. I enter the building and walk to my office. As I wait for my psychotherapy patient to arrive, my smartphone beeps. 'Running a few min late' reads the text message, an unfortunate reminder of the time I forgot to block caller ID when using my personal mobile phone to contact her. With some unexpected time, I check my email: a Facebook friend request from a young man with schizophrenia who participates in a support group that I lead. I delete the request, aware of the threat of boundary violations yet hoping it will not hurt his feelings. I wonder if I can adjust my privacy settings to be more difficult to locate on the Internet. I am thankful for my common name and the relative anonymity it offers. Next, a hospital administrator's email reminds residents not to store protected health information on USB flash drives; I recall frantic colleagues scouring resident workrooms and computers for these devices. I delete this email, and open a training video that I need to complete before beginning my research. My learning is interrupted by a knock on my office door. The patient enters and sits across from me. I set my smartphone on silent mode

How to Succeed in Psychiatry: A Guide to Training and Practice, First Edition.
Edited by Andrea Fiorillo, Iris Tatjana Calliess and Henning Sass.
© 2012 John Wiley & Sons, Ltd. Published 2012 by John Wiley & Sons, Ltd.

and close the video. 'Hi, Dr Davis. Sorry I'm a bit late. Let me tell you about my last week. . .'

Introduction

Today we are living during a period of revolution: the 'digital revolution'. Economists and sociologists have dubbed it the 'third industrial revolution'; in other words, computer technology and informatics today hold the same cultural significance and economic potential that mechanization, electrification and mass production represented for the 'first' and 'second' industrial revolutions that occurred from the eighteenth to the nineteenth and during the twentieth centuries, respectively. Of course, the relationship between human beings and technology is not new. Since human kind's first attempt to produce tools, we have ventured to overcome the topological limits of the human body and mind by enhancing, creating, reducing or abolishing human characteristics (to facilitate the ease and speed of accessing action/knowledge). However, some of the characteristics of the 'digital revolution' are different from those observed in previous periods of technological advancement. The twenty-first century is clearly dominated by a human culture that has a 'bidirectional' relationship with technology: human creates technology, and technology, in turn, shapes the human. After six centuries, the Cartesian distinction between *res cogitans* and *res extensa* seems now, more than ever, out of date.

For early career psychiatrists, the relation between technology and clinical practice perhaps represents an even more crucial frontier than it does for other medical specialties. More than other disciplines, psychiatry is most sensitive to societal and individual changes, and the digital revolution has already had an impact on psychiatry's object. In the last decades, human beings have been exposed to a huge amount of previously unavailable (at least on a world-scale and in real time) information, and the internet has already changed the way we read, think and remember. Consequently, we no longer perform certain cognitive operations (due to the so-called 'technological delegation') and different models of social interaction have arisen. In this sense, cognition, reasoning, perception and the mind itself have been dramatically changed by recent technologies. A survey of 400 US neuroscientists showed that 81 % of respondents believe that use of the internet has enhanced human intelligence and that changes in brain structure, function and plasticity may occur depending on such technological advancements. If the human mind has been so modified by the use of technology, how can the doctors of the mind not be expected to keep up with such changes?

The aim of the present chapter is not to thoroughly reconcile all of the above issues; even a book devoted solely to the topic would likely be insufficient. Without attempting to be comprehensive, we seek to highlight the main technological advancements in the field of psychiatry that might imply direct changes for psychiatric practice and research; we will also attempt to unveil the new changes and, at the same time, foresee the possible risks connected to the use of such new technologies in psychiatry.

In detail, within this chapter, we try to highlight technological advancements relevant to psychiatry that might imply direct changes for psychiatric practice and research and to discuss changes and anticipate risks connected to the use of such technologies in psychiatry. Furthermore, we provide insights into how recent technological developments have produced new approaches to psychiatric diagnosis and treatment that may be of particular relevance to early career psychiatrists, and suggest ways to optimize internet use for professional purposes. Finally, we highlight mental health problems connected to the misuse of the internet and describe new models of computer-assisted psychiatry.

Digital tools in psychiatry: who needs them?

Digital technology has already had a substantial impact on psychiatry. However, this has happened (and is happening) at different levels and varying rates, depending on the diverse profiles of technology users within our discipline. Some 'digital changes' already have a direct influence on psychiatric practice; others remain confined to research, but will probably exert a direct influence on psychiatric practice in the near future. Others are influenced by the health-care systems in which psychiatry is embedded.

Non-psychiatrists

Digital tools are increasingly being utilized by different professionals who do not directly belong to psychiatry, but surround it and have a substantial impact on it.[1] One example is commercial information providers. As long as psychiatrists need access to online scientific information, those who are selling such information have explored more ways to deliver it. Scientific information is easier to obtain, manipulate and distribute in electronic form. The success of the portable document format (PDF, an open standard for document exchange, consisting of a two-dimensional file that contains information on the text, fonts, images and vector graphics) is an example of how information provision necessitates new technologies. The same concept applies to the growing number of journals that ensure electronic information provision as a basic feature of their editorial policy, and to those that only support electronic publication of their scientific papers.

Another example of how psychiatry might be influenced by changes connected to the use of digital technology outside its field is commercial health-care providers. Clearly, the management of medical information is essential to analyse costs and determine quality standards and the efficacy and efficiency of medical procedures. Many companies now monitor such procedures and standards in terms of cost-effectiveness by collecting data in digital databases and using sophisticated software to analyse the data. Also, individual health-care providers are relying more on technology for reaching patients, providing services, or simply completing daily tasks more efficiently. Consequently, any doctor is expected to consult the internet to answer a questionnaire on his/her practice or to update his/her schedule by email alerts.

Clinical psychiatrists

One of the main challenges for clinical psychiatrists is to objectify subjective constructs and experiences (e.g. those concerning an individual's mood, thinking, perception, behaviours, personality, etc.). Many different rating scales have been developed with this specific purpose. They now constitute a 'clinical standard' in many therapeutic and rehabilitation settings. However, they can be time consuming, and tracking scores and changes over time presents a challenge. Computer-administered versions of formerly clinician-administered scales are now available for the assessment of most psychiatric symptoms, allowing for spare time to obtain more objective and reliable evaluations, and easy access to previously recorded information.[2] Patients' reactions to these scales have generally been positive. Although computer-administered rating scales have many advantages, they also have limitations.[3] Computers can only establish rapport with patients to the extent that they are programmed to do so (i.e. by their developers); other disadvantages of computer interviews include limited ability to process non-verbal information, and inability to tailor the wording of items to particular patients to ensure that questions are understood. In this sense, digital versions of such instruments will probably remain a useful aid to the psychiatrist as a supplement to clinician evaluations. Another relevant and recent application of digital technology to psychiatric practice is the development of digital tests aimed to assess specific brain functions such as memory, attention or executive functions for specific clinical populations (mostly dementia and schizophrenia patients). Such tests have the same reliability as paper-and-pencil tests but have several advantages (such as the exploration of a wider range of ability, the minimization of floor and ceiling effects, the provision of a truly standardized format, and the higher accuracy and sensitivity of recording the performance of tests).[4]

Psychiatric researchers and neuroscientists

During the last decades, digital technology has had a constantly growing impact on research in psychiatry and neuroscience. First, we have to consider that psychiatric researchers need digital technology to rapidly access the constantly growing body of published scientific evidence, to communicate in real time with colleagues at long distances, and to publish their findings. Given the substantial advantages of digital communication, it is not surprising that, nowadays, telephone conferences among researchers are managed via computers, digital scientific articles are available long before their printed counterparts, and searching among a million references takes a few seconds. For the same reasons, the internet now represents the largest source of information about medical and scientific topics.

Second, digital technology has been increasingly applied to develop newer and more complex research paradigms to be administered to psychiatric patients and used to record and analyse data concerning brain functioning. Perhaps one of the biggest challenges in psychiatry and behavioural sciences is to visualize the activity of the brain *in vivo* while performing a certain task, or to characterize a dysfunctional mental activity. This is now possible through neuroimaging technology. The term 'neuroimaging' refers to the use of various techniques to, directly or indirectly, image the structure and/or function of the brain.[5] Neuroimaging techniques have existed for many decades and are routinely used in clinical psychiatric practice (often to exclude the presence of a primary medical condition); however, recently, the evolution of magnetic resonance (MR) apparatus and newer electrophysiological methods has enabled a significant shift forwards in the use of such techniques. On the one hand, modern MR machines allow for the acquisition of multiple images faster than in the past, without losing the high spatial definition that is typical of the technique. On the other hand, imaging methods based on the electroencephalogram (EEG) – once seen as a unique source of information (because, unlike methods based on regional blood-flow changes, it provided 'direct' information about brain activity in real time) but with very low spatial resolution – have been recently refined to enable the identification of cortical electrical generators of scalp-recorded activity with a satisfying spatial resolution, without losing its optimal temporal resolution. One hundred years ago, no psychiatrist would have imagined seeing brain areas activated by a schizophrenic patient when hallucinating, yet this has already been achieved more than 10 years ago (as an example, see Figure 7.1).

Preliminary accounts of how functional imaging may predict response to treatments are growing in number; such methods will likely allow clinicians to tailor pharmacological and psychological treatments to individual

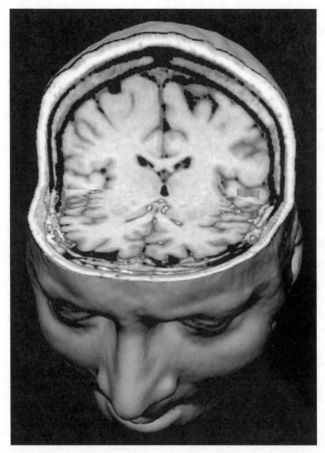

Figure 7.1 Neuroimaging of actively hallucinating patients with schizophrenia. Reprinted from Dierks T, Linden DE, Jandl M *et al.* Activation of Heschl's gyrus during auditory hallucinations. *Neuron* 1999 Mar;**22**(3): 615–621, with permission of Elsevier.

psychiatric patients in the foreseeable future. Moreover, the scope of neuroimaging research will probably expand beyond neuroscience and into clinical psychiatry. However, we have to consider that we are not yet at the point of implementing any technological procedure to diagnose a mental disease or to clearly predict an individual's response to a certain treatment.

Recent technologies have ushered in the 'genomic era', and its implications for psychiatry are significant.[6] However, even within this field, new technological tools have also brought new challenges: no single genetic study has clarified the true heritability of psychiatric disorders, and, thus, recent claims of 'genetic counselling' for schizophrenia should be considered with caution. In the USA, several private companies offer services to people who may have inherited schizophrenia or who may pass schizophrenia on to their children to assess 'recurrence risk'; however, we should remember that genetic counselling is complex and not entirely reliable if a well-known pattern of inheritance is not established.

Still, some technological advances have already made an impact on psychiatric theory and practice. Our expanding knowledge of pharmacogenomics has allowed researchers to partially predict the efficacy of antipsychotic drugs for various symptomatic domains of psychopathology, taking into account the wide inter-individual variability in clinical response and tolerability. Such approaches are likely to drive choices of psychoactive drugs for an individual based on the patient's genetic profile.[7] We are now more aware of the subtle interaction between environment and genome, and the study of epigenetics (i.e. the covalent modification of DNA due to the interaction with the specific social and psychological milieu in which each individual lives) will probably help in more precise definition of the impact of such factors on inter-individual behavioural trajectories and on the rise of mental illnesses.[8] Finally, let's consider that psychiatrists in court are already using neuroimaging evidence to assess psychopathology[9] – although the Iowa Supreme Court and the Oklahoma appeals court recently dismissed 'brain fingerprinting' (an EEG-based technique to assess the suspect's response to short questions covering neutral and incriminating topics) as unacceptable/unreliable evidence; however, the Indian courts convicted two suspected murderers based on the evidence provided by an analogous technique (namely, the 'Brain Oscillations Signature', or BEOS). Furthermore, functional magnetic resonance imaging (fMRI)-based neuroimaging research has recently been used in courts of various countries to demonstrate the presence or absence of 'psychopathic' characteristics in a single individual or to assess 'objectively' the ability to stand in court or the responsibility for a crime.[10] Unfortunately, none of these technological advancements has allowed for meaningful modifications in the way psychiatrists assess mental functions or diagnose psychiatric disorders, and so-called 'neuro-law' still represents a complex and tangled interface between medical professionals, neuroscientists and the legal system, which should be evaluated with caution since it could represent a valid tool to integrate standard psychiatric evaluation and help forensic psychiatrists to critically think about their work.[9]

However, hope remains that, in the near future, advances in neuroscience and genomics, their integration, the combination of such knowledge with evidence from large longitudinal and population-based studies, and the achievement of innovative conceptualizations of mental illnesses will identify more precise risk and protective factors and aid in the development of more informed and specific diagnostic, intervention and prevention strategies.

Digital treatments

The twentieth century witnessed the development of numerous pharmacological, somatic and psychological treatments for mental illnesses. Despite the great advances in psychiatric therapy with respect to the past, we are still far from achieving optimal treatments. Even the most effective antidepressant or antipsychotic drug has significant side effects, and some psychiatric cases still prove refractory to the most grounded and evidence-based psychotherapy. Even the most experienced doctor cannot always predict the best treatment for a specific patient, and a significant percentage of patients are left with unsatisfactory therapeutic results in spite of the best integration of currently available therapies. Moreover, after such an initial 'wave of innovation' in the first half of the twentieth century, research in psychopharmacology and psychotherapy seems, at present, less active than in the past. However, it is also true that the availability of new technologies has brought new ideas into the field and that, in the last few decades, new treatment modalities for psychiatric illnesses have been proposed. At present, not all these new treatments have received official endorsement from national/international bodies, and some still need to be supported by a larger evidence base although most are often used in clinical practice. We present below a brief summary of basic principles, main applications and caveats of the digital psychiatric treatments that currently seem to be the most promising.[11]

Transcranial magnetic stimulation and transcranial direct current stimulation

Transcranial magnetic stimulation (TMS) is a non-invasive method that causes the regional depolarization of neurons by means of an electromagnetic induction of weak electric currents due to a rapidly changing magnetic field (Figure 7.2). In a TMS machine, a bank of capacitors is rapidly discharged into an electric coil, which produces an intense magnetic field pulse. When the coil is placed near a subject's head, the magnetic field penetrates the brain and induces an electrical field in the underlying region of the cerebral cortex; if such an electrical field is of sufficient intensity, it will depolarize cortical neurons, generating action potentials. These then propagate to exert their biological effects. This can cause (de)activation of specific regions of the brain. For example, TMS over the left motor cortex causes action potentials that propagate through the corticospinal tract, causing twitches in contralateral skeletal muscles.

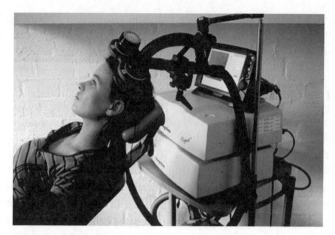

Figure 7.2 Direct electromagnetic stimulation of the brain.

Similar to TMS, transcranial direct current stimulation (tDCS) employs low-intensity electrical (not magnetic) impulses delivered directly to the area of interest via positive and negative scalp electrodes. tDCS has two directions of current that cause different effects. Although the method by which biological effects (i.e. increases or decreases in neuronal activity) are induced differs from that of TMS, the general principles of tDCS as well as its advantages and disadvantages are similar. Increased and decreased neuronal activity is induced in repetitive TMS by using a higher or lower frequency, respectively.

In psychiatry, TMS and tDCS have primarily been used as treatments for major depression (in particular, a repetitive application of TMS of the left dorsolateral prefrontal cortex might become a safe, non-convulsive alternative to electroconvulsive treatment in depression and has been shown to be superior to placebo). Most studies indicate that slow-frequency repetitive TMS (rTMS) and higher frequency rTMS have a clinical use in the treatment of mania, obsessive-compulsive disorder, post-traumatic stress disorder and schizophrenia.[12]

Vagus nerve stimulation

Vagus nerve stimulation (VNS) employs a small device that sends mild electrical impulses to the brain via the vagus nerve, which is the cranial nerve that carries information to and from the brain to the larynx, heart, stomach, lungs and oesophagus. But researchers think it is also connected to the limbic structures, which are associated with the regulation of mood and emotions. Unlike other nerves, the vagus nerve has few pain fibres; therefore, it can deliver electricity to targeted areas without requiring surgery on the brain.

To implant the device, surgeons make small incisions in the neck and below the collarbone. Once the battery-operated electrical-pulse generator is implanted, a flexible, insulated plastic tube containing electrodes is run under the skin to the vagus nerve on the left side of the neck. The generator delivers 30-second pulses of electricity to the vagus nerve every 5 minutes. The use of VNS in psychiatry is particularly attractive for patients suffering from treatment-resistant depression[13] as a therapeutic alternative especially to electroconvulsive therapy (which carries the risk of short-term memory problems). The possible risks of VNS include injury to the vagus nerve, which can lead to a hoarse speaking voice, coughing or difficulty in swallowing. Other complications include injury to the carotid artery or internal jugular vein.

Neurofeedback

Neurofeedback (NFBK) is a specific type of biofeedback that can be defined as the process of becoming 'aware' of physiological functions by means of digital instruments that provide information on the activity of such systems; once the subject is aware of his/her own biological responses, he/she might be able to manipulate them at will. Biofeedback can be applied to many biological parameters (heart rate, skin conductance, etc.); when it is applied to brain waves, it is called NFBK, also known as 'EEG biofeedback' or 'neurotherapy'.

Neurofeedback provides subjects with real-time feedback on their brain activity; after training, they are able to control their central nervous system activity. One of the most popular applications of NFBK is an increase in activity in the 12–18-Hz band (the so-called sensorimotor rhythm, SMR) and a decrease in the 4–8-Hz (theta band) and in the 22–28-Hz band (beta band) to treat anxiety. Although the range of applications of the technique is rapidly expanding and encompassing many mental and brain disorders (especially anxiety and affective disorders; for a review, see ref. 14), and the number of practitioners using it to treat patients is constantly growing, further controlled trials are needed to definitively validate the therapeutic use of NFBK in psychiatry.

Information technology and psychiatry

In 1958, when the US government established the Information Processing Technology Office (IPTO), probably no one could have imagined that such a 'secret' military network, intended to ensure a nationwide interconnection between a few military computers, would have such a deep impact on worldwide communication and lifestyles in the twentieth century. Only 30 years later, in 1989, Tim Berners-Lee already envisioned the 'world wide web', a network of networks, in turn composed of personal computers interconnected to each other. Today, the 'net' is not only one of the most relevant and fastest forms of mass media, but it also represents a resource for medical information, a communication medium, a possible source of 'addictions', a tool for delivery of medical treatments, and numerous other functions.

Thus, it is not surprising that the internet today represents a possible focus of interest for psychiatry too. The relationship between psychiatry and the new information technologies (IT) is manifold and complex, ranging from the clinical to the research arenas, from web-based educational events to the information available to our patients, which is too often misleading.

Psychiatrists who are in an early phase of their careers may interact daily with their peers using social networks; they will probably learn from 'virtual teachers', who will deal with specific, IT-related psychiatric disorders.

Medical information online: what, where and how to search

Medicine is a career that demands lifelong scholarship because advances are frequent and numerous. After physicians have been licensed and board certified, learning continues. Yet editing a book often takes several months; books are more or less 'out of date' right after they have been printed. Sometimes the publication of good and timely journal articles is also delayed for editorial reasons. However, the internet enables publication almost in real time, giving life to an idea long before it can be printed on paper.[15] In this respect, the internet might be considered the perfect medium to disseminate medical information. However, the information about medicine (including psychiatry) on the internet is heterogeneous and requires honed search techniques to produce reliable, accurate results.

Before an internet search, we should focus on 'what' we are looking for as well as 'if', 'where' and 'how' it could be found.[1] Essential explanations of the basic concepts related to IT are reported in Table 7.1.

The first major internet search criterion is to decide whether 'free' or 'structured' information is needed. New information may come first from unofficial sources (newspapers, blogs, etc.), but sparse and occasional sources are less reliable than official ones (e.g. an online journal or the official website of a professional association). However, even in the latter case, another issue may limit your search: the constant update of web material implies that information is continually published on and removed from the net (we might not find what we were looking for although it was there not long ago). Also, remember that the amount of information on medical and psychiatric issues far exceeds the average user's needs. Thus, simply starting your search with your favourite search engine may not

Table 7.1 Glossary of basic IT concepts.

Term	Definition
HTML	Hypertext markup language – the predominant language for writing web pages.
HTTP	Hypertext transfer protocol – a standard request–response protocol for client (e.g. a web browser)–server (e.g. a computer hosting the website) computing.
Hyperlink, hypertext	Reference to a web document that is followed automatically or that the reader can follow; *hypertext* is a text with hyperlinks.
Internet (or the 'Net')	Global data communications system comprising hardware and software infrastructure that provides connectivity between computers.
Intranet	A network of computers; mainly used within an organization to facilitate communication and access to information, usually with access restricted to employees/members of that organization.
Link	A set of characters (most frequently a word) that connects the reader to another page or point of a hypertext.
Protocol	Set of rules for communicating.
Uniform Resource Locator (URL)	A string of characters that specifies where an identified 'resource' (e.g., a web page) is available on the internet.
World Wide Web (www or 'Web')	One of the services communicated via the internet; a collection of interconnected documents and resources.

be useful. Rather, a *medical internet database* may be considered a virtual medical library.

The most widely known medical electronic database is probably the National Library of Medicine (NLM) of the US National Institutes of Health (NIH), which allows users to search an electronic scientific reference archive known as PubMed (http://www.ncbi.nlm.nih.gov/pubmed). PubMed is a free-access virtual portal where searchers may find all relevant sources of information concerning biomedical knowledge, ranging from the archive of all biomedical journals to all materials published for a specific gene or peptide. The most relevant application of PubMed for a young psychiatrist is undoubtedly MEDLINE, a virtual library comprising more than 19 million citations of biomedical articles that have been published in almost 5000 scientific journals from 1966 to today (or even 'tomorrow', since MEDLINE provides access to materials – so called *in process* and *publisher supplied* articles – that will be published in the future); the database comprises scientific articles within the major fields of science and covers medicine, psychology, veterinary medicine and preclinical sciences. Citations include titles, authors' names and affiliations, bibliographic references, the abstract of the paper (when available) and, eventually, a direct link to the publisher's website (this allows registered users to directly download the PDF version of the paper). This information may be read on the screen or printed, but it can also be exported and consulted later. Documents may be retrieved by author's name, journal title, publication date or (more relevant) keywords. MEDLINE uses MeSH (Medical Subject Headings; http://www.ncbi.nlm.nih.gov/mesh), which is a structured vocabulary (more properly, a 'metadata' system) comprising more than 24 000 biomedical terms used for indexing articles; these have been hierarchically organized and developed to ensure a univocal representation of biomedical concepts. The use of MeSH terms, instead of common ones, avoids the need to try different terminologies for the same concepts and helps the user create an effective search. Another relevant tool is the 'clinical query' option (http://www.ncbi.nlm.nih.gov/sites/pubmedutils/clinical); this function refines the results by limiting them to specific evidence-based 'clinical areas' only. The results of a query will include only systematic reviews, meta-analyses, guidelines or articles relative to aetiology, diagnosis, prognosis or therapy of the chosen medical condition.

On the PubMed home page, tutorials and FAQs introduce the reader to all the 'secrets' of this virtual library. A quick search strategy guide to PubMed has been provided in Table 7.2.

Besides MEDLINE, many other biomedical databases currently exist.[16] There is no perfect, comprehensive database; all have advantages and disadvantages. Which database(s) should be used for a literature search is an individual choice. In Table 7.3, we summarize the characteristics of some of the most popular and widely used ones.

Resources for early career psychiatrists

Among the vast amount of medical web resources are clinical and educational materials (including freely distributed articles on psychiatric practice and clinical guidelines), psychiatric journals – most scientific papers are now distributed in PDF format, and nearly all psychiatric journals provide electronic tables of contents (or TOCs) – and psychiatric e-books (freely consultable and/or downloadable). For researchers, statistical tools are also available online.

Beyond general internet resources that might be of interest for any psychiatrists, some websites that may be of specific interest to early career psychiatrists are listed in Table 7.4.

Table 7.2 PubMed 'tricks'.

'Cubby' strategy	The 'My NCBI' option allows registered users to link from MEDLINE abstracts only to online journals to which they are subscribed; it also permits users to store keyword searches for future use.
'Explode' function	Will automatically expand your search to all headings and subheadings related to the chosen MeSH term.
'Related Articles' function	Enables quick selection of all articles related to the MeSH of your main hit.
Break It!	Break your topic into separate concepts and search for them in MEDLINE; to associate or exclude concepts, use Boolean operators (AND, OR, etc.)
Clinical queries	Choose this strategy when looking for a specific pathological condition; the scope of the search might be 'narrow' (i.e. more specific) or 'broad' (i.e. more sensitive, but possibly including less relevant papers).
MeSH terms	First check within the MeSH database and then choose the most appropriate heading for your search; avoid unusual words; always check MeSH subheadings.
Use 'Limits'	To refine your search, use age and language (English) limits; also, 'type of publication' may be useful.

Communication technology for early career psychiatrists

In recent decades, communication modalities have changed significantly. However, some changes remain of particular interest for early career psychiatrists because they allow individuals, at only minor cost, to interact with patients and colleagues over long distances and in real time. These tools have had a great impact on associations of young psychiatrists and the building of peer relationships (Figure 7.3). An overview of the most innovative and relevant applications within this field are provided in Table 7.5.

Telepsychiatry

Telepsychiatry refers to the provision of mental health care from a distance, including clinical work with the patient, as well as educational and administrative activities related to mental health care delivery. Although previous studies have demonstrated the high reliability, technical feasibility, improvements in access to care, satisfaction and acceptance by both patients and providers, and the cost-effectiveness of telepsychiatry, the potential of psychiatric videoconferencing has not been as fully explored and exploited in Europe as it has in North America and Australia (where telepsychiatry has been developing since 1959). However,

Table 7.3 Biomedical databases.

MEDLINE	The most famous and used biomedical database; free with many search options. The large number of references may make it difficult for an inexperienced user to find what he/she is looking for. www.ncbi.nlm.nih.gov/pubmed/
OLDMEDLINE	Also created by the US National Library of Medicine, it has features similar to MEDLINE but is devoted to scientific articles published before 1966. No MeSH terms and abstracts are available. http://www.nlm.nih.gov/databases/databases_oldmedline.html
Ovid	Only registered users may use OVID. Search results may be saved and sent by email. MeSH terms are available to define a narrower search strategy. 'In-process' articles are also available. Major flaws are the update process (annually) and the small number of older (pre-1966) citations. gateway.ovid.com
Scopus	Developed by a private company (Elsevier), it is 'free access', updated daily, and available in 10 languages. References dating pre-1995 have limited availability. www.scopus.com/scopus/home.url
EBSCO	One of the most commonly used databases, especially by university students, because of its simple and user-friendly interface. No in-process citations available. www2.ebsco.com/it-it/Pages/index.aspx
PsychINFO	Database dedicated to psychiatry, psychology and related sciences dating back to 1887. This service is provided to subscribers by the American Psychological Association. http://www.apa.org/pubs/databases/psycinfo/index.aspx
Google Scholar	Developed by Google, it's a free collection of academic materials (including official documents, published studies, books, theses, unpublished data, etc.) from different research and educational fields; users provide published materials on a voluntary basis. May be less reliable compared to other biomedical databases. www.scholar.google.com

in the last decade, relevant activities related to telepsychiatry have also taken place in some European countries, such as the UK, Spain and the Scandinavian countries. This is not happening by chance. Telepsychiatry has become more affordable for and accessible to a broad spectrum of users.[17] Many countries worldwide face resource shortages within various mental health settings, which result in significant gaps in psychiatric care provision. As a tool capable of building bridges over those gaps, telepsychiatry offers a number of solutions regarding more effective and efficient mental health care delivery without compromising the quality of care. Both professionals and non-professionals who have direct or

Table 7.4 Web resources for early career psychiatrists.

AYPAP	Newly established association of the African Young Psychiatrists and Allied Professions (www.africanyoungpsychiatrists.org)
EFPT	The European Federation of Psychiatric Trainees is the historical reference for residents in psychiatry across Europe. In addition to its activities and online discussions, a collection of 'statements' forwarded to the European Union of Medical Specialties (UEMS) and covering psychiatric training issues is available. (www.efpt.eu)
EPA Early Career Psychiatrists	Official website for the Early Career Psychiatrists of the European Psychiatric Association. A list of major organizational and educational activities and a glance at the special events and awards for the annual European Congress of Psychiatry are provided. (www.europsy.net/what-we-do/early-career-psychiatrists/)
National associations of psychiatric trainees	Many national associations of psychiatric trainees exist. The most active and representative are:
Croatia	(mladi.psihijatrija.hr)
France	(www.affep.net)
Germany	(www.dgppn.de)
Ireland	(www.irishpsychiatry.ie/Postgrad_Training.aspx)
Italy	(www.sipgiovani.it)
UK	(www.rcpsych.ac.uk/specialtytraining.aspx)
USA	(www.psych.org/resources/EarlyCareerPsychiatrists.aspx)
WAYPT	The World Association for Young Psychiatrists and Trainees (WAYPT) is an association of psychiatric trainees and psychiatrists who completed psychiatric training no more than 5 years ago that aggregates its members from all over the world on a voluntary basis. (www.waypt.org)
WPA Early Career Psychiatrist Council	The World Psychiatric Association (WPA) has recently appointed an official junior representative for each national Member Society, supported special grants and approved an 'action plan' for early career psychiatrists. (www.wpanet.org)

indirect contact with mental health services (Box 7.1) would benefit from becoming more familiar with telepsychiatry. During the last decade, interesting new research fields and clinical applications have been developed in Europe.[18] 'Cross-cultural telepsychiatry' refers to the use of telepsychiatry in the assessment and/or treatment of ethnic minorities via their respective mother tongue in situations when access to bilingual clinicians is limited. Every national telepsychiatry network should develop its own

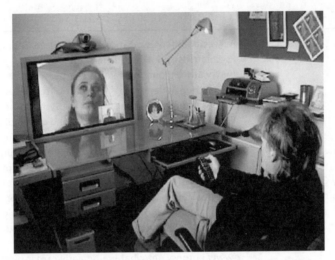

Figure 7.3 New communication technology. A typical telepsychiatric videoconference setting enables psychiatric assessment in real time, despite the distance.

telepsychiatry applications, but developing such national, and especially international, networks needs clear legal, regulatory and ethical guidelines that have yet to be agreed upon. Recently published guidelines drafted by the American Telemedicine Association[19] might be useful to read prior to potential establishment of a telepsychiatry service within public health care.

The use of video recording for training of young professionals within mental health care is an increasingly common way of supervision, particularly in psychotherapy. Sessions are video-recorded and viewed by the supervisor for comments and suggestions, with the advantage of being able to pause or skip to different sections in the video clip. Telepsychiatry, in contrast, is a real-time video transmission. It can be used in order to supervise residents/trainees in real time as they treat patients. One potential scenario is a 'meet the experts' video-conference, where a trainee can learn from experienced colleagues around the world. As telecommunications technologies continue to improve, new educational techniques are sure to be explored and developed.

The internet and the dangers for mental health

Harry S. Truman once said: 'There are dangers in religious freedom and freedom of opinion. But to deny these rights is worse than dangerous, it is absolutely fatal to liberty.' Had he been alive today, he may have had a similar opinion about the internet. As the most recent, uncontrollable

Table 7.5 New communication media for early career psychiatrists.

Chat	A form of synchronous conferencing (usually text-based) over the internet; one-on-one or group interactions can occur. E.g. webmessenger.msn.com.
Newsgroup	Usually described as a specific email application that allows registered users to participate in online discussion groups about specific topics (all members can receive emails from and send emails to all other members). Sometimes the term also identifies a sort of online repository, in which messages posted from registered users are stored for public consultation. European psychiatric trainees may subscribe to the mailing list of EFPT from its homepage (www.efpt.eu).
Virtual phone	A less expensive alternative to landline phones. With call forwarding, call diversion, phone conference and video conference (if a webcam is on the computer), it can be connected with social networks or personal web dialler. The most widely used software for voice calls over the internet is Skype (www.skype.com); this software is freely downloadable and provides many additional features (such as instant messaging, file transfer and video conferencing).
Virtual community	A social network in which individuals interact through specific media, crossing geographical and political boundaries. A typical aspect of the virtual community is the possibility for users to build their own homepage (blog). An example of a virtual community of mental health professionals can be found on the About.com website (mentalhealth.about.com/od/professional/For_Mental_Health_Professionals.htm).
Blog	Blog is short for 'web-log', a specific type of website (or a part of a website) that may be regularly updated with commentaries, descriptions of events or other material. Many blogs serve as personal online diaries whereas others provide commentary or news on a particular subject. Many are dedicated to mental health; examples include: social-psychiatry.com; adventuresintele psychiatryblog.patrickbarta.com; www.telehealth.net/blog/; http://voyagerllc.blogspot.com.
Social network	A social structure comprising individuals or organizations ('nodes'), connected by some interdependency (e.g. friendship, kinship, financial exchange, relationships, beliefs, knowledge or prestige).

(continued overleaf)

Table 7.5 (Continued)

	Among the most famous are Facebook (www.facebook.com) and twitter (twitter.com); the latter is considered a 'microblogging service' – users send/read messages (i.e., 'tweets' of up to 140 characters). All messages posted on a user's homepage are displayed on the author's profile page and are visible to all or select users. In addition to contact with professionals within our field, several Facebook pages are publicly dedicated to famous psychiatrists (e.g. www.facebook.com/pages/Freud/23223649358?ref = search) or official psychiatric organizations (e.g. www.facebook.com/psychiatry24x7?ref = search), and special interest groups are devoted to well-established or innovative psychiatric theories. Some other social networks share content such as videos (youtube.com) or music and videos (myspace.com).
Distance learning	Because congresses and frontal teaching are expensive, time consuming and limited by the availability of local experts, major medical organizations have taken advantage of new media to implement online education, which may also grant Continuing Medical Education credits. One of the first websites dedicated to this kind of activity is Medscape (www.medscape.com), which provides its registered users with educational online events, according to users' preferences, in addition to other services (such as videos, slideshows, etc.). Medscape also offers a special service dedicated to psychiatry and mental health (www.medscape.com/psychiatry).
Podcast	A 'webcast' is the virtual procedure by which a single media file (audio or video) is broadcast to many simultaneous listeners/viewers through the Net, either 'live' or 'on demand'. A 'podcast' is a 'non-streamed' webcast (i.e. a series of digital media files, episodically released and often downloaded through the Net). Podcasting usually requires software like iTunes, Juice or Doppler. Once downloaded, podcasts can be consulted (even offline). A large collection for psychiatrists is available at Podcastdirectory.com (www.podcastdirectory.com/podcasts/19505).
RSS feed	A web feed (or 'news feed') is a data format for providing subscribed users with frequently updated content from a website. An RSS (acronym for 'Really Simple Syndication') is a family of web feed formats used to publish frequently updated works (e.g. blog entries, news headlines, audio and video) in a standardized format. Syndication is the process by which website material is made available to multiple other sites upon subscription.

(continued overleaf)

Table 7.5 (Continued)

	Usually, RSS feeds are read using dedicated software ('RSS reader'), which can be web, desktop or mobile-device based and uses the standardized XML file format. RSS feeds for psychiatry are available at the US National Institute of Mental Health website (www.nimh.nih.gov/site-info/subscribe-to-nimh-rss-updates.shtml) or at CurrentPsychiatry.com (www.currentpsychiatry.com/pages_rss.asp).
Wiki	This designates websites that can be openly modified or updated by users in real time; all of these events are recorded in a 'log' file. This knowledge-sharing modality is rapidly expanding: the most brilliant example is doubtlessly Wikipedia (www.wikipedia.org), the free, collaborative, multilingual encyclopedia project.

and 'free' form of mass media, the internet is susceptible to abuse. In recent years, expressions like 'cyberchondria', 'social network addiction', 'online gaming addiction' and 'online gambling addiction' have appeared in newspapers, television reports and even scientific journals.[20] Although no such disorder has officially been listed in any current psychiatric diagnostic manual, internet addiction has repeatedly been proposed for inclusion in the forthcoming fifth edition of the *Diagnostic and Statistical Manual of Mental Disorders* (DSM-5).[21] Since 1997, anecdotal cases worldwide indicated that the typical 'Net addict' is a teenager (now extended up to early 30s), usually male, with little or no social life, and little or no self-confidence. Affected subjects are typically characterized by excessive or poorly controlled preoccupations, urges or behaviours regarding computer use and internet access that lead to impairment or distress. Some of the most interesting research on internet addiction has been published in South Korea, where internet addiction has become one of the most serious public health issues; according to 2006 data, approximately 210 000 South Korean children (21 %; aged 6–19 years) are afflicted and require treatment.[22] Besides different estimates in different countries, the condition has increasingly attracted attention both in the media and scientific world. An aetiological explanation for the phenomenon is still needed but the mechanism behind it seems to arise from the search for stimulation or from the need to escape real-life difficulties. It appears that many individuals have become addicted to the internet in the same way that others become addicted to drugs or alcohol.[23] The consequences of internet addiction should be seen in the light of common consequences of almost any other type of addiction. There are also physical and academic

Box 7.1 Advantages of telepsychiatry

- Team-based treatment in many foreign languages (including sign language).
- Rapid and effective consultations.
- Increased speed and accuracy of psychiatric diagnoses and treatments.
- Acute psychiatric assessments, follow-up, and discharge planning in remote locations.
- Increased access to child, adult, geriatric, forensic and deaf services specialty staff.
- Increased collaboration among general practitioners, and staff within primary care service and mental health service.
- Second-opinion service made more easily available.
- Increased continuity of care and professional contact.
- Psychoeducation of family members made more easily available.
- Improved online education (distance learning via case conferencing and best-practice demonstration; distance supervision, and staff consultation).
- Increased efficiency and effectiveness through improved performance.
- Reduced staff costs: travel time, staff time.
- Decreased number of inappropriate admissions and readmissions into the acute sector.

risks. Frequent use of the mouse may lead to physical pain. Students may surf irrelevant websites, participate in chat rooms, converse with internet friends, and play interactive games at the cost of productive academic activity. Internet misuse among employees is a serious concern in the corporate world; time surfing the internet on non-business purposes may diminish employees' effectiveness at work. Family life can be affected as the ability to carry out romantic and sexual relationships online further erodes the stability of real-life couples. Additionally, the social consequences of internet gambling addiction are tremendous.

Psychological (mostly cognitive behavioural) approaches may be helpful, but there are no clear indications for the use of psychotropic drugs. A self-imposed ban on computer use and internet access has been reported as necessary in some cases. Unfortunately, internet addiction seems to be resistant to treatment, entails significant risks and has high relapse rates. Moreover, it also makes comorbid disorders less responsive to therapy. Thus, such conditions need to be better explored, understood and treated.

Ethical considerations of technology in psychiatry

Although technology facilitates easy access to patients' medical and psychiatric histories, enables psychiatrists to provide care to patients in remote areas, allows immediate communication with colleagues in any part of the world, and distributes pioneering research in almost real time, a number of ethical considerations arise. Imprudent and careless use of technology can threaten patient privacy, increase practitioner liability, and blur the boundaries between patient and provider.

Patient privacy should be a primary concern for contemporary practitioners. The patient should fully understand the risks of communicating over unsecure connections like email or text message. When sending personal medical information like lab results or treatment plans to a patient via email, the physician should first remind the patient that the physician is unable to control the security of the patient's email server. Some psychiatrists may wish to have their patients sign a legal agreement that gives the physician permission to communicate with the patient by email. By extension, physicians should use only encrypted connections, with USB/security software for personal digital assistant (pda) devices, virtual private networks (VPNs), etc. Additionally, all medical professionals should avoid using unsecure forms of data storage like USB flash drives, which may be easily forgotten at a public computer.

Psychiatrists must use their discretion when distributing personal contact information and should be careful to block phone numbers when calling patients from mobile phones or other personal lines. In some cases, patients who were raised in the digital era may be most comfortable with non-verbal forms of communication like email and text message; and although physicians will likely need to learn to accommodate such mainstream types of communication, they should also exert caution so as not to blur the ethical boundary between patient and provider. In addition to these digital communication issues, social networking on websites such as Facebook and LinkedIn poses a threat to that ethical boundary.

Conclusions

In this chapter we have tried to describe the most recent and relevant current technological trends of interest for early career psychiatrists, with an awareness that many technologies will be replaced by improved versions or superseded in the next months or years. For example, the changes that characterize 'Web 2.0' (i.e. the evolution of the internet from a 'passive' medium into a highly interactive one, in which users can easily communicate by means of information sharing, interoperability, user-centred design and collaboration with website owners) will probably be irrelevant in a few months for the virtual community, which is already looking at newer applications that will push the Web another step forward.

Importantly, from this chapter, the reader should be warned about the need for the modern psychiatrist to be up to date and to remain open to the future. Having easier access to scientific information, understanding patients' concerns about their 'virtual lives', or communicating in real time with colleagues on the other side of the world seem to be essential for a psychiatrist in the twenty-first century. New technologies resemble a double-edged sword, bringing new possibilities but also new problems and/or dangers. The psychiatrist of the future will have to be familiar with new psychopathologies specifically related to emerging information technology, and be able to diagnose and cure some clinical cases using informatics. Clinical practice will hopefully always remain a human interaction, but machines can greatly help; a good practitioner should know how to make best use of them and to lower the risks associated with their use. In the coming years this interaction between doctors and machines will probably become a crucial issue for all of medicine. Finally, we hope this chapter will leave the reader with the sense of what Pablo Picasso condensed in the motto 'computers are useless... they provide you only with answers'. It is up to the new generations of psychiatrists to ask the right questions.

References

1. Stone J, Sharpe M. Internet resources for psychiatry and neuropsychiatry. *J Neurol Neurosurg Psychiatry* 2003; **74**: 10–12.
2. Erdman HP, Klein MH, Greist JH. Direct patient computer interviewing. *J Consult Clin Psychol* 1985; **53**: 760–773.
3. Miller M, Hammond K, Hile M (eds). *Mental Health Computing*. New York: Springer, 1996.
4. Wild K, Howieson D, Webbe F, Seelye A, Kaye J. Status of computerized cognitive testing in aging: a systematic review. *Alzheimers Dement* 2008; **4**: 428–437.
5. Bassett DS, Bullmore ET. Human brain networks in health and disease. *Curr Opin Neurol* 2009; **22**: 340–347.
6. Merikangas KR, Risch, N. Will the genomics revolution revolutionize psychiatry? *Am J Psychiatry* 2003; **160**: 625–635.
7. Foster A, Miller del D, Buckley P. Pharmacogenetics and schizophrenia. *Clin Lab Med* 2010; **30**: 975–993.
8. McGowan PO, Szyf M. Environmental epigenomics: understanding the effects of parental care on the epigenome. *Essays Biochem* 2010; **48**: 275–287.
9. Aggarwal NK. Neuroimaging, culture and forensic psychiatry. *J Am Acad Psychiatry Law* 2009; **37**: 239–244.
10. Müller JL. Psychopathy – an approach to neuroscientific research in forensic psychiatry. *Behav Sci Law* 2010; **28**: 129–147.

11. George MS, Aston-Jones G. Noninvasive techniques for probing neuro-circuitry and treating illness: vagus nerve stimulation (VNS), transcranial magnetic stimulation (TMS) and transcranial direct current stimulation (tDCS). *Neuropsychopharmacology* 2010; **35**: 301–316.
12. López-Ibor JJ, López-Ibor MI, Pastrana JI. Transcranial magnetic stimulation. *Curr Opin Psychiatry* 2008; **21**: 640–644.
13. Rado J, Janicak PG. Vagus nerve stimulation for severe depression. *J Psychosoc Nurs Ment Health Serv* 2007; **45**: 43–51.
14. Hammond DC. Neurofeedback with anxiety and affective disorders. *Child Adolesc Psychiatr Clin N Am* 2005; **14**: 105–123.
15. Taubes G. Science journals go wired. *Science* 1995; **271**: 764–766.
16. Falagas ME, Pitsouni EI, Malietzis GA, Pappas G. Comparison of PubMed, Scopus, Web of Science, and Google Scholar: strengths and weaknesses. *FASEB J* 2008; **22**: 338–342.
17. Hailey D, Roine R, Ohinmaa A. The effectiveness of telemental health applications: a review. *Can J Psychiatry* 2008; **53**: 769–778.
18. Mucic D. Telepsychiatry in Denmark: mental health care in rural and remote areas. *J eHealth Technol Applic* 2007; **5**: 3.
19. Yellowlees P, Shore J, Roberts L. *Practice Guidelines for Videoconferencing-based Telemental Health.* American Telemedicine Association, 2009.
20. Block JJ. Pathological computer game use. *Psychiatr Times* 2007, **1**: 49.
21. Beard KW, Wolf EM. Modification in the proposed diagnostic criteria for Internet addiction. *Cyberpsychol Behav* 2001; **4**: 377–383.
22. Choi YH. Advancement of IT and seriousness of youth Internet addiction. In *2007 International Symposium on the Counseling and Treatment of Youth Internet Addiction.* Seoul, Korea:National Youth Commission, 2007, p. 20.
23. Shaw M, Black DW. Internet addiction: definition, assessment, epidemiology and clinical management. *CNS Drugs* 2008; **22**: 353–365.

CHAPTER 8

Portrayals of mental illness in different cultures: influence on training

Joshua Blum[1] and Sameer Jauhar[2]
[1]Department of Psychiatry, University of Massachusetts Medical School, Worcester, MA, USA
[2]Sackler Institute of Psychobiological Research, Institute of Neurological Sciences, Southern General Hospital, Glasgow, UK

Introduction

This chapter is not designed to be a treatise on cultural psychiatry. There are many other book chapters and entire volumes on this subject. Nor is this chapter designed to provide specific information on what to say or do to bridge the gap between mental health professionals and patients from other cultures. To make these presumptions would be overly ambitious and a disservice to the specialty itself. Although there are a few examples of how mental illness is interpreted and expressed in various cultures, they are included as examples of how the setting can determine the phenotype of the illness. This chapter is designed to be a practical guide to the subject and give trainees and young psychiatrists food for thought when meeting patients from a different culture.

The caveat to the statement above is that (too often) we forget that 'culture' does not only apply to those of a different culture to ours, but rather is something that is part of simply being human. Everyone has a culture, and many people likely belong to more than one. Human behaviour is inseparable from culture. It is the substrate in which the biological, environmental and psychological factors that determine it exist. Since behaviour in large part influences health, the cultural substrate of an individual is important to consider when judging the expression of illness.

How to Succeed in Psychiatry: A Guide to Training and Practice, First Edition.
Edited by Andrea Fiorillo, Iris Tatjana Calliess and Henning Sass.
© 2012 John Wiley & Sons, Ltd. Published 2012 by John Wiley & Sons, Ltd.

The anthropology of psychiatry

What exactly is culture? In the broadest sense, it consists of the elements that describe a group of human beings that live and/or function together – for example, the social relationships, beliefs, values, knowledge base and ways of interacting.[1] It is something that is absorbed from an early age, from those who grow up in a particular culture, or is passed down from one generation to the next – though at some point, there will be inevitable changes to the culture that may render it outwardly different. It is important to note that everyone belongs to a culture of some kind. Although 'culture' tends to evoke images of people from different geographical locations than your own, many different cultures can exist within the same geographical area. Anything that can bring people together, such as music, sports, sexual identity and political affiliation, can also bring the ingredients needed for a culture.

Although culture and ethnicity are sometimes used interchangeably, ethnicity is more specific, referring to a group identity of people who share a common heritage, cuisine, dress, language and belief system. It is thus more closely tied to biology and geography. The term 'race' is again often used interchangeably with ethnicity, but denotes the outward phenotype of a person that belongs to a particular ethnicity. It is pseudo-scientific at best, although in medicine often it becomes part of a patient's identifying data, along with age, occupation, marital status and religious preference.[1,2] Therefore, in short, culture may be defined as a society's way of life, ethnicity as a group's cultural heritage, and race as its outward appearance.[1,2]

Cultural psychiatry in the context of globalization

Any discussion of culture in the modern era would be remiss for not acknowledging the role of globalization. Globalization has been defined in many ways and in many different contexts. Broadly, it can be seen as 'a process in which the traditional boundaries separating individuals and societies gradually and increasingly recede'.[3] This is exemplified by enhanced communication technologies, easier travel and economic deregulation, with effects on society in general. Whilst a discussion of the philosophical and moral underpinnings of this is beyond the scope of this chapter, it is worth reflecting on the possible influences globalization has on mental health. An example would be the process of urbanization, where people gravitate to more urban environments, with recognized effects on mental health. Examples of such effects include decreased social support, increased stressors and subsequent increases in rates of mental illnesses, such as depression. For early career psychiatrists, it is probably worth appreciating that, as globalization increases, cultural factors may increasingly contribute to the way in which patients will present.

Migration in the context of psychiatry

Within the context of globalization, and particularly in areas such as Western Europe, rates of migration are increasing significantly, with a consequent increase in the burden of mental illness. Migration has been defined as 'the process of societal change whereby an individual moves from one cultural setting to another for the purposes of settling down either permanently or for a prolonged period'.[4] Bhugra and Jones[4] identify three stages: pre-migration, the process of migration itself, and post-migration. Each has its own set of stressors, relating to the individual and the society they are entering. For example, an individual or family may have to migrate as a result of stressors in their home environment, such as war or for political reasons. The process of migration itself may be stressful, and assimilation into another culture will have its own set of challenges. Amongst these and a myriad of other factors, studies on migrants and psychiatric illnesses and psychological disturbance have taken place for decades. Young psychiatrists should be aware of the influence of migration on mental health, and we will use the example of schizophrenia to illustrate this. As far back as 1932, Odegaard noted increased rates of schizophrenia in Norwegians emigrating to the USA, approximately 10–12 years after migration. The increased rates of schizophrenia in those of African Caribbean descent in the UK had frequently been ascribed to possible racism on the part of doctors, misdiagnosing these patients, though the AESOP systematic multi-site study suggested otherwise, with this population having a nine-fold increase in incidence of schizophrenia (relative risk of 5.8) compared to the white British population, while those of south Asian descent had a relative risk of only 1.8.[5] Various factors have been used to explain this, though the weighting of the evidence has favoured social isolation and exclusion in this population. This evidence adds to other data on social factors in schizophrenia, where urban environment has been shown to increase the incidence by 1.7, and deprivation has been associated with a slightly increased prevalence of the illness.

Classifications around the world

Despite these different rates of incidence of mental disorders, the existing classification systems aim to provide patients and practitioners with a common language.[6] Ideally, this could lead to improved treatment and prevention of disease. Unfortunately, that is not entirely what has happened. Because the location and culture can determine how an illness is portrayed or expressed in a given culture, it can be difficult to create a set of universal criteria that apply to all people. Nonetheless, highlights of some popular classification systems are provided in the next sections.

The International Classification of Diseases (ICD) system

The first edition of the ICD can be traced to 1853, when William Farr and Marc d'Espine were commissioned to prepare a uniform system of nomenclature for tabulating the causes of death between countries. The first International Classification of Causes of Death was adopted in 1893 and, now known as the International Classification of Diseases, is in its 10th revision. Psychiatric disorders were first included in the sixth revision (1948), are currently found in Chapter 5, and are coded with the letter F (F0–F9). It is currently accepted for use by many countries around the globe, especially for research and statistical reporting. The ICD-10 is the official classification system of the World Health Organization and of the World Psychiatric Association. To better meet the needs of local populations, annotations and additions of the ICD-10 are in circulation. One such example is the DSM.[10]

The Diagnostic and Statistical Manual (DSM) system

When the ICD-6 came out in 1948, there were numerous psychotic, neurotic and charactereological classifications, but there was not widespread international use. Only the UK, Finland, New Zealand, Peru and Thailand made official psychiatric use of it. Dementias, adjustment disorders and some personality disorders were notably absent. This widespread lack of use led the World Health Organization to ultimately commission the American Psychiatric Association to publish a revision of the ICD-6 mental disorder chapter for use in the USA. The DSM-1 was published in 1952.[10] The third revision of the DSM introduced the idea of the biopsychosocial multiaxial evaluation system, with five different axes. Axis I comprises all clinical disorders, except disorders thought to be part of one's substrate (personality disorders and mental retardation), which are on Axis II. Axis III is for general medical conditions relevant to the patient's psychiatric disorder; Axis IV includes psychosocial factors influencing Axis I and II disorders; and Axis V gives comments on overall functioning with its 100-point global assessment of functioning scale.

The Chinese Classification of Mental Disorders (CCMD) system

Because China has so much of the world's population, it is important to consider how the Chinese have conceptualized mental illness. When creating the CCMD, Chinese psychiatrists tried to blend terms being used worldwide with more traditional terms.[8] One of the historical problems the Chinese people have faced over the centuries is how to deal with the country's vast size and heterogeneity in terms of language and traditions, and this was true while creating this text as well. The current edition, the CCMD-3, has the dichotomy of being heavily influenced by the ICD-10 and DSM-IV while maintaining local features, such as *qi-gong induced mental disorder* – a condition believed to arise from the inappropriate practice of *qi-gong* (a traditional Chinese martial art centred around the cultivation of *qi*, the life force) – or *travelling psychosis*, which is an acute psychotic episode with anxiety, impulsivity and potential for self-harm seen in rural migrant workers who travel long distances in severely cramped trains in search of work.[1,8] There were also some sections seen in Western systems that were omitted in previous versions of the CCMD (though they have since returned). The rationale at the time was that certain personality disorders, such as avoidant and dependent, were not viewed as pathological in Chinese culture, as the main traits – preoccupation with being criticized or rejected and putting others' needs before one's own – are inherently part of Confucianism. In addition, the whole idea of a personality disorder is based on the (largely Western) view that certain behaviours are considered socially unacceptable.[8] Borderline personality disorder was also excluded since some of its main traits, emotional dysregulation and impulsivity, were considered aspects of bad behaviour and should not be medicalized. In general, because deviant behaviour in China is mostly dealt with via the penal system, Chinese psychiatrists are less involved in diagnosing personality disorders.[7,8]

Examples of culturally specific syndromes

As seen above, culture not only determines what is considered an 'appropriate' behaviour, but also determines how the disease will look and be thought of. In the following paragraphs some examples of syndromes that describe patterns of behaviour seen in various cultures are provided. There are potential explanations to these syndromes according to the ICD or DSM criteria, but the value in examining them is not in trying to fit them into the lens of our experience, but in viewing them as examples of how the culture expresses illness.

Neurasthenia

This disorder is currently listed in both the ICD-10 and the CCMD-3.[9] Interestingly, the syndrome was first described in the late 1800s by an American, Dr George Beard, who called neurasthenia a constellation of symptoms, such as headaches, irritability, insomnia, gastrointestinal discomfort and a number of other somatic symptoms.[9] In many cases, it would meet DSM criteria for a somatoform, mood or anxiety disorder on Axis I and/or a chronic fatigue-like syndrome such as fibromyalgia on Axis III.[2] No longer part of the DSM, it is, however, a common diagnosis in China, where the theory of 'nerve weakness' mirrors Dr Beard's original theory of exhaustion of the nervous system.[9] It provides a perhaps more culturally acceptable way to treat mental illness, given that it is mainly somatic in nature. Because mental illness has traditionally been a taboo subject in China, one also wonders if the expression of mental distress via somatic means allows one to receive treatment with less stigma.

Ataque de nervios

In Spanish, this literally means 'an attack of the nerves' and generally refers to the various manifestations of stress. It is an acute stress reaction, which is generally out of one's control. It has been described amongst the Latin populations of the Caribbean and Latin America, as well as in the Mediterranean populations.[9] The symptoms are generally self-limited and are pseudoepileptiform, somatoform, dissociative and panic-like in nature, with trembling, crying, difficulty in moving limbs, poor memory or apparent loss of consciousness, shouting, striking out, then falling to the ground.[2,9] It seems similar to the DSM description of panic disorder, but with a dissociative element.

Amok

This culture-bound syndrome has elements of mental distress found in many cultures. Essentially, a cross between the berserker rage of Norse mythology and 'going postal', it has been incorporated into the English language ('run amuck' or 'run amok').[2,9] A pattern of behaviour primarily described in Southeast Asia, it is a syndrome characterized by initial brooding followed by a rampage of violent and/or homicidal behaviour, typically in men after perceived personal insults, often with paranoid persecutory ideas and other psychotic symptoms, amnesia of the event, and a return to premorbid functioning afterwards.[2,9] One also wonders if patients who experience so-called 'blackouts' when in fits of rage are experiencing some variation of this disorder. Historically, the US Army encountered Filipino Moro tribesmen, who in addition to running *amok* into battle, were often high on psychoactive substances. US soldiers found that the calibre .38 revolver that was then standard issue didn't fire a round with enough stopping power to halt the Moros. The Army ended up switching to the larger calibre .45 bullet, and this incident ultimately led to the development of the Colt 1911 .45 automatic, one of the most influential handgun designs in the world.[7,8] Unfortunately and ironically, incidences of sudden mass violence take on new meaning when the weapons that can be used increase in lethality.

Generalized effects of culture on psychopathology

Although the above syndromes are striking examples, we would like to emphasize that culture will (understandably) have effects on psychopathology, and that early career psychiatrists should be aware of this. An example would be the difference in incidence of depressive symptoms between cultures shown in the WHO's investigation in the late 1970s and early 1980s, where guilty feelings were present to twice the extent in subjects from Switzerland compared to those from Iran, and somatic symptoms were twice as prevalent in the Iranian population of depressed patients compared to the Canadian cohort.[12] Other observations have included 'pathoplastic' effects, where culture affects the content of psychopathology (e.g. auditory hallucinations); 'patho-facilitative' effects, where the incidence of a psychiatric disorder can increase in certain cultures (e.g. anorexia in Western culture); and 'pathoreactive' effects, where the behavioural response to a mental illness is affected by cultural factors (e.g. post-traumatic stress disorder after war) – the societal response to these effects will influence an individual's behaviour.[13]

Culture in clinical practice

History-taking and treatment in a culturally aware fashion requires many of the principles of good psychiatric practice, though the following specific issues (some of which form part of the cultural formulation – see below) have to be taken into consideration:

1. Being aware of *one's own cultural background*. As alluded to above, we all have our own unique cultural makeup, and this undoubtedly has effects on our understanding of patients, their mental problems, and how this impacts on their daily functioning. In a study of US residents (house officers), Rousseau et al. (1995)[11] showed that residents tend to base transcultural perceptions on their own cultural background, as opposed to the experience of patients from differing backgrounds.
2. Being aware of *how patients' culture affects their illness (and vice versa)*, in biological, psychological and social domains.

Corroborative information

A corroborative history from an informant, family member or statutory organization is obligatory in most psychiatric assessments, but it is essential in patients from differing cultural backgrounds. Understanding the context in which a patient presents will not only help from a diagnostic viewpoint, but also inform treatment plans.

Use of interpreters

Given the nature of psychiatry, being able to understand clearly what a patient is trying to communicate is a prerequisite. Moreover, symptom recognition in patients from different cultural backgrounds is clearly improved when speaking in their own language.[14] Often, when a patient is unable to understand the native language (or communicate in this language), family members or a spouse will offer to 'translate'. We would guard against this practice, as it can complicate interpersonal relationships, and it can be difficult to know how accurate translation can be. If at all possible, a professional translator should be sought, and in most metropolitan hospitals this can be arranged. However, problems still exist in the use of interpreters in psychiatric practice, the main points being summarized below:[14]

1. *Omission* – some issues may not be mentioned by the interpreter, particularly if of a sensitive nature (e.g. financial or sexual in nature).
2. *Addition* – information not given by the patient is included by the interpreter.
3. *Condensation* – a complicated phrase and response is paraphrased into a simple answer that fails to convey the full meaning of what the patient has said.
4. *Role exchange* – the interviewer adopts the role of the doctor.
5. *Normalization* – specifically occurring in psychiatric settings, the interpreter normalizes the patient's responses, and therefore the phenomenological value of what the patient is saying is lost.

Possible solutions to these problems include meeting with the interpreter beforehand, speaking slowly and clearly, using simple terms, speaking to the patient directly and not to the interpreter, asking for a verbatim response when unsure, and asking the translator whether the form of conversation is normal/coherent. Since interpreters may feel the need to clarify or paraphrase to make sense of a patient's speech, it can be helpful to tell the interpreter to inform you exactly what the patient is saying, even if it does not make sense. This is especially true if you are concerned about delirium or a formal thought disorder. There still may be aspects of the patient's expressive emotional prosody and speech that are lost in translation, but you are more likely to pick it up if you can use the interpreter's puzzlement to your advantage. It is also helpful to make sure to allot extra time and lower expectations for what can be covered in a given time for interviews requiring translators.

Cultural case formulation/explanatory models

In 2002, the American Psychiatric Association (APA)[15] proposed the following five elements of a cultural formulation, in an effort to formalize a cultural understanding of patients: (i) cultural identity of the individual; (ii) cultural explanations of the individual's illness; (iii) cultural factors related to psychosocial environment and levels of functioning; (iv) cultural elements of the relationship between the individual and the clinician; (v) overall cultural assessment for diagnosis and care.

Keeping all these factors in mind, we are also reminded that often patients (and their families and communities) will give different explanations to their psychiatrists and mental health professionals for their problems. Dealing with their explanations of illness, and what this means for them, is essential for maintaining a therapeutic relationship. This may not always be easy, as Bhui and Bhugra point out,[16] but the general tenets of empathy and respect will undoubtedly help what may be a difficult situation. The reader is asked to think of these issues when considering the case scenario shown in the box.

Case Example

This case involves a 30-year-old primarily Mandarin-speaking married female, formerly an architect in China, with a past psychiatric history of paranoid schizophrenia and past medical history of gastroesophageal reflux disease (GERD) who was in the USA temporarily while accompanying her husband, a diplomat. She had an extensive treatment history in China with several inpatient admissions, at least one suicide attempt, and a trial of ECT. However, prior to her relocation, she had been stable for some time on risperidone 5 mg daily. But, with the move to the USA, had wanted to try a newer 'American' antipsychotic and, under the treatment of a local psychiatrist, switched to quetiapine. She was still in the midst of quetiapine titration when she decompensated, with paranoia that people were after her and contaminating her food and water. These delusions extended to her husband, whom she felt was trying to murder her or leave her for another woman. She denied perceptual abnormalities, suicidal or homicidal thoughts, and the rest of her review of systems was otherwise negative. Although the patient was able to speak some English, a Mandarin translator was used for communication.

Interestingly, she did not present to the hospital due to paranoia but because she was having headaches on quetiapine and wanted to get the dose adjusted. Given that her husband felt unsafe with her at home in her current state, medication adjustment could not be done in the emergency room (ER) with adequate follow-up, and her outpatient psychiatrist could not be contacted the night she presented, so she was admitted to an inpatient psychiatric unit.

She was initially very angry at her husband for 'abandoning' her in the hospital, as family members are often allowed to stay in the hospital in China, and on his first visit the day after her admission, she slapped him in the face before staff could stop her. Soon after, on her first meeting with the attending psychiatrist on the unit, she got down on her hands and knees and, repeatedly bowing down to touch her head to the ground, begged the doctor to make her better, behaviour that her treatment team initially interpreted as further evidence of psychosis, though after discussion it was seen as an aspect of her background meant to convey sincerity. She met with the treatment team daily with the assistance of a Mandarin interpreter. Unfortunately, although she achieved some symptom remission on quetiapine, she continued to have the side effects of dizziness and headaches, which prevented further titration. She was ultimately transitioned back to risperidone, with a final dose of 4 mg daily, which was successful in minimizing the severity of her delusions. Her relationship with her husband gradually improved, and she was set up to see an outpatient psychiatrist who, luckily, was fluent in Mandarin and could provide psychotherapy and medication management for the duration of her stay in the USA.

After her discharge from the inpatient unit, she started weekly psychotherapy with her new doctor and worked, over the course of months, to improve her understanding of what it meant to have schizophrenia and how this affected some long-standing difficulties she had with her family as well as the relationship with her husband. There were occasions when she would present with psychosomatic complaints and then express paranoid thoughts about her headaches or other physical discomforts. By the end of her stay in the USA, she was better able to redirect herself and had come to the realization that there was no basis for people wanting to harm her.

Discussion
This case illustrates a number of challenges. It is an example of an intelligent, high-functioning woman who was a stranger in a new country where the customs and language were different. In terms of biological predisposing factors, she had an extensive treatment history back in her home country, and she was in the midst of a medication change. Interestingly, she had the idea that medication and medicine in general were more advanced in the USA, hence the desire to try a newer, 'more advanced' antipsychotic. She shared with her inpatient treatment team and outpatient psychiatrist how

mental illness was viewed in her own country, which made her feel ashamed. As a result, her coping mechanisms regarding how to deal with her illness were limited. Furthermore, there were varied psychosocial factors that compounded her presentation; these included not only the new country and language barrier, but the increased amount of time she had at her disposal now that she was not working. China, like many non-Western countries, is more group-oriented, and this patient not only had a strained relationship with her biological family but was physically displaced from them. When she was admitted to the inpatient unit, she was under the impression that her husband, her only family in the USA, would be able to stay and/or play a more central role in her treatment. He was told on admission that she would be taken care of and went back home, which his wife felt was a form of abandonment. In addition, her way of conveying her sincerity and a desire for help (essentially prostrating herself) was strange to the largely US treatment team. In this case, there were hospital Mandarin-speaking interpreters as well as staff members who were able to provide both language and cultural interpretation, though that was partially through luck. Although language interpretation would have been possible even if there had been no in-house interpreter – via a national telephonic language line – had the patient been from a culture that staff had been less familiar with, no cultural interpretation would have been possible. Should that have been the case, the team would have needed to ask the patient herself to help bridge the gap. In the end, it is always the patient who must do so, since every patient is different.

It is important to keep in mind that a full knowledge of all cultures is impossible. There is no way to guarantee that physicians will know what the culturally appropriate things to say or do are in all situations, and it is unreasonable to be held to such a standard. Even if a psychiatrist knows something about a patient's culture, a little knowledge can be a dangerous thing, as it can lead to stereotyping and overgeneralization. This is one of the reasons why our current level of knowledge about ethnopsychopharmacology is often of limited clinical use, since the data we have are about small demographic groups, which minimizes the heterogeneity apparent within ethnic labels.[6] One practical answer is to meet the individual where he or she is, something that sounds obvious but can be practically difficult, given the constraints of clinical practice. It is always helpful to consider what expectations the patient has given her or his background. In this case, for example, asking our patient what her experience of living in the USA had been like so far, what she expected, and what differences there were from her own country would have been a good place to start. It would have let her know that her treaters were being honest about where their knowledge ended and were open to learning. That opens the door for a discussion about potentially differing points of view. That is the basis for diplomacy between countries and can be applied to individuals as well. Clearly, it is something that is easier said than done, and adopting an open and curious frame of mind cannot always prevent misunderstandings. It just allows for a more open forum for discussion when misunderstandings occur, as they inevitably do.

Treatment

Obviously, the provision of equitable and culturally sensitive mental health services is important (especially n the modern era of globalization), though for this chapter we will focus on treatments for the individual patient (interested readers are directed to the relevant books).

Ethnopsychopharmacology principles

A multitude of factors will influence a patient's response to a drug, and a cultural awareness of these can be helpful (and in some cases avoid disastrous consequences). Readers are reminded that the majority of our evidence base on psychopharmacology relates to Caucasian patients without a history of substance misuse, from North America and Western Europe, and that differences exist in people of different ethnic backgrounds. The largest difference is in relation to pharmacokinetics, specifically drug metabolism. As pointed out by Yu et al.,[17] the cytochrome P450 system has been the most studied in drug metabolism, and within this, the CYP2D6 enzyme has clear genetic variations in its levels, affecting metabolism of a variety of tricyclic antidepressants, selective serotonin reuptake inhibitors (SSRIs) and antipsychotics (e.g. clozapine). There are ethnic variations in CYP2D6 enzyme activity, depending on allelic variants, causing some populations to be poorer metabolizers of drugs used by the CYP2D6 system.[3,17] Certain Asian populations have a 50 % prevalence of the allelic variant causing decreased CYP2D6 enzyme activity, and hence are poorer metabolizers of drugs utilizing this system (compared to Caucasian populations who have a negligible prevalence of this variant).[17] Pharmacodynamics also differ amongst ethnic groups, with increased prolactin levels noted in Asian patients when given haloperidol, taking into account confounding factors.[3,17] To date, this work has not been translated into clear guidance that we are aware of, though we would urge early career psychiatrists to be aware that patients from differing cultures may be more sensitive to side effects of psychotropic medication, and that the maxim of 'start low, go slow' clearly applies here. Furthermore, psychiatrists should be aware of cultural factors regarding the use of psychotropic medications, and that levels of concordance may vary as a result – a problem helped by a non-judgmental approach.

Conclusions: is there a role for training in cultural psychiatry for young psychiatrists?

In short, yes! A number of training curricula from different countries have acknowledged the importance of cultural (or 'transcultural') psychiatry, including the Royal College of Psychiatrists. Despite this, it remains a fairly difficult task to accomplish in isolation. There is no substitute for the kind of learning that happens when actually confronted by a patient from a different culture. In other words, early career psychiatrists can learn all theoretical bases for transcultural practice, but there is no substitute for practice. In many ways, that is not as difficult as one might think. As mentioned before, your office or hospital does not have to be the relocation site for the latest local refugee group to get practice in transcultural psychiatry. Everyone has certain beliefs, whether religious, societal or familial, that can be thought of as aspects of culture.[2] Therefore, early career psychiatrists can practise asking after aspects of the cultural formulation when taking the social histories of their patients. The use of interpreters is another skill that, while initially cumbersome, becomes easier with practice and may be very helpful. Because we tend to learn well through good modelling, try to watch as many of your supervisors as possible practise these skills so you can see different styles. And, if you happen to get the opportunity to travel to a different culture (or country), it can be a very eye-opening experience. The goal of putting yourself in these situations is just that – to open your eyes, expose yourself to new situations, and introduce you to different ways of practising.

References

1. Favazza A. 4.1 The Psychiatric Scientist and the Psychoanalyst. In: Sadock BJ and Sadock VA, Eds. *Kaplan & Sadock's Comprehensive Textbook of Psychiatry*, 8th edn. New York: Lippincott Williams & Wilkins, 2005; pp 598–623.
2. Griffith EH and Gonzalez CA. Essentials of cultural psychiatry. In: Hales RE and Yudofsky SC, Eds. *Synopsis of Psychiatry*. Washington, DC: American Psychiatric Press, 1996; pp. 1283–1306.
3. Bhugra D, Mastrogianni A. Globalisation and mental disorders: Overview with relation to depression. *Br J Psychiatry* 2004; **184**: 10–20.
4. Bhugra D, Jones P. Migration and mental illness. *Adv Psychiatr Treat* 2001; **7**: 216–223.

5. Morgan C, Dazzan P, Morgan K *et al.* First episode psychosis and ethnicity: initial findings from the AESOP study. *World Psychiatry* 2006; **5**: 40–46.
6. Herrera JM, Lawson WB, Sramek, JJ. *Cross Cultural Psychiatry*. Chichester: Wiley, 1999.
7. San Juan E. *The Philippine Temptation: Dialectics of Philippines-U.S. Literary Relations*. Philadelphia: Temple University Press, 1996.
8. Stein G and Wilkinson G, Eds. *Seminars in General Adult Psychiatry*. Trowbridge, UK: Cromwell Press, 2007.
9. Trujillo M. Culture-bound syndromes. In: Sadock BJ and Sadock VA, Eds. *Kaplan & Sadock's Comprehensive Textbook of Psychiatry, 8th edn*. New York: Lippincott, Williams & Wilkins, 2005; pp. 2282–2292.
10. Zimmerman M and Spitzer RL. 9.1 Psychiatric Classification. In: Sadock BJ and Sadock VA, Eds. *Kaplan & Sadock's Comprehensive Textbook of Psychiatry, 8th edn*. New York: Lippincott, Williams & Wilkins, 2005; pp. 1003–1034.
11. Rousseau C, Perreault M, Leichner P. Residents' perceptions of transcultural psychiatric practice. *Comm Ment Health J* 1995; **31**: 73–85.
12. Sartorius N, Davidian H, Ernberg G *et al.* Depressive disorders in different cultures: report on the WHO collaborative study on standardized assessment of depressive disorders. Geneva: World Health Organization, 1983.
13. Tseng W. Culture and psychopathology. In: *Textbook of Cultural Psychiatry*. Bhugra D, Bhui K (Eds) Cambridge: Cambridge University Press, 2007; pp. 95–113.
14. Farooq S, Fear C. Working through interpreters. *Adv Psychiatr Treat* 2003; **9**: 104–110.
15. American Psychiatric Association. *Cultural Assessment in Clinical Psychiatry*. Washington, DC: American Psychiatric Press, 2002.
16. Bhui K, Bhugra D. Communication with patients from other cultures; the place of explanatory models. *Adv Psychiatr Treat* 2004; **10**: 474–478.
17. Yu S, Liu S, Lin K. Psychopharmacology across cultures. In; *Textbook of Cultural Psychiatry*. Bhugra D, Bhui K. Cambridge: Cambridge University Press, 2007; pp. 402–14.

Further reading

Bhugra D, Bhui K (eds). *Textbook of Cultural Psychiatry*. Cambridge: Cambridge University Press, 2007.
This textbook, edited by two experts in the field, offers more in-depth examination of this topic. The chapters, written by a panel of international experts, are well edited and encompass both theoretical and clinical perspectives.

CHAPTER 9

Recruitment of medical students into psychiatry

Adriana Mihai,[1] Otilia Butiu[1] and Julian Beezhold[2]
[1]Psychiatric Department, University of Medicine and Pharmacy Tg Mures, Romania
[2]Norfolk and Waveney Mental Health NHS Foundation Trust, United Kingdom University of East Anglia, Norwich, UK

Recruitment issues

Psychiatry is a relatively new field of medicine,[1] and recent studies have shown that the demand for psychiatrists,[2] or at least for psychiatric services,[3] is consistently growing, in particular in developing countries.[4,5] Several signals concerning the lack of psychiatrists have been raised in the last 30 years.[5-8] Different ways have been adopted to measure the recruitment of physicians into psychiatry. Two directions are evident, one evaluates the quantitative shortage, and the other the qualitative issues.

The quantitative deficit could be expressed as an under-representation of psychiatrists in the physician workforce throughout the world and an increasing number of vacancies in psychiatry.[9] In the UK, the number of students interested in psychiatry has been consistently low[10,11] (Figure 9.1).

The shortage in this field of medicine leads to the obvious question: 'What workforce is necessary in psychiatry?' The answer varies from country to country and depends on the type of approach – community-based mental health or psychiatry mostly based in hospitals. Ethical issues arise in relation to patients who do not have self-awareness of their illness. Medicine, including psychiatry, has in recent decades moved towards a greater emphasis on self-care and patient choice.[12] A huge number of patients remain undiagnosed and untreated because of the multiple filters that intervene between the patient and psychiatric services.[13]

How to Succeed in Psychiatry: A Guide to Training and Practice, First Edition.
Edited by Andrea Fiorillo, Iris Tatjana Calliess and Henning Sass.
© 2012 John Wiley & Sons, Ltd. Published 2012 by John Wiley & Sons, Ltd.

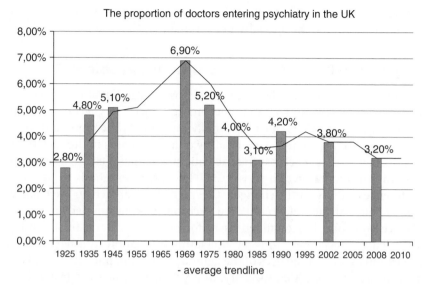

Figure 9.1 The proportion of doctors entering psychiatry in the UK. Drawn using data from Brockington and Mumford[10] and Lambert et al.[11]

In 2008, UK graduates applying for psychiatry specialist training comprised only 14 % of total applicants for psychiatry, the lowest proportion of all specialty fields. Specialty popularity was correlated with predicted income ($p = 0.006$).[14] In this situation, the vacancies were filled with candidates from abroad. The highest proportion of overseas applicants was in psychiatry, being 86 % of the total number of applicants.[15] In the USA, the proportion of overseas graduates taking up psychiatric residency has been limited and estimated to be no more than 30 %.[16] International candidates usually choose psychiatry because of the perceived availability of vacancies and relative chance of success.[14] A consequence of the free movement of the workforce within the European Union is the loss of qualified doctors from the medical systems of the country of origin.

Regarding the qualitative issues relating to recruitment, some authors maintain that international medical graduates are more likely to obtain the lowest average scores than other specialties or local graduates, probably because of challenges in understanding the care system and guidelines used. Further postgraduate training in legislative, ethnic, social and cultural differences for overseas applicants seems necessary.[17-20]

Another problem is the low retention rate in psychiatry. In Romania the problem is not with numbers entering training in psychiatry, but rather with retaining these doctors in training or after completing specialist training. The huge differences between working conditions and salaries (six to ten times more) from one country to another stimulate many young doctors to emigrate. In other countries low retention rates are caused by changing the specialty or working in other domains.

Why is psychiatry facing recruitment problems?

Recruitment shortage is affecting not only psychiatry but also many other specialties.[10,15] The motivation for becoming a doctor has become less one of taking care of others, altruism or saving people, but more and more the prospect of a good job, a good salary or a good status in the society. In a consumer society, each psychiatric patient becomes a client, a user or a customer of mental health services.[12] The shift in emphasis to patients' preferences has recently changed the medical approach in psychiatry, from a paternalistic style to a shared decision-making approach.[21]

Once someone has qualified as a doctor, their criteria for choosing a particular specialty seem to be the status in relation to other medical professionals, and in the eyes of the general public and politicians, and the available resources in that specialty. In psychiatry, some specific items are also involved: the challenges of dealing with patients with poor insight, the threats of suicide/homicide made by patients, the false belief that 'psychiatry is an unscientific and conceptually weak' medical discipline and that 'psychiatric disorders are not really treatable'.[22]

Perceived stigmatization of psychiatrists, mental health professionals and mental health patients by medical colleagues is a common observation. The low status of psychiatry in many cases is due to low salaries, stigma and lack of respect from other physicians, family and friends.[15,23] The low status of psychiatry and the unsympathetic attitude and lack of respect shown by other medical professionals and faculty members could be important factors in explaining the recruitment problems in the mental health field.

Other factors leading to poor recruitment include the perceived lack of evidence-based treatments and the perceived poor prognosis of mentally ill patients.[15] Moreover, 'biological reductionism, neglect of individual responses to treatment, massive propaganda from the pharmaceutical industry, misleading effects of psychometric theory on clinical assessment, and lack of consideration of multiple therapeutic ingredients and of the role of psychological well-being are identified as major sources of an intellectual crisis in psychiatric research'.[6]

Others consider that only certain types of doctors choose psychiatry, and different authors have tried to find which features are associated with the decision to become a psychiatrist, including mental disturbances, particular personality traits, social status, lifestyle or gender. Some suggest that psychiatrists enter this discipline because of personal concern for persons with mental disorders (e.g. they may have family members with psychiatric disorders or they may have personally experienced psychiatric problems in the past). The hypothesis that psychiatrists are more vulnerable to psychiatric illnesses was not proved in studies in which they were compared to doctors from other specialties.[24] Eagle and Marcos[25] postulate that psychiatry is more attractive for students who are from a lower social class, from an urban background, who are single and politically liberal. Fazel and Ebmeier (2009) argued that the choice of a given specialty depends also on lifestyle, personality and gender, among other factors.[15]

Some students find psychiatry too slow moving, with too few tangible results, and feel that the disorders are manageable, but not reversible. Some authors consider that recruitment problems could be caused by stressful working conditions, describing psychiatric patients as 'aversive, anxiety provoking, unpleasant, untrustworthy, and disabled'.[26] In some countries, diagnosis, assessment and treatment of psychiatric disorders are to some extent performed in primary care or in neurology settings. Certain treatments of mild psychiatric disorders are provided more frequently in private practice settings. In many countries there is pressure to restrict the public sector to 'the most seriously ill', the chronic psychotic patients or to those needing hospital admission.

In some places the role of psychiatrists is taken over by general practitioners, social workers, medical prison staff, educators, psychologists, neurologists and internal medicine physicians. Lay associations may play a significant role in helping people with addictions and other psychiatric disorders, for example in support groups for relatives or patients with acute or chronic illness. When should these problems be tackled by psychiatrists? Where is the place of psychiatry? Who needs psychiatric services – whether patients, relatives or society? Is psychiatric treatment a luxury for well-being? Some other questions arise about the role of psychiatrists, and need urgent answers.[27] Brockington and Mumford[10] consider that psychiatrists should diagnose and prescribe pharmacological treatment, but should not be involved in psychological treatment, like psychotherapy, which could be provided by nursing staff, psychologists, social workers and others. The European Federation of Psychiatric Trainees (EFPT),[28] in line with the Union of European Medical Specialists (UEMS),[36–30] considers that each psychiatrist should have at least a minimal knowledge of psychotherapy. In some countries, like Germany and Switzerland, psychiatrists are considered the coordinators of care planning, not only as regards biological and pharmacological treatments, but also the psychotherapeutic ones.

All these questions have stimulated an intense debate, both among mental health policy-makers and the main psychiatric associations (World Psychiatric Association, European Psychiatric Association, UEMS and EFPT). Particular emphasis and attention has been devoted to psychiatrists' role and profile.[28,31]

How to improve recruitment into psychiatry?

Several solutions have been proposed to improve recruitment of medical doctors into psychiatry. One is to increase the number of medical students. However, recruitment depends on judgments made about psychiatry's role. Students' opinions are not fixed, being formed in a period of discovery and development, and even after students are enthused about psychiatry during their undergraduate psychiatric training, they may often change their opinion.[10] A number of countries have increased medical school places to address shortages in the number of graduates training in certain specialties.[32,33] This method risks an eventual oversupply of medical graduates, who may then be unable to find a work. In the UK there has been a very significant increase in the number of medical school training places. Indeed, in 2011 some newly qualified UK doctors were initially unable to find jobs within the National Health Service due to oversupply of graduates.

Another proposal is to enhance psychiatry and related disciplines during medical teaching. The importance of undergraduate education in choosing psychiatry as a specialty has been recently highlighted.[15] A counter-argument is that students on clinical attachments in psychiatry may 'be exposed to wards which are often dirty, unpleasant, frightening and understaffed. They see a service that is underfunded and, subsequently, staff members with low morale and burnt-out.... Attractive conditions might also reduce stigma, further contributing to recruitment'.[34,35]

Sierles[36] mentions the important role of the directors of medical student education, stating that 'two of the three best predictors of career choice in psychiatry are the academic rank of the director and whether he or she had won an award in teaching. The importance of a positive training experience, initially at undergraduate level but also at later stages in a doctor's career, is emphasised. An enthusiastic teacher is particularly seen as a strong motivator to entering psychiatry'. A counter-argument is that the highest recruitment into psychiatry in the USA was in the 1950s, when psychiatry had a minor role in the curriculum.

Psychiatry residents may appreciate the holistic approach and the opportunity to know patients in depth. Even in the 1960s, psychiatrists advocated the study of psychology and sociology as part of preclinical teaching. Behavioural science courses in the preclinical teaching period, modules of training in psychiatry and a special emphasis on giving students some clinical responsibility, for example in the liaison psychiatry module, are recommended for improving the recruitment potential of psychiatry. Yet, the increasing duration of undergraduate training in psychiatry seems not to have delivered the expected increase in accessing the postgraduate specialist training in psychiatry. The recruitment deficits persist despite the increasing role of psychiatry in new undergraduate curricula. Some evidence shows that a 6-month psychiatry post in a general medicine rotation is an important source of recruitment.[10] The national application system and competition for places in medical specialty training introduced in the UK in 2007 has attempted to balance the demand for places between the different medical specialties.[15]

Personality traits, such as being more reflective and responsive to abstract ideas, a liking for complexity, tolerance of ambiguity, preference for a non-authoritarian attitude, open-mindedness, interest in theoretical and social welfare issues, and a preference for aesthetic values, seem to be qualities favourable for choosing psychiatry as a career. Attitude and ability are considered important factors for choosing psychiatry, more than in any other specialty.[10]

There is a significant difference between Western and Eastern European countries in the frequency with which career choices change. In the UK, historically 41 % of doctors change their first choice after 5 years and 69 % after 11 years; moreover, 9 % of doctors change their career choice at least four times.[10] This is likely to have been significantly reduced as a result of recent changes to the process and structure of postgraduate training. In other countries, such as Romania, it is difficult to change specialty during training because of strict rules and difficult admission exams. Financial issues also motivate trainees to minimize the duration of training because their salary is much lower than that of a specialist. It is quite rare to change specialty after finishing training in psychiatry.

The following recommendations have been made in order to improve recruitment into psychiatry:[10]

1. To recruit medical students who have an interest in psychology, sociology and in a broad understanding of their patients.
2. To promote research during the training period and more interest in the field.
3. To be from the same cultural background as the patients, which may contribute to better understanding of patients' beliefs and behaviours.

Brown *et al.*[14] emphasized the top five factors that may increase recruitment in psychiatry: (i) interest in, and concern for, mentally ill persons; (ii) a greater interest in people than in diseases; (iii) a greater interest in social aspects of medicine; (iv) the ability to tolerate ambiguity;

and (v) good undergraduate exposure to psychiatry. Gender balance is also important to ensure that psychiatry adequately meets patients' needs.

Older trainees may choose psychiatry because of earlier work in a different specialty, such as general practice. In Romania this was not possible in the past because, once a specialty was chosen, it was compulsory to complete a number of years working in that field. In the last few years, however, this situation has been changing, and the trainees can now switch specialty if they pass a new national exam.

The World Health Organization (WHO) has expressed its concerns regarding recruitment from developing countries, which already have a shortage of psychiatrists and other doctors. For example, India, where after training many doctors leave the country and go to work in high-income countries, has approximately one psychiatrist per 500 000 inhabitants.

> Most developing countries need to increase and improve training of mental health professionals, who will provide specialised care as well as support the primary health care programmes. Most developing countries lack an adequate number of such specialists to staff mental health services. Once trained, these professionals should be encouraged to remain in their country in positions that make the best use of their skills. This human resource development is especially necessary for countries with few resources at present. Though primary care provides the most useful setting for initial care, specialists are needed to provide a wider range of services. Specialistic mental health care teams ideally should include medical and non-medical professionals, such as psychiatrists, clinical psychologists, psychiatric nurses, psychiatric social workers and occupational therapists, who can work together toward the total care and integration of patients in the community.
>
> Community care has a better effect than institutional treatment on the outcome and quality of life of individuals with chronic mental disorders. Shifting patients from mental hospitals to community care is also cost-effective and respects human rights. Mental health services should therefore be provided in the community, with the use of all available resources. Community-based services can lead to early intervention and limit the stigma of taking treatment. Large custodial mental hospitals should be replaced by community care facilities, backed by general hospital psychiatric beds and home care support, which meet all the needs of the ill that were the responsibility of those hospitals. This shift towards community care requires health workers and rehabilitation services to be available at community level, along with the provision of crisis support, protected housing, and sheltered employment.

World Health Organization[37,38]

Finally, some advocate advertisement campaigns aimed at promoting the value of psychiatry as a career and at eliminating the stigma associated with mental health as an aid to attract new recruits.[39]

Who is responsible for recruitment?

Workforce planning in psychiatry in Europe is a responsibility of different stakeholders. Political organizations may take specific measures, such as limiting the number of places in other specialties and using national exams for starting training in psychiatry, as a means for matching availability of and demand for training places. An advantage could be that all medical students could find a place of work and be trained, while a disadvantage could be that some specialties may be 'chosen' because of ranking, not representing a real first option.

Morreale et al.[23] remarked that the directors of medical student education are exposed to double, if not multiple, loyalties and demands, and that recruitment should be left to the leadership of the residency training programme (and other faculties), and the directors of medical student education in psychiatry should be left 'to teach principles of good psychiatric care to all future physicians'.

The World Health Organization recommends that 'Mental health policy, programmes and legislation are necessary steps for significant and sustained action. These should be based on current knowledge and human rights considerations. Most countries need to increase their budgets for mental health programmes from existing low levels. Some countries that have recently developed or revised their policy and legislation have made progress in implementing their mental health care programmes. Mental health reforms should be part of the larger health system reforms. Health insurance schemes should not discriminate against persons with mental disorders, in order to give wider access to treatment and to reduce burdens of care'.[37]

Conclusions

Modern mental health systems should be based on specific local needs and demands, and on respect for human rights. Today the role of psychiatrists in society greatly depends on their status among other medical professionals, the general public and politicians, as well as on available economic and social resources. Research in mental health could reduce stigma and increase respect from other medical professionals. Promoting education of the general population about mental disorders may increase demands on mental health services. When people can express their needs without shame or fear of being stigmatized, politicians will fight for recognition of those needs and will help to find the appropriate resources. Good working conditions and a good salary could be crucial factors in improving the recruitment process in psychiatry, by enhancing the motivation of medical doctors to join this profession.

Keeping in mind the success and the problems of psychiatry, and learning from our past, specialists, associations, politicians and community representatives should work together to find the correct way to further develop and improve this amazing science.[40-42]

References

1. Marneros A. Psychiatry's 200th birthday. *Br J Psychiatry* 2008; **193**: 1–3.
2. Workforce Review Team, NHS. Workforce summary – General psychiatry. Available at: www.wrt.nhs.uk.
3. Vernon DJ, Salsberg E, Erikson C *et al*. Planning the future mental health workforce: with progress on coverage, what role will psychiatrists play? *Acad Psychiatry* 2009; **33**: 187–191.
4. Patel V. The future of psychiatry in low and middle-income countries. *Psychol Med* 2009; **39**: 1759–1762.
5. Kasching H. Are psychiatrists an endangered species? Observation on internal and external challanges to the profession. *World Psychiatry* 2010; **9**: 21–28.
6. Fava GA. The intellectual crisis of psychiatric research. *Psychother Psychosom* 2006; **75**: 202–208.
7. Editorial. The crisis in psychiatry. *Lancet* 1997; **349**: 965.
8. Oxtoby K. Psychiatry in crisis. *Brit Med J* 2008; classified suppl: 27 August. Available at: http://careers.bmj.com/careers/advice/view-article.html?id=3050.
9. Rao NR. Psychiatric workforce: past legacies, current dilemmas and future prospects. *Acad Psychiatry* 2003; **27**: 238–240.
10. Brockington I, Mumford D. Recruitment into psychiatry. *Br J Psychiatry* 2002; **180**: 307–312.
11. Lambert TW, Goldacre M, Turner J. Career choices of United Kingdom medical graduates of 2002. *Med Educ* 2006; **40**: 514–521.
12. Lazarescu M. *Psihiatrie, Sociologie, Antropologie* [*Psychiatry. Sociology. Anthropology*]. Brumar, 2002 [in Romanian].
13. Thornicroft G, Tansella M. *The Mental Health Matrix: A Manual to Improve Services*. Cambridge: Cambridge University Press, 1999.
14. Brown TM, Addie K, Eagle JM. Recruitment into psychiatry: views of consultants in Scotland. *Psychiatr Bull* 2007; **31**: 411–413.
15. Fazel S, Ebmeier KP. Specialty choice in UK junior doctors: is psychiatry the least popular specialty for UK and international medical graduates? *BMC Med Educ* 2009; **9**: 77.
16. Salsberg E, Rockey PH, Rivers KL *et al*. US Residency training before and after the 1997 balanced budget act. *JAMA* 2008; **300**: 1174–1180.

17. Woolf K, Cave J, Greenhalgh T *et al.* Ethnic stereotypes and the underachievement of UK medical students from ethnic minorities: qualitative study. *Br Med J* 2008; **337**: 1220–1222.
18. Dorsey ER, Jarjoura D, Rutecki GW. Influence of controllable lifestyle on recent trends in specialty choice by US medical students. *JAMA* 2003; **290**: 1173–1178.
19. National Resident Matching Program. Charting Outcomes in the Match: Characteristics of applicants who matched to their preferred specialty in the 2007 NRMP Main Residency Match. National Resident Matching Program and the Association of American Medical Colleges, 2007. Available at: http://www.nrmp.org/data/chartingoutcomes2007.
20. Zulla R, Baerlocher M, Verma S. International medical graduates (IMGs) needs assessment study: comparison between current IMG trainees and program directors. *BMC Med Educ* 2008; **8**: 42.
21. Mihai A. The patient's participation at the elaboration of the therapeutic plan. In: Covrig C, Zichil G, Turcu I, Chirita R, Lazarescu M, Chirita V (eds) *Quality of Life in Psychiatry*. Vicovia, 2006; pp. 63–68.
22. Issa BA, Adegunloye OA, Yussuf AD *et al.* Attitudes of medical students to psychiatry at a Nigerian medical school. *Hong Kong J Psychiat* 2009; **19**: 72–79.
23. Morreale MK, Balon R, Roberts LW. Directors of medical student education in psychiatry and recruitment into psychiatry: an ethical issue? *Acad Psychiatry* 2009; **33**: 177–179.
24. Mowbray RM, Davies BM, Biddle N. Psychiatry as a career choice. *Aust NZ J Psychiatry* 1990; **24**: 57–64.
25. Eagle PF, Marcos LR. Factors in medical students for choice psychiatry. *Am J Psychiatry* 1980; **134**: 423–427.
26. Tucker GJ, Reinhardt RF. Psychiatric attitudes of young physicians: implications for teaching. *Am J Psychiatry* 1968; **124**: 986–991.
27. Engels GL. The needs for a new medical model: a challenge for biomedicine. *Science* 1977; **196**: 129–136.
28. Mihai A. Education in psychiatry across Europe. EFPT Statements, Sinaia 2002. Tg Mures: UMF, 2002.
29. Union of European Medical Specialists Section of Psychiatry/European Board of Psychiatry. European framework for competencies in psychiatry. UEMS, 2009. Available at: www.uems.net.
30. Union of European Medical Specialists Section of Psychiatry/European Board of Psychiatry. Charter on training of medical specialists in the EU: requirements for the specialty of psychiatry. UEMS, 2003. Available at: www.uems.net.
31. Union of European Medical Specialists Section of Psychiatry. The profile of a psychiatryist. UEMS, 2005. Available at: www.uems.net.
32. Joyce C, Stoelwinder J, McNeuk J *et al.* Riding the wave: current and emerging trends in graduates from Australian university medical schools. *Aust Med J* 2007; **186**: 309–312.
33. Howe A, Campion P, Searle J *et al.* New perspectives – approaches to medical education at four new UK medical schools. *Br Med J* 2004; **329**: 327–331.

34. O'Gara C, Sauer J. Recruitment and retention in psychiatry. *Br J Psychiatry* 2002; **181**: 163.
35. Clarke-Smith L, Tranter R. Recruitment and retention in psychiatry. *Br J Psychiatry* 2002; **181**: 163.
36. Sierles F. Medical school factors and career choice of psychiatry. *Am J Psychiatry* 1982; **139**: 1040–1042.
37. World Health Organization. The way forward. WHO, 2001. Available at: http://www.who.int/mental_health/.
38. Gadit AA, Khalid N. Human rights and international recruitment of psychiatrists: dilemma for developing countries. *J Pakistan Med Assn* 2006; **56**: 474–476.
39. Oxtoby K. Psychiatry in crisis. *Br Med J Careers* 2008. Available at: http://careers.bmj.com/careers/advice/view-article.html?id = 3050.
40. Pichot P. The history of psychiatry as a medical profession. In: Gelder MG, Lopez-Ibor JJ, Andreasen N *et al.* (eds) *New Oxford Textbook of Psychiatry*, 2nd edn. Oxford: Oxford University Press, 2009; pp. 17–27.
41. Poole R, Bhugra D. Should psychiatry exist? *Int J Soc Psychiatry* 2008; **54**: 195–196.
42. Baker M, Menken M. Time to abandon the term mental illness. *Br Med J* 2001; **322**; 937.

CHAPTER 10

Not quite there yet? The transition from psychiatric training to practice as a psychiatric specialist

*Florian Riese,[1] Virginio Salvi,[2] Paul J. O'Leary[3]
and Corrado De Rosa[4]*
[1]Psychiatric University Hospital Zurich, Switzerland
[2]Mood and Anxiety Disorders Unit, Department of Psychiatry, University of Turin, Italy
[3]Department of Psychiatry, Emory University, Atlanta, Georgia, USA
[4]Department of Psychiatry, University of Naples SUN, Naples, Italy

Introduction

As in any other context, the term 'transition' refers to a process of change from one state to another. For the scope of this chapter, the two states under examination are the late phase of psychiatric training and the early stages of more or less independent practice as a psychiatric specialist. There is no clear consensus about how long this transition process usually takes, and even less about how long it should ideally take. However, it appears safe to say that it starts before formal qualification and certification as a specialist in psychiatry. It then continues for the first months – if not years – of independent practice in the field until the new specialist has fully embraced his or her professional identity. The term 'transition' does not immediately imply whether the process is goal-oriented, purposeful and active by nature, or 'if it just happens to happen'. In fact, a lack of reflection on the nature of this process as much among late-stage trainees as well as among health care authorities may contribute to the difficulties encountered during that period. On the part of senior psychiatric faculty, the transition from psychiatric trainee

How to Succeed in Psychiatry: A Guide to Training and Practice, First Edition.
Edited by Andrea Fiorillo, Iris Tatjana Calliess and Henning Sass.
© 2012 John Wiley & Sons, Ltd. Published 2012 by John Wiley & Sons, Ltd.

to specialist is often disregarded with 'benign neglect',[1] while anxiety prevails on the part of the late stage trainee.[2]

Similar to the transition from medical student to specialty training, completing psychiatric training and becoming a psychiatric specialist is a period when everybody has the same needs – guidance in job selection, counselling for job interviews, supervision in the first steps as an independent practitioner, etc. – and is a major step in professional development. However, while there has been some research on the first phase, for example investigating variables influencing career choices for specialty training among medical students[3,4] and the impact of psychiatric residency on trainee personality,[5] the range of available studies on the transition from psychiatric training into independent practice is very limited. This is surprising since, while the first transition determines how many potential future specialists enter into a field, the second transition determines how these specialists are allocated within the field. Both phases therefore seem to be equally important for planning health service provision.[6] For example, if psychiatric teaching facilities do not adequately prepare trainees for positions in community mental health services in rural areas, trainees may be less likely to apply for such positions even though their expertise would be highly welcome in that field of psychiatry.

The final years of training

As mentioned before, the transition to independent practice begins long before certification as a specialist in psychiatry. Several steps taken by late-stage trainees before graduation were identified in a study based on interviews with psychiatric residents from a major US training programme.[2] According to this study, these steps usually include: (i) acknowledging and undertaking the task of choosing a practice; (ii) defining personal, professional and family issues; (iii) establishing minimal requirements and reward priorities (e.g. choosing between academic and financial rewards); (iv) determining a professional presentation; (v) inquiring about practice opportunities in the professional market; (vi) interviewing for positions; (vii) negotiating the employment terms; (viii) committing to a practice; (ix) preparing for practice and (x) using decision-making facilitators.

From this list it becomes clear that the preparation for transition is a complex task with an ultimately unknown outcome. It is therefore not surprising that a high percentage of residents in the study reported symptoms of anxiety and depression, with 25 % reporting an unusual physical illness during the transition period. Of note, a study of how US residents graduating from psychiatry training programmes perceived their level of preparedness for clinical practice found a subjective perception of a high degree of preparedness for diagnosing and treating all major psychiatric conditions.[7] One may therefore conclude that the insecurity associated with the transition to independent practice is based mainly on a lack of preparation for the transition process rather than lack of knowledge or skills in psychiatry itself.

Unfortunately, it is currently largely unknown how satisfied early career psychiatrists are with the training they received, and how well they feel prepared in different aspects of psychiatry. In a survey conducted among graduates of US child and adolescent psychiatry programmes, the overall quality of residency training was rated high.[8] However, the areas that respondents felt least prepared for were administration and leadership skills, medical economics and business skills, arguably areas that become highly relevant when practising independently.

Various attempts have been made to address this lack of preparation, although these efforts were not part of broader strategies across psychiatry, but rather initiatives of individual teaching institutions. In the 1970s, a six-session weekly seminar called 'The transition into practice' was introduced into the training curriculum of a major US psychiatric residency programme.[1] Tellingly, the seminar was commonly referred to as 'reality rounds' among residents, as a major part of the seminar consisted in giving trainees the opportunity to talk directly to psychiatric practitioners about what their 'reality' was like. More recently, another structured attempt in a major US teaching centre was reported.[9] Here, a 32-week practice management course was established for third-year postgraduate psychiatric residents, which was designed to prepare them for the 'real world'. Indeed, the reality in many countries for future psychiatric specialists may be discouraging. They face the situation that jobs in their desired area of the country, in the desired field of psychiatry or in the desired institutional setting may not be available. In some countries, there may even be a period of mandatory involuntary placement to underserviced regions. Early career psychiatrists may also have to accept temporary positions, including fellowships, substitute positions (e.g. to cover maternity leaves), locum positions or on-call services. Only with time may it then be possible to move on to a permanent position.

For the public mental health sector, the average time between training completion and employment varies greatly between countries (Table 10.1). In some countries, the process of getting a job in the public sector is fast and fluid: in some cases, such as Belarus and the Czech Republic, early career psychiatrists become employed immediately after having passed board examinations. In other countries, such as France, Finland, Israel, Portugal, Slovenia and Switzerland, young specialists can immediately obtain a temporary position, which is usually converted to a permanent position in the public sector either immediately – due to shortage of

Table 10.1 Job transition in 12 countries.

Question	Belarus	Czech Rep.	Finland	France	Israel	Italy	Lithuania	Portugal	Slovenia	Spain	Switzerland	USA
How long is the time between end of training and employment in public MHC?	Immediately	Short time	Immediately	Immediately	Short time	Short time	1 month	1 month	0–3 months	Short time	Immediately	Immediately
How long does an ECP usually wait for a permanent job?	Immediately	3 months	Immediately	Immediately	2 years	Months to years	3 months	1 year	Immediately	Months to years	10 years	Immediately
Can ECPs continue with research activities once they are employed for another agency?	Sometimes	Sometimes	Sometimes	Usually not	Yes	Usually not	Yes	Yes	Yes	Usually not	Sometimes	Usually not

	R1	R2	R3	R4	R5	R6	R7	R8	R9	R10	R11	R12
What are the main problems addressed by ECPs in the first years after finishing training?	Bureaucratic overload and responsibilities Few opportunities in continuing education	Work overload Low salary Few opportunities in continuing education	Bureaucratic responsibilities Few opportunities in continuing education Private vs public sector choice	Work overload Lack of psychotherapy training Public vs private sector choice	–	Work overload Bureaucratic overload and responsibilities Difficulties in finding permanent jobs	No place to work in our country Low salary Professional stigma	Work overload Low salary Workplace distant from home	Bureaucratic responsibilities	Work overload Lack of psychotherapy training	Bureaucratic overload and responsibilities Cost of psychotherapy training	Getting registered as a preferred provider by insurance companies Collecting fees from insurance and patients Setting up a referral base
What are the pros and cons of working with more experienced colleagues?	Pros: learning with older's experience	Pros: learning with older's experience, clinical support	Pros: learning with older's experience	Pros: learning with older's experience	–	Pros: learning with older's experience	Pros: learning with older's experience	Pros: learning with older's experience	Pros: learning with older's experience; involvement in research	–	–	Pros: learning with older's experience

(continued overleaf)

Table 10.1 Job transition in 12 countries.

Question	Belarus	Czech Rep.	Finland	France	Israel	Italy	Lithuania	Portugal	Slovenia	Spain	Switzerland	USA
	Cons: none	Cons: higher competition	Cons: none	Cons: conform to old and conservative ways of working		Cons: conform to old and conservative ways of working	Cons: conform to old and conservative ways of working	Cons: conform to old and conservative ways of working	Cons: none			Cons: Placed at lower level with less flexibility than older colleagues
Are the characteristics of patients in MHC different from those attending university settings?	Yes	No	No: public MHS usually provides treatment on less complicated cases	Sometimes	No	Yes	No	Yes	Yes	No	No	No
Do ECPs receive specific training on professional responsibility in psychiatry?	No	No	No	Yes	Yes	No	Yes	No	No	No	No	Yes
On average how many colleagues are involved in a work shift?	3–4	2	1–2	1–2	1–4	2	2	1–3	1–2	1 in rural regions; 2–3 in main cities	1	1–2

Are ECPs immediately involved in routine activities in MHC?	Yes	Yes (with few exceptions)	Yes	In maximum 2 days	Yes	Yes	Yes	Yes	Gradually	Yes	Yes	Yes
Do ECPs usually prefer to work in community MHC or in hospital-based services?	Hospital-based services (considered more interesting and prestigious)	Hospital-based services (we almost have only hospital-based services)	Hospital-based services	Variable; it depends on the interest of the YP	Variable; it depends on the interest of the YP	Hospital-based services	Hospital-based services	Hospital-based services	Variable; it depends on the interest of the YP	Variable; it depends on the interest of the YP	Hospital-based services	Variable; it depends on the interest of the YP

YP, young practitioner.

psychiatry specialists, such as in France, Finland and Slovenia – or within 2 years, such as in Israel and Portugal. As in the USA there is a shortage of psychiatrists, finding a job is almost a certainty, and most young psychiatrists have secured a job before they graduate. In other countries, such as Italy or some regions of Spain, it may take years to become employed by the public sector, and sometimes it may even be difficult to get a temporary position, especially in rural, poor or less organized regions. Needless to say, waiting or interim periods prolong the transition phase and may be accompanied by high levels of stress for early career psychiatric specialists.

In some countries, it may be easier and quicker to gain employment in the private sector (see also Chapter 12). Facilities such as rehabilitation clinics or nursing homes may offer recently specialized psychiatrists jobs immediately after completing training, without substantial waiting time and sometimes even with better salaries. In the USA, the complexity of constraints in private sector psychiatry imposed by medical insurance providers or managed care providers may lead to frustration about denial of treatment and poor reimbursement if early career psychiatrists are not properly informed.

Obtaining a research position at a university hospital is usually very difficult, and frequently requires a doctoral and/or a postdoctoral degree (research career opportunities are outlined in Chapter 2 of this book). Therefore many young psychiatrists will be forced out of research activities that they started during training. In some countries, such as Israel, Lithuania, Portugal and Slovenia, the lack of separation between medical schools or universities and community hospitals may make it feasible for some early career psychiatrists to continue research projects started during their training (Table 10.1).

The initial period as a specialist in psychiatry

Once engaged in the new job, a new psychiatrist may feel great relief. He or she has successfully managed to survive medical and specialty training. The prospect may be of a stable working position and therefore a stable living situation for the first time. Professional status improves and usually the salary increases. Young psychiatrists have gained the freedom to structure their work according to their own priorities and preferences more than ever before. On the other hand, new psychiatrists have to come to terms with themselves, if their actual work matches their expectations: Is this the kind of psychiatry they envisioned? Can they make use of their new position to shape how psychiatry is practised in their environment? Do they still allow themselves to be learners or do they have to know everything? How does it feel to be perceived by patients much more as individual physicians rather than as part of a larger health care institution? Will they see their new responsibilities as a burden or as an opportunity? And, equally important, can they establish a sustainable work-life balance? These issues, among many others, shape the professional identity of psychiatrists.

The difficulties for early career psychiatrists in forming a professional identity may be seen as a reflection of what psychiatry as a whole is exposed to. The leading paradigms of psychiatry have been evolving continously.[10] Psychiatry has for years been considered an instrument for maintaining political order or a vehicle for protecting society from insanity. It has been practised with either a strong philosophical or biological focus, predominantly in either community settings or large asylums. Now, research in neuroscience, molecular biology, behavioural economics, psychotherapy and social sciences is again reshaping the field.[10] These advances are mirrored in the evolving nosology of psychiatry,[11] with the definition of new disorders, such as those related to the use of internet. Economic and political pressures are imposed on the field, which may eventually lead to the dangerous replacement of psychiatrists by psychologists, social workers or nurses (at least in some parts of the world). Considering the entire picture, the notion of what 'psychiatry really is' seems to be subject to constant change. Likewise, it is a complex task for early career psychiatrists to define their position in the psychiatric field, which, for the above-mentioned reasons, may be even more difficult than in other medical specialties.

Notably, building an identity as a psychiatrist may also mean dealing with some negative aspects of it, such as professional stigma. Some people still view psychiatry as a low-prestige medical career, based on weak scientific assumptions and practised by physicians who are often seen as 'odd' or 'neurotic' themselves; in several countries, families and friends discourage medical students from choosing psychiatry as a career.[12] Even colleagues from other medical specialties may consider psychiatrists as less important physicians with a non-scientific background. Reducing professional stigma should therefore be regarded a key issue, not only for improvement of patient care but also for the professional development of young psychiatrists.

On the practical side of the transition, a mismatch between preparation during training and the reality of psychiatric practice may become apparent. Early career psychiatrists may have to face their own professional inadequacies. They may lack sufficient skills in leadership or management, but also the specific kind of hands-on expertise that is required in a new work setting that usually has a smaller workforce and less specialization. For example, psychiatry schools often do not teach residents how to set up rehabilitation projects, or how to deal with patients affected more by social than psychopathological problems. On many occasions, training also fails to teach how to perform various certifications, such as those requested by courts or disability commissions. Finally, many residency schools do not request trainees to perform on-call night shifts, which on the contrary are very often essential when working in community services.

As a further complication, patients seen during residency are sometimes different from those who are referred to community settings. While the former, who are often referred to tertiary clinics specialized in assessment and 'fine tuning', are perhaps more complex from a psychopathological and clinical standpoint, the latter are more often low-income patients with long-term mental illnesses and challenging social problems, such as unemployment and homelessness, whom early career psychiatrists may not be adequately prepared to approach. In countries where psychiatric education relies heavily on short rotations through different services, the early career psychiatrist may have found it difficult to develop a real sense of responsibility for the long-term well-being of patients and the improvement of functioning of the service institution itself.[13]

Professional responsibility and liability are clearly key issues of clinical practice that early career psychiatrists have to deal with, but for which they may not be completely prepared. During residency, young doctors are caught in an ambiguous position, since they are considered as students by their teaching facilities and as doctors by the court, meaning that they are fully responsible and liable for their acts by judges. However, during training, young doctors are under the supervision of a tutor. Professional liability is therefore quite rare during the residency years and usually shared with mentors, if not with the whole team. On the contrary, once employed, early career psychiatrists are fully responsible for their acts and omissions, which depend solely upon them. The majority of European early career psychiatrists report the lack of specific training in professional responsibility (Table 10.1), which clearly needs to be taken into account in order to improve the doctors' self-confidence when treating difficult patients and dealing with difficult situations. On the other hand, in the USA most residents in psychiatry receive some training about risk reduction. Also, most malpractice insurance providers give courses about how documentation can reduce liability. However, these programmes focus on the ideals and rarely discuss the realities of a busy practice, leaving many young psychiatrists feeling overwhelmed by the requirements and vulnerable to malpractice lawsuits, even if they are practising good medicine.

A survey carried out on a random sample of recent graduates from psychiatric training programmes in the USA[14] showed how stressful the first steps as a psychiatric specialist can be. Among the 273 respondents, 73 % reported anxiety as a problem, ranging from moderate to incapacitating;

66 % had difficulties with patients; 45 % reported stress in their marriage; and 14 % had undergone separation or divorce. Despite the many challenges and clearly elevated levels of stress in the lives of these early career psychiatrists, the respondents most strongly endorsed statements underlining feelings of personal growth, mastery of the subject, maturity, support by loved ones and happiness to be out of training. Also, the overall contentment with their lives was found to be between moderately and very happy. When asked for coping strategies, the respondents most frequently stated emotional support from spouse or loved one, play and recreation, and ad hoc consultation with colleagues. It therefore seems, that, at least in this study population, the transition to the new professional role is successful for most psychiatrists, albeit not without difficulties. Consequences of a difficult transition may be burnout of the invididual (well described in Chapter 19) and practice of defensive medicine.

Burnout of early career psychiatrists may set in if coping strategies for the new demands are insufficient. It may ultimately lead to personal problems and the loss of their job. In a recent multicentre study conducted in Italy,[15] the main sources of stress reported by psychiatrists were the inadequacy of health-care facilities and the excessive workload. It is conceivable that at least in some cases insufficient coping leading to burnout is not due to individual variables, but to the characteristics of the job itself. Early career psychiatrists often lack the control of the resources they need to provide adequate care and may yet carry the entire responsibility for structurally inadequate care. Too many difficult-to-treat patients on the one hand, and an ever increasing bureaucracy on the other, can create a workload that is impossible to handle for the new psychiatrist alone. In several European countries, such as the Czech Republic, France, Italy, Portugal and Spain, work overload is regarded as the biggest problem encountered in the first years after training (Table 10.1). One way of overcoming the initial challenge of feeling overwhelmed might be continued supervision by more experienced colleagues. However, new psychiatrists are often left alone by senior colleagues, either because they lack time to look after young doctors or because they expect that young colleagues will relieve them of the most wearing duties. Even when young psychiatrists do have the chance to work with more experienced colleagues, there may be drawbacks, such as the need to adapt to more conservative or old-fashioned views of psychiatry.[16]

On the level of psychiatry as a whole, a failure to assume the professional identity of an independent psychiatrist may encourage 'defensive medicine', whose practice includes ordering tests or procedures or admitting patients to hospitals mainly for the purpose of protecting the physician from criticism or legal prosecution rather than for the patient's benefit. The tendency to practise defensively may stem from the attitudes of the mass media, the increased attention of courts and judges to the practice of physicians, and the increasing number of financial compensation cases, among other factors. Furthermore, so-called 'frivolous lawsuits' (i.e. charging someone without any grounds but lured by the possibility of compensation) towards doctors are becoming increasingly frequent in several countries. Other factors contributing to defensive medicine are specific for psychiatry, for example the particular characteristics of some mental disorders that may lead to conflicts with patient autonomy. Junior psychiatrists were found to be particularly prone to practise defensively when compared with psychiatrists at other career stages,[17] which was supposedly attributable to their lack of confidence and experience or, in other words, to an incomplete formation of their professional identity. Open discussion and ideally specific training for early career psychiatrists on this issue could therefore be highly beneficial not only for the individual psychiatrist, but also for the entire psychiatric profession.

Recommendations for a better transition

The challenges and difficulties in the transition process that are outlined in this chapter may vary greatly between countries as well as within a country. Indeed, most of the cited literature stems from English-speaking countries and – within these countries – frequently from the leading teaching institutions. The available literature by no means covers all the various circumstances under which early career psychiatrists are working. Thus, it is difficult to draw a conclusive picture of early career psychiatrists as a whole. However, at least some of the challenges described here are likely to be common to all psychiatric trainees who become psychiatrists. Still, the following recommendations are tentative and should eventually be appropriately tested.

In order to facilitate the transition from psychiatric training to independent practice the following recommendations should be considered:

1. The transition phase is a complex task. It is frequently accompanied by high levels of stress. Junior psychiatrists should reflect on the difficulties they are facing. Senior psychiatrists should help junior colleagues with this task.
2. Preparation for the transition phase should be considered a priority both for the individual psychiatrist and for the involved health-care institutions and authorities. Difficulties related to the transition may lead to burnout and to an increase in defensive practices in psychiatry.
3. Skills that are relevant in the 'real world of psychiatry' should be identified and included into psychiatric training curricula. These skills clearly go beyond classical psychiatric expertise into fields like leadership,

management and health. It is essential to integrate instruments of quality control into psychiatry teaching, in order to continually modify curricula alongside the evolving demands.

4. The knowledge base about this phase of career development in psychiatry should be increased. Only US psychiatry seems to be sensitive to the issue of transition, and much of the relevant literature is outdated.
5. The professional identity of psychiatrists should be continually reviewed. To this aim, the active involvement of early career psychiatrists in the national and international psychiatric organizations seems crucial.
6. Stigma against psychiatric patients and against psychiatry as a profession has to be identified, prevented and counteracted, as it is a major factor leading to poor working conditions for psychiatrists and to poor treatment for patients.
7. Before the transition occurs, it is essential for psychiatric trainees to create opportunities to discuss with 'real-world practictioners'. After the transition has occurred, early career psychiatrists should try to overcome isolation by continuing existing mentor/mentee relationships and by creating new professional support networks, wherever possible.

Conclusions

In conclusion, the transition into independent practice is an important step in the personal and professional development of any physician. The difficulties that may arise during this process have been largely neglected by teaching services and health-care authorities, but also by trainees and senior colleagues themselves. It has recently been suggested[18] that psychiatry should find a new identity in order to survive. In no other phase of a psychiatric career is this need for definition of a professional identity more pressing than during the transition from trainee to psychiatrist. The vitality in the practice of psychiatry, i.e. the caring, curious and ethically inspired attitude towards mentally ill patients, ultimately depends on the success of this transition. Colleagues who are in transition should therefore receive the strongest possible support from mentors, senior colleagues and professional associations.

References

1. Borus JF. The transition to practice seminar. *Am J Psychiatry* 1978; **135**: 1513–1516.
2. Borus JF. The transition to practice. *J Med Educ* 1982; **57**: 593–601.
3. Sierles FS, Taylor MA. Decline of U.S. medical student career choice of psychiatry and what to do about it. *Am J Psychiatry* 1995; **152**: 1416–1426.

4. Gowans MC, Glazier L, Wright BJ *et al*. Choosing a career in psychiatry: factors associated with a career interest in psychiatry among Canadian students on entry to medical school. *Can J Psychiatry* 2009; **54**: 557–564.

5. Pasnau R, Bayley SJ. Personality changes in the first year of psychiatric residency training. *Am J Psychiatry* 1971; **128**: 79–84.

6. Brockington I, Mumford D. Recruitment into psychiatry. *Brit J Psychiatry* 2002; **180**: 307–312.

7. Blumenthal D, Gokhale M, Campbell EG *et al*. Preparedness for clinical practice: reports of graduating residents at academic health centers. *JAMA* 2001; **286**: 1027–1034.

8. Stubbe DE. Preparation for practice: child and adolescent psychiatry graduates assessment of training experiences. *J Am Acad Child Psychiatry* 2002; **41**: 131–139.

9. Wichman CL, Netzel PJ, Menaker R. Preparing psychiatric residents for the "real world": a practice management curriculum. *Acad Psychiatry* 2009; **33**: 131–134.

10. Fiorillo A. L'identità dei giovani psichiatri. In: Fiorillo A, Bassi M, Siracusano A (eds) *Professione psichiatra: guida pratica alla formazione, all'inserimento lavorativo e all'aggiornamento*. Rome: Il Pensiero Scientifico Editore, 2009; pp. 1–14.

11. Cassano G. La psichiatria nel 21° secolo. *Giornale Italiano di Psicopatologia* 2000; **6**: 2.

12. Roberts LW. Stigma, hope, and challenge in psychiatry: trainee perspectives from five countries on four continents. *Acad Psychiatry* 2010; **34**: 1–4.

13. Bernabeo EC, Holtman MC, Ginsburg S *et al*. Lost in transition: the experience and impact of frequent changes in the inpatient learning environment. *Acad Med* 2011; **86**: 591–598.

14. Looney JG, Harding RK, Blotcky MJ *et al*. Psychiatrists' transition from training to career: stress and mastery. *Am J Psychiatry* 1980; **137**: 32–36.

15. Bressi C, Porcellana M, Gambini O *et al*. Burnout among psychiatrists in Milan: a multicenter survey. *Psychiatry Serv* 2009; **60**: 985–988.

16. De Rosa C. Primi passi in un Dipartimento di Salute Mentale. In: Fiorillo A, Bassi M, Siracusano A (eds) *Professione psichiatra: guida pratica alla formazione, all'inserimento lavorativo e all'aggiornamento*. Rome: Il Pensiero Scientifico Editore, 2009; pp. 137–150.

17. Passmore K, Leung W-C. Defensive practice among psychiatrists: a questionnaire survey. *Postgrad Med J* 2002; **78**: 671–673.

18. Katschnig H. Are psychiatrists an endangered species? Observations on internal and external challenges to the profession. *World Psychiatry* 2010; **9**: 21–28.

CHAPTER 11

When things go wrong: errors, negligence, misconduct, complaints and litigation

Julian Beezhold,[1,2] Stavroula Boukouvala,[1] Nya Maughn[1] and Kate Manley[1]

[1]Norfolk and Waveney Mental Health Care NHS Foundation Trust, Hellesdon Hospital, Norwich, UK
[2]University of East Anglia, Norwich, UK

Introduction

Have you ever made a clinical error, or been the subject of a complaint, or been accused of professional misconduct, or had to defend yourself against litigation in court? Medicine in general, and psychiatry in particular, are scientific and professional disciplines that are subject to constant change as new treatments and understandings are developed, tested and introduced into clinical practice. Yet there is also change in many non-clinical aspects of medicine and psychiatry.

The increasing complaints and litigation culture is one of these aspects that often causes great difficulties, anxieties and significant amounts of stress to psychiatrists, who, like all doctors, are on the receiving end of these actions. Many early career psychiatrists will not have experienced being the subject of a complaint or of litigation – yet it is statistically inevitable that sooner or later most or all will have to deal with one or more of these unwelcome intrusions into our day-to-day clinical work.

All early career psychiatrists will have made errors, even if trivial, because of human fallibility. How to minimize and prevent human

How to Succeed in Psychiatry: A Guide to Training and Practice, First Edition.
Edited by Andrea Fiorillo, Iris Tatjana Calliess and Henning Sass.
© 2012 John Wiley & Sons, Ltd. Published 2012 by John Wiley & Sons, Ltd.

errors, and the consequences thereof, has been increasingly recognized as presenting one of the greatest challenges for medicine in modern times.

In recent years there has been an increasing focus in medicine on error prevention. This has followed from acknowledgement that simple improvements in clinical equipment and systems may be able to significantly reduce the risk of errors that result from our common human fallibility.

The National Clinical Assessment Service (NCAS), which advises the National Health Services (NHS) in the UK on the management of performance concerns in doctors and dentists, has reported high rates of referrals for performance concerns in psychiatrists relative to other specialties in medicine.[1] Data on complaints regarding psychiatrists reveal that they are about as likely as other physicians to prescribe drugs inappropriately, including making drug errors. Psychiatrists have been over-represented among physicians investigated for inappropriate personal relationships with patients.[2-4]

Other major causes of action that may be brought against a psychiatrist include negligent diagnosis, abandonment from treatment, various intentional and quasi-intentional torts (assault and battery, fraud, defamation, invasion of privacy), failure to obtain informed consent, and breach of contract. Areas of liability specific to psychiatry include harm caused by organic therapies – electroconvulsive therapy (ECT), psychotropic medication – breach of confidentiality, failure to control or supervise a dangerous patient or negligent release, failure to protect third parties from potentially dangerous patients, false imprisonment and negligent infliction of mental distress.[5]

Malpractice can be thought of as comprising different types of conduct. These could include negligence on the one hand and unprofessional behaviour on the other.

This chapter will deal separately with negligence and unprofessional conduct, as well as with the possible consequences, including complaints and litigation. We will describe in detail what these issues are, use case examples to illustrate key points, look at how this affects professional practice, provide pointers on how to deal with and manage complaints and litigation should they occur, and also examine some simple steps that early career psychiatrists and hospitals can take to either prevent or reduce the severity of complaints and litigation.

Error

An error is defined as the failure of a planned action to be completed as intended or the use of a wrong plan to achieve an aim. Errors can include problems in practice, products, procedures, and systems.

Quality Interagency Coordination Task Force (2000)[6]

Medical error is different to error in most other contexts. Doctors making errors tend to affect patients and their families and may lead to disability or death. This contrasts with many other industries where the impact of error may be inconvenience rather than a matter of life or death.

In 2000 in the USA, the Institute of Medicine (IoM) published a report that pulled together a wide ranging collection of data and research regarding medical error entitled *To Err is Human: Building a Safer Health System*.[7] This report drew the compelling conclusion that up to 98 000 American deaths were caused annually by preventable errors. It highlighted the fact that, even using much more conservative figures, medical error amounted to the eighth leading cause of death for Americans. This ranked ahead of motor vehicle accidents, AIDS and breast cancer. The IoM report went on to conclude that at least 50 % of all adverse events in medicine were a consequence of some form of medical error that was preventable. There was a huge economic, health and social burden resulting from medical errors. It estimated that the economic burden alone for disability, healthcare costs and lost productivity was likely to be some $29 billion per year in the USA. The report tried to examine why this high rate of medical errors was occurring. It acknowledged that substandard performance by individual doctors was important, but stated that it was in fact systems rather than individuals that led to most medical errors. In other words, it concluded and made the case that medical errors could potentially be dramatically reduced by improving and redesigning systems. This drew attention to the dangers inherent in simply blaming individuals for medical error. Humans are fallible and will therefore make errors. A blame approach to medical error, whereby individuals are 'named and shamed' or penalized or punished, is more likely to create an incentive for doctors to hide error. When errors remain hidden or otherwise undetected, society is deprived of the opportunity to learn from the error and also cannot use the error information to make changes that design-out the possibility for such an error to recur.

One of the most important early studies that examined medical errors was the Harvard Medical Practice Study by Leape *et al.* and by Brennan *et al.*, the main findings of which were published in two papers in the *New England Journal of Medicine* in 1991.[8,9] This was a very large study that scrutinized 30 195 health-care records that were randomly selected from 51 different hospitals in the state of New York. This study found that adverse events occur in 3–4 % of all inpatients.[9,10] Medication errors alone accounted for 19 % of all the adverse events found, and the study concluded that 45 % of these were a result of medical error. Of even more concern was the finding that 30 % of those patients who had suffered a medication adverse event had died. The researchers concluded that an astonishing 58 % of all the adverse outcomes such as death or injury that had been caused by medication mistakes were preventable.[8,9]

The report from the Institute of Medicine[7] estimates that at least 7000 Americans die every year as a result of preventable medication errors. This is more than those killed by injuries at work. Medication errors, according to this report, also lead to an estimated extra cost of $2 billion to the economy because of the additional treatment required as a consequence of the injury caused by these errors. Researchers estimated that about 10 % of all hospital admissions in the USA resulted from medication errors, with a significant negative impact on overall morbidity and mortality.[11]

At around the same time as the Institute of Medicine report was published, the Chief Medical Officer for the UK, Liam Donaldson, led a working group on adverse events in medicine that culminated in the publication in 2000 of *Organisation with a Memory*.[12] This report estimated that around 10 % of all people admitted to hospital in the UK would experience a medical error. This amounted to around 850 000 individual patients every year. The report went on to estimate that about 1 % of these errors would be classified as very serious with a consequence of death or permanent injury. This meant that as many as 34 000 patients were dying every year, and 40 000 sustaining a permanent injury as a result of the actions of healthcare staff including doctors.[12]

Many other industries, for example the motor, airline and banking industries, have made great progress in using design to reduce error. They share certain common factors with the healthcare industry. For example, they all deal with complex transactions and interactions between people and technology. But there is a very important difference that makes the challenge of error reduction in medicine a far more difficult task. This difference is that healthcare is far more complex, involving the interactions between often many different people, different systems and different technologies. This is well illustrated by research done in an intensive care unit that found that patients on average have 178 different actions performed each day.[13]

There is a minimum of five separate but interdependent steps involved in the process of prescribing, through to the patient successfully taking the medication: prescription, transcribing, dispensing, delivering and administering.[6] Leape and colleagues looked at this process in more detail and found that as many as 78 % of medication errors could be ascribed to system failures.[13]

An interesting perspective was provided by Millenson,[14] who stated that the amount of information and knowledge required to carry out health care safely and effectively is such that the human brain cannot cope due to a lack of storage capacity. Leape drew an interesting comparison between the airline industry and medicine by examining error rates. He found that each patient in an intensive care unit (ICU) experienced just short of two separate errors in their treatment every day, of which 20 % were grave enough to be potentially fatal. He used these data to calculate that the error rate in the ICU was roughly 1 %. He then went on to make the dramatic point that if the airline industry had an error rate one-tenth of this, at 0.1 %, this would lead to the equivalent of two dangerous landings per day at O'Hare International Airport.[15]

Psychiatric care itself is complex and fragmented, which in turn contributes to the difficulties faced by psychiatrists when attempting to even recognize the problem of medical errors. There are many local, regional, national and international differences in systems, terminology, technology, health records and treatment practices. Other factors that add to the challenge of error prevention and reduction in psychiatry include:

- Many healthcare systems and institutions do not yet use robust and effective error-reporting systems.
- Poor links and communications both within mental healthcare organizations and between mental health and other medical, social and health disciplines result in difficulties in transmitting and implementing changes in practice.
- There is a wide variety of settings in which psychiatrists practise (such as hospitals, outpatient clinics, community settings, prisons, private practice).
- Patients respond differently to identical interventions and treatments. The treatments themselves are not universally effective. Because we expect this, it can be hard to recognize errors.
- The pervasive blame culture within medicine, whereby errors are seen as the fault of the individual doctor leading to a disciplinary action as the remedy, acts as a disincentive to error reporting, and therefore deprives us of the opportunity to learn from mistakes.
- It can be difficult to see trends in medical errors when the healthcare system tends to look at adverse events as one-off incidents that affect only one patient at a time, and are then analysed in isolation from other similar events, if at all.
- Misplaced concern relating to patient confidentiality can also inhibit error reporting and learning.
- Personal, local, regional and national pride can lead to difficulties in reporting and acknowledging errors.
- International communication of good practice and error reduction strategies may be hampered by the issue of multiple different languages and access to information.

Negligence

Negligence is relatively common in medicine. The Harvard medical practice study[9] estimated that '27179 injuries, including 6895 deaths and 877 cases of permanent and total disability, resulted from negligent care in New York in 1984'. Overall, they found that 27.6 % of adverse events were caused by negligence.

Negligence, amounting to malpractice in medicine, including psychiatry, has a very specific definition in most legal jurisdictions. There are generally four critical elements that each separately have to be proved in order to establish that a doctor has been negligent:

1. There must be a doctor-patient relationship, which establishes a duty of reasonable care.
2. There must be a breach of this duty of reasonable care.
3. Harm must have occurred that involves physical, emotional, financial or other forms of damage.
4. A causal link must be demonstrated between the negligence and the harm or damage suffered.

In order for negligence to have taken place, a psychiatrist must breach this duty to provide a reasonable standard of care. Yet, it is often unclear what this standard is. There is frequent disagreement between expert witnesses who testify during malpractice litigation even though in theory they are all informed by the same research literature, guidelines and codes of practice.

Discussing the role of forensic psychiatrists, Stone[16] has pointed out that 'the standard of care in psychiatric treatment, which is the central question in malpractice cases, is by no means the "natural" province of the subspecialty of forensic psychiatrists'. Proving that the harm was actually caused by the alleged breach of duty of care can be very difficult. Many other factors may lead to the harm occurring. A brief look at a number of hypothetical cases can help illustrate some of the difficulties involved in the determination of negligence and malpractice. Which, if any, of the following may amount to negligence or malpractice? Each case will be followed by some discussion of the issues raised.

Case studies

Case 1

John was very agitated and disturbed in hospital. He was sedated using intravenous haloperidol as follows – an initial dose of 2 mg followed by repeated doses every 15–20 minutes while agitation persisted. Each repeat dose was double the previous dose. John developed a ventricular tachyarrhythmia and died.

This case involves the issue of what is a 'reasonable standard' of care. The dosage regime described is one officially recommended by the Society of Critical Care Medicine in the USA as recently as 1995 and 2002.[17,18] Another official guideline, the British National Formulary, states that the maximum recommended intravenous dose should not exceed 18 mg daily.[19] This contradiction between different guidelines obviously places the clinician in a very difficult position when having to make clinical decisions in day-to-day practice.

A number of legal principles have been developed that attempt to deal with the issue of determining what an acceptable and reasonable standard of care may be. The following discussion will generally use British legal cases to illustrate these issues, but the essence of these is reflected in most jurisdictions.

The most famous case is that of *Bolam v Friern Hospital Management Committee*. This case led to the so-called 'Bolam test' for reasonable standard of care as 'If a doctor reaches the standard of a responsible body of medical opinion, he is not negligent'. This test means that where a doctor, effectively a person with better than average skills at medical procedures and treatments, practises in accordance with a responsible body of (even minority) opinion, then he is not negligent even if the practice of others is different.

Mr Bolam was admitted voluntarily to hospital and agreed to have electroconvulsive therapy treatment. This was administered without muscle relaxant or restraint and Bolam suffered a number of injuries, including serious fractures, during the treatment. He sued, alleging negligence for failure to use muscle relaxants, failure to restrain him and failure to warn him of the risks involved.

Mr Justice McNair, in the Bolam case, noted that expert witnesses had confirmed that it was common practice to not use relaxant drugs or restraints, and also to not warn patients of the treatment risks unless the patient asked. He stated that common practice was very relevant to determining the reasonable standard of care. He went on to state 'I myself would prefer to put it this way, that he is not guilty of negligence if he has acted in accordance with a practice accepted as proper by a responsible body of medical men skilled in that particular art. . . . . .Putting it the other way round, a man is not negligent, if he is acting in accordance with such a practice, merely because there is a body of opinion who would take a contrary view. At the same time, that does not mean that a medical man can obstinately and pig-headedly carry on with some old technique if it has been proved to be contrary to what is really substantially the whole of informed medical opinion. Otherwise you might get men today saying: ''I do not believe in anaesthetics. I do not believe in antiseptics. I am going to continue to do my surgery in the way it was done in the eighteenth century.'' That clearly would be wrong'.[20]

Another case, the Hedley Byrne case,[21] created the rule of 'reasonable reliance' by the claimant on the professional judgment of the doctor. 'Where a person is so placed that others could reasonably rely upon his judgment or his skill, or upon his ability to make careful inquiry, and a person takes it upon himself to give information or advice to, or allows his information or advice to be passed on to, another person who, as he knows or should know, will place reliance upon it, then a duty of care will arise'.[21]

The Hedley Byrne case relates to the communication of all forms of advice and information about diagnosis, treatment options and prognosis, including the information required for the purpose of obtaining informed consent. The Bolam case relates to all the acts and omissions that form part of diagnosis and treatment.

The case of *Barnett v. Chelsea & Kensington Hospital* illustrates the importance of causation. Three people who presented at the local casualty department were not seen by the doctor there, who was feeling unwell. He did advise that they go home and see their own doctors. One of the three died shortly afterwards and was found on post mortem to have arsenic poisoning. Expert evidence was that had he been examined and treated at the casualty department there would still have been almost no chance that he would have recovered. The court held that there was negligence (failure to examine), but that there was no evidence that this caused the deceased's death.[22]

The case of *Sidaway v. Bethlem Royal Hospital Governors* further developed the law on informed consent and reasonable standard of care. The patient gave consent for a cervical cord decompression. However, the surgeon did not discuss the less than 1 % chance of paraplegia resulting from the operation. The patient sued after developing paraplegia during the operation. The court rejected her claim on the basis that a very detailed explanation of very unusual side effects was not required. It is worth noting the dissenting judgement from Lord Scarman, who stated that a doctor should indeed tell the patient of any 'inherent and material' risk involved in the proposed intervention.[23]

The Bolitho case further defined the legal test for reasonable standard of care. A doctor was sued for allegedly negligently failing to attend a 2-year-old boy who suffered brain damage and cardiac arrest secondary to airway obstruction. Five expert witnesses gave evidence that they would not have intubated the boy, whereas one testified that he would have intubated him. The House of Lords held that there had to be logical reasoning behind the decision not to intubate that involved weighing the risks and the benefits. This meant that the court could reject expert opinion where it was 'logically indefensible'.[24]

In the case of *Fv.R*, Chief Justice King stated, 'In many cases, an approved professional practice as to disclosure will be decisive. But professions may adopt unreasonable practices. Practices may develop in professions, particularly as to disclosure, not because they serve the interests of the clients, but because they protect the interests or convenience of members of the profession. The court has an obligation to scrutinize professional practices to ensure that they accord with the standard of reasonableness imposed by the law. A practice as to disclosure approved and adopted by a profession or section of it may be in many cases the determining consideration as to what is reasonable. On the facts of a particular case, the answer to the question whether the defendant's conduct conformed to approved professional practice may decide the issue of negligence, and the test has been posed in such terms in a number of cases. The ultimate question, however, is not whether the defendant's conduct accords with the practices of his profession or some part of it, but whether it conforms to the standard of reasonable care demanded by the law. That is a question for the court and the duty of deciding it cannot be delegated to any profession or group in the community.'[25]

Case 2

Jane is a psychiatrist who fully believes in the importance of physical health issues. Her routine practice with new outpatients is to perform a full physical examination that includes testicular examination on all male patients.

This case again would revolve around issues of reasonable standard of care and informed consent. However, there is another dimension. Is this a case where the conduct of the doctor is either so unusual or motivated by personal issues that it may amount to misconduct? What if the psychiatrist was male and insisted on an internal vaginal examination for all female patients?

Perhaps the key point here is that all interventions and treatments should be tailored to the needs of the individual patient, rather than a blanket one-size-fits-all approach. Also, where one's practice differs significantly from that of most psychiatrists, then there should be clear and acceptable reasons for this in every case.

> **Case 3**
>
> Edwin has a psychotic illness that you have diagnosed as schizophrenia. He has a delusional belief that he can fly and was brought to your outpatient clinic after being found on the roof of his house 'about to take off'. Despite your thorough explanation of all the appropriate information regarding the proposed antipsychotic medication he does not wish to take any medication. You explain that if he does not take the medication he will be detained in hospital. Edwin is now scared and 'agrees' to take the medication.

This case goes to the heart of the legal issue of informed consent and the criteria that should be satisfied to demonstrate that informed consent has been appropriately obtained from the patient. The requirements in English law, but reflected in most jurisdictions, for a consent decision to be valid are that it should be voluntary, informed and made by a competent person.

Voluntary means free from any form of coercion, whether overt or implied, direct or indirect. However, even this simple concept gives rise to potential conflict in practice. In the Case 3 scenario above, the psychiatrist has a duty to give information, so that the patient is fully informed. Yet the information that the psychiatrist is considering the use of legal powers of detention, should the patient not take the medication, may at the very same time be perceived as a form of coercion.

In English law, all persons over the age of 16 are presumed to be competent unless the contrary be proved. There are specific statutory criteria for testing competence where this may be in doubt. These are: (i) is there disturbance or impairment in the functioning of mind or brain; (ii) does the patient understand the information relevant to the decision, including the consequences of decisions for or against or of not deciding, *and* can that patient use or weigh that information as part of the process of making a decision, *and* can the patient retain the information long enough to make a decision, *and* can the patient communicate the decision? Only if the patient both satisfies criterion (i) and fails to satisfy one or more of the components of criterion (ii) may they be deemed to lack the capacity to make a specific decision.[26] It should also be noted that capacity is a decision-specific issue. A patient may simultaneously have capacity to make one decision, whilst at the same time lacking capacity to make another.

The law in England also clearly specifies that the more grave and more serious the decision, the more certainty and expertise is required to establish whether or not capacity is present in cases where there is doubt. It goes on to make clear that in life-or-death situations involving uncertainty about capacity that the first priority should be to preserve life pending the final determination regarding the presence or absence of capacity.

Case 4

Mr X attended his outpatient appointment and informed his therapist that he was planning to kill a third party, Miss T, when she returned from a summer in Brazil. The therapist informed the authorities, who took no further action. However, neither Miss T nor her family were informed of the patient's statement by the therapist or the authorities. Miss T then returned from Brazil and was killed by Mr X.

This case revolves around the conflict between two duties, namely the duty of confidentiality and the duty to protect third parties.

The case in 1976 of *Tarasoff v. Regents of the University of California*, which was reviewed by the California Supreme Court, resulted in a closer look at the duty of mental health professionals to protect or warn potential victims from harm caused by their patients. The case involved a psychiatric outpatient who had told his therapist that he was planning to kill Tatiana Tarasoff, when she returned home from spending the summer in Brazil. The therapist decided to inform the authorities, who found him not dangerous and no further actions were taken. Neither Ms Tarasoff nor her parents were warned or notified of the threats made by the patient. In due course the patient returned and murdered Ms Tarasoff. Her parents filed suit alleging that the involved therapists failed to warn them or their daughter of the threats.

The duty to warn third parties about threats made by a patient who has expressed specific threats of violence against them is fortunately an infrequent cause of litigation. Despite the fact that the frequency of these events is relatively rare, they constitute one of the most complicated duties for psychiatrists.

Before 1970, this was not a legal issue for psychiatrists. However, with the Tarasoff ruling in 1976, a legal responsibility was established for therapists, and subsequently all psychiatrists, to protect certain individuals who were not their patients. The Court stated 'In this risk-infested society we can hardly tolerate the further exposure to danger that would result from a concealed knowledge of the therapist that his patient was lethal'.[27] The difficulty for psychiatrists lies in understanding exactly which third parties need to be protected and how the psychiatrist is supposed to protect them. All psychiatrists practising in a Tarasoff jurisdiction should understand the implications for their clinical practice.

Following the Tarasoff ruling, which is law in most US states, decisions in similar cases have been confusing and interpretations vary widely, with the majority of courts recognizing a duty to warn only when the victim is 'foreseeable'. The Tarasoff duty is often misunderstood as a duty to warn, when in fact it is a duty to protect. Even courts have misunderstood this; for example, in 2001 a court in California gave incorrect instruction to the jury on this point, leading eventually to attempts to amend the statute law to define this duty more explicitly.[28]

Most jurisdictions will require two criteria to be met before making a finding of negligence in this type of case: firstly that the psychiatrist recognized or should reasonably have recognized that the patient presented a risk to one or more third parties, and secondly that the psychiatrist failed to take reasonable action to protect the parties involved.

Misconduct

Misconduct is defined, for the purposes of this chapter, as any conduct likely to lead to censure or disciplinary action against the doctor concerned. This broad definition therefore includes a range of behaviours varying from substandard performance to substance misuse and addiction problems through attitudinal problems and wilful and deliberate failure to follow policies and protocols and on to outright criminal behaviour.

Morrison and Morrison examined the records of 584 cases of physicians who were disciplined by the California Medical Board over a 30-month period. This equated to about 0.25 % of all licensed physicians in California – all the physicians disciplined during this period. They compared the findings from this group with a control group of physicians who had not been subject to disciplinary action and a control group comprising only psychiatrists.[2]

Morrison and Morrison found that 12.8 % of the disciplined sample were psychiatrists, compared to 7.2 % of the sample of non-disciplined physicians. Amongst physicians who had surrendered their licences whilst under investigation, 13.2 % were psychiatrists. The authors found that psychiatrists were significantly more likely to be disciplined for sexual boundary violations compared to non-psychiatrists. Female psychiatrists were under-represented in the disciplined group. Rates of discipline for negligence or incompetence were about the same as for other specialties. There were no demographic differences, other than gender, between the disciplined and non-disciplined psychiatrists. Morrison and Morrison speculated that 'Several factors could increase psychiatrists' risk of sexual boundary violations. They often work in isolation, out of view of other professionals. Also, psychiatrists have more personal contact, longer and more sessions with individual patients, hence more opportunity to become intimate with them.'

Other studies have found that psychiatrists are about as likely to make medication errors as other specialists.[3,4] The National Clinical Assessment Service (NCAS) was established in the UK in 2001 in order to manage performance concerns regarding doctors working in the National Health Service (NHS) in a fairer and more effective manner. Data from the first eight years of the NCAS suggest that roughly '1 in every 190' doctors will be referred to the NCAS each year. About 33 % will have been suspended or excluded from their employment. The male:female ratio is just over 4:1, showing a strong over-representation of men. The number of white doctors is almost exactly the same as the number of ethnic minority doctors who are referred, showing a disproportionately high referral rate for ethnic minority doctors.[1]

During this period, 541 doctors working in psychiatry were referred, comprising 12 % of all referrals. This is a very significant over-representation compared to other medical specialties. However, this may be almost entirely accounted for after controlling for the far higher number of ethnic minority and non-UK medical graduates who work in psychiatry. The NCAS report analysed 1472 cases who were referred between December 2007 and March 2009 to elicit the reason for referral showing:

Clinical concerns	54 %
Governance/safety	36 %
Misconduct	33 %
Behavioural concerns	29 %
Health problems including substance misuse	24 %
Work environment influences	11 %
Personal circumstances (not ill health)	5 %

The NCAS also did some interesting work looking at 567 doctors who had been excluded or suspended from work. They found that 72 were psychiatrists, versus an expected number of about 35 if proportional to their ratio in the medical workforce. Female doctors were under-represented, with fewer than 52 excluded versus a predicted 132.[1]

Complaints

There appears to be an inexorably rising tide of complaints in medicine. Acquiring skills in complaint investigation and management has now become an essential requirement for all early career psychiatrists.

Dealing with complaints can take a disproportionate amount of time, and can exact a heavy toll in stress on the clinicians concerned, especially when handled in a suboptimal way. The number of complaints in the NHS that were officially recorded grew from 90 081 in 2006–7 to 101 077 in 2009–10. There was an average overall growth rate of 1 % per annum in the number of complaints over the period 1997–2010. Of these, 44 % related to medical staff, 42 % to all aspects of clinical service, and around 9 % related to mental health services including psychiatry.[29]

Ingram and Roy examined all 68 specific complaints made against psychiatrists in a geographical area of England over a 5-year period.[30] This study found that complaints could be classified as follows:

Failure to discuss or inform	29 %
Treatment plan issues	26 %
Discharge or placements	22 %
Attitudes and availability	15 %
Suicide	3 %
Medications	0 %

Litigation

A number of authors have found that psychiatrists are less likely to be sued for malpractice than many other medical specialists.[31–33] However, the amount of litigation continues to increase rapidly (Figures 11.1 and 11.2).

The main causes of litigation include suicide, non-fatal self-harm, diagnostic errors, medication issues and electroconvulsive therapy (ECT). The standard of proof required to succeed in civil litigation is described as follows: 'For these purposes, the evidence produced by the claimant must satisfy the burden of proof which, in a civil case, is the balance of probabilities. Hence, the burden is satisfied and negligence is proved if there is greater than 50 % chance that the claim as argued is correct, i.e. the duty was owed and the breach caused the injury. So the question of law is based on assessing the medical chances of recovery. If, given proper treatment, the claimant's chances of avoiding the current level of injury were anything less than 50 %, he or she will not be awarded any damages at all. There is no right to damages for the loss of the prospect of recovery if the chance of that recovery was less than probable'.[34]

Expert witnesses may give evidence that is flawed. Knoll and Gerbasi[35] provide several examples of this:
• Some errors were made by Dr Liptzin when treating a patient who went on to kill two strangers and wound a police officer. When the patient sued Dr Liptzin for alleged negligent treatment, the lower

court erroneously found against him, but the verdict was overturned on appeal because the 'psychiatrist's alleged negligence was not the proximate cause of the plaintiff's injuries'.

• A patient with diabetes insipidus was admitted with acute psychosis, but unfortunately died because the hospital pharmacy ran out of vasopressin and neither the pharmacy nor the nursing staff notified the psychiatrist of this. An academic neuropsychiatrist who specialized in neuroendocrine disorders gave evidence that the psychiatrist was negligent in failing to sufficiently educate the nursing staff about the importance of not omitting the vasopressin. This was held to be a higher than reasonable standard of care for the psychiatrist concerned.

• A patient presented in some distress and agitation about four months after the death of her father. The psychiatrist noted that the patient 'denied suicidal ideation' but failed to fully consider all the circumstances including some behaviour suggestive of depressive psychosis, and also failed to obtain collateral history from the patient's husband that would have revealed even more worrying behaviour such as being rescued after twice 'walking into heavy traffic' in the past two weeks. Expert witness evidence that it was reasonable practice to assess and document suicide risk in this way was deemed unsatisfactory as it failed to consider the full circumstances.

An interesting approach to controlling the spiralling cost of malpractice litigation is the use of 'no-fault' compensation schemes, such as that introduced in New Zealand in 1972. This avoids the need for costly court

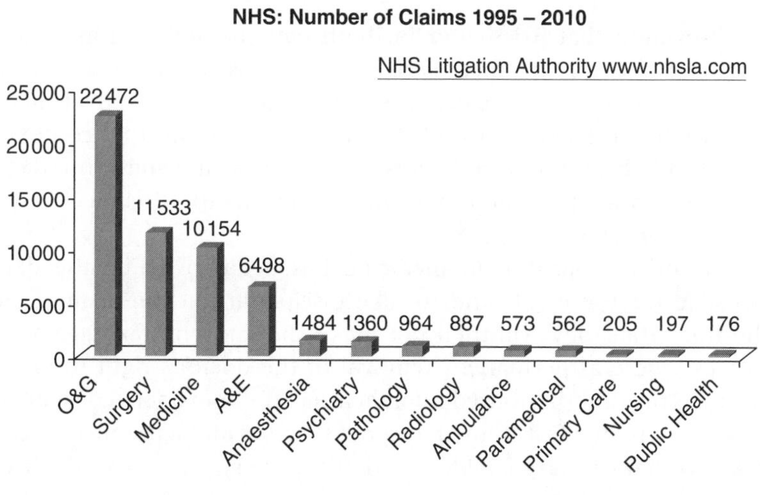

NHS: Number of Claims 1995 – 2010

Figure 11.1 NHS: number of claims 1995–2010. Source: NHS Litigation Authority (www.nhsla.com).

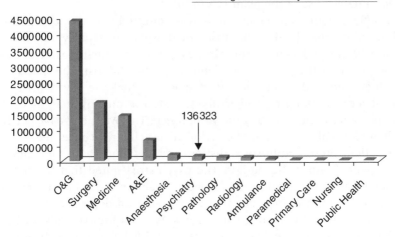

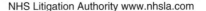

Figure 11.2 NHS: value of claims 1995–2010 (£000). Source: NHS Litigation Authority (www.nhsla.com).

procedures and for the requirement for negligence to be proven while ensuring that injured patients are fairly compensated.

Prevention

It is self-evident that it is better for both patients and doctors to avoid making mistakes in the first place. Yet there is a huge contradiction being played out within medicine everywhere, as we try to deal with the inevitable consequences of human fallibility in the context of medical care. This is the clash between two contrasting and contradictory approaches towards the improvement of the quality of clinical care by reducing error rates.

The historical approach in medicine has been to blame the doctor responsible for the error, and to take disciplinary action against them in the hope that they will then not make the same mistake again. This can be as severe as permanent removal of the doctor's right to practise medicine. This time-honoured approach has the inevitable consequence that doctors are in effect trained to conceal errors and ignorance, because they know that they are fallible and that discovery may mean the loss of their livelihood.

There is a somewhat newer method of reducing and minimizing medical error based on a systems design approach. The essence of this is that errors and mistakes are valued as providing an opportunity to learn from and eventually redesign the system in a way that makes it more difficult for errors to occur. The origins of this systems approach go back a long way within medicine. For example, Semmelweis dramatically reduced rates of perinatal maternal mortality in nineteenth century in Vienna by insisting that medical staff wash their hands thoroughly.[36]

Systems approaches try to design out possibility for error and often use a 'no blame' mechanism for encouraging error reporting. By contrast, personal approaches tend to 'blame' the individual and often use education and disciplinary action to try to reduce error rates. There is strong evidence both from within medicine, such as work from Lucian Leape and David Bates, and from other industries, that a systems-driven approach to error reduction can produce dramatic benefits for patients.[11,14]

The number of deaths caused by road traffic accidents has reduced from 18 per 100 million vehicle miles travelled (VMTs) in 1925, to 1.28 per 100 million VMTs in 2008 – a reduction of well over 90 %.[37,38] This astonishing reduction in deaths really gained pace in the 1960s when Dr William Haddon, a public health physician, became the founding director of the National Highway Safety Bureau, and introduced a systems-based approach to motor vehicle safety. Examples of features introduced as a result of this approach include seat belts, head-rests, shatter-resistant windscreen glass, impact-absorbent steering wheels, air bags, reflective road markings, centre line stripes, improved lighting and guardrails.

Another example from a different setting comes from the airline industry. In 1949 there were 998 deaths among 27 million airline passengers, yet this had reduced to 654 fatalities among 2.3 billion passengers in 2009. This is a 130-fold improvement in safety.[39]

There are several examples within medicine of the success of the same approach. Anaesthesia has dramatically improved its safety record, achieving a near seven-fold reduction in error rates. According to Orkin, 'The first step in reducing surgical anesthesia error rates was the collection of data that permitted a systems analysis of errors, rather than a hunt for "responsible" individuals. Through teamwork, practice guidelines, automation, procedure simplification, and standardization of many functions, anesthesiologists demonstrated that a properly designed system can either prevent mistakes or prevent mistakes from doing harm'.[40] The WHO Surgical Checklist, using a simple list of fewer than 20 questions routinely asked before and after surgery, has reduced surgical mortality by 50 %.[41]

President Clinton established the Quality Interagency Coordination (QuIC) Task Force to report on how to reduce medical errors and improve quality of medical practice. The Task Force[6] highlighted important characteristics of error-reducing industries including:

- Not tolerating high error rates, and setting ambitious targets for error reduction initiatives.
- Developing tracking mechanisms that expose errors.
- Relying on the abundant reports of errors and 'near misses'.
- Thoroughly investigating errors, including a root causes analysis.
- Focusing on systems solutions that do not seek to find individual fault and blame.
- Recognizing that solutions often come from unexpected sources, 'out of the box' thinking, and new combinations of disciplines (e.g. human factors psychology with aeronautical engineering).

The QuIC also focused on obstacles to quality improvement and error reduction including:

- Lack of awareness that a problem exists.
- A traditional medical culture of individual responsibility and blame.
- The lack of protection from legal discovery and liability, which causes errors to be concealed.

Conclusions

In Box 11.1 we report some practical suggestions on how to avoid errors, negligence, misconduct, complaints and litigation in psychiatry. The readers should keep in mind that the clinical approach to the symptoms of a patient with psychiatric problems should always be holistic and not focused narrowly on psychiatric aspects. Psychiatric patients may have associated medical problems; and indeed medical conditions, such as subdural haematoma, encephalitis and AIDS sometimes present with primarily psychiatric symptoms.

Box 11.1 Some practical suggestions

1. Talk to the patient... and listen.
2. Talk to relatives and carers... and listen.
3. Talk to staff... and listen.
4. Write it down.
5. Write down reasons for decisions.
6. Communicate decisions and changes of plan, including to the patient and family where appropriate.
7. After the event – talk to patient, family, carers.
8. Apologize for distress and suffering.
9. Be honest about things that have gone wrong – this does *not* mean that you admit liability.

Medical evaluation, in addition to the psychiatric evaluation, is more than fundamental in order to assess for underlying medical causes. This includes evidence of adequate and appropriate examination accompanied by laboratory and radiological investigations. Proper supervision of junior colleagues and adequate medical/neurological training for psychiatrists-in-training and adequate psychiatric training for medical staff are essential.

The importance of a successful relationship between psychiatrists and patients and their families is an integral part of the Good Psychiatric Practice guidance from the Royal College of Psychiatrists, and cannot be overemphasized.[42] Appropriate record keeping is recognized as an important component of professional standards and of medico-legal evidence. Finally, prompt, honest and sensitive communication with patients, staff, families, and other teams and professionals will in many cases avoid any unnecessary complaints and litigation.

References

1. NCAS (2009). *NCAS Casework: The first eight years*. London: National Clinical Assessment Service.
2. Morrison J, Morrison T. Psychiatrists disciplined by a State Medical Board. *Am J Psychiatry* 2001; **158**: 474–478.
3. Bloom JD, Williams MH, Kofoed L, Rhyne C, Resnick M. The malpractice claims experience of physicians investigated for inappropriate prescribing. *Western J Med* 1989; **151**: 336–338.
4. Kofoed L, Bloom JD, Williams MH, Rhyne C, Resnick M. Physicians investigated for inappropriate prescribing by the Oregon Board of Medical Examiners. *Western J Med* 1989; **150**: 597–601.
5. Firestone M., Sandar SS. *Psychiatry Malpractice, Medical Malpractice Survival Handbook*. Schaumburg, IL: American College of Legal Medicine, 2007.
6. Quality Interagency Coordination Task Force. *Doing what Counts for Patient Safety: Federal Actions to Reduce Medical Errors and their Impact*. Washington DC: Quality Interagency Coordination Task Force (QuIC), 2000.
7. Institute of Medicine. *To Err is Human: Building a Safer Health System*. Washington, DC: National Academy Press, 1999.
8. Leape LL, Brennan TA, Laird N *et al*. The nature of adverse events in hospitalized patients: Results of the Harvard Medical Practice Study II. *New Engl J Med* 1991; **324**: 377–384.
9. Brennan TA, Leape LL, Laird NM. Incidence of adverse events and negligence in hospitalized patients. Results of the Harvard Medical Practice Study I. *New Engl J Med* 1991; **324**: 370–376.
10. Thomas EJ, Studdert DM, Newhouse JP *et al*. Costs of medical injuries in Utah and Colorado. *Inquiry* 1999; **36**: 255–264.
11. Bates DW, Cullen DJ, Laird N *et al*. Incidence of adverse drug events and potential adverse drug events: Implications for prevention. ADE Prevention Study Group. *JAMA* 1995; **274**: 29–34.

12. Donaldson L. *Organisation with a Memory*. London: The Stationery Office, 2000.
13. Leape LL, Bates DW, Cullen DJ *et al.* Systems analysis of adverse drug events. *JAMA* 1995; **274**: 35–43.
14. Millenson ML. *Demanding Medical Excellence*. Chicago: University of Chicago Press, 1997.
15. Leape LL. Error in medicine. *JAMA* 1994; **272**: 1851–1857.
16. Stone A. The forensic psychiatrist as expert witness in malpractice cases. *J Am Acad Psychiatry Law* 1999; **27**: 451–461.
17. Jacobi J, Fraser GL, Coursin DB *et al.* Clinical practice guidelines for the sustained use of sedatives and analgesics in the critically ill adult. *Crit Care Med* 2002; **30**: 119–141.
18. Shapiro BA, Warren J, Egol AB *et al.* Practice parameters for intravenous analgesia and sedation for adult patients in the intensive care unit: an executive summary. Society of Critical Care Medicine. *Crit Care Med* 1995; **23**: 1596–1600.
19. *British National Formulary* 61. BMJ Group and Pharmaceutical Press, 2011 (http://bnf.org/bnf/).
20. *Bolam v. Friern Hospital Management Committee* [1957] 1 WLR 583.
21. *Hedley Byrne & Co. Ltd. v. Heller & Partners Ltd.* [1964] AC 465.
22. *Barnett v. Chelsea & Kensington Hospital* [1968] 1 All ER 1068.
23. *Sidaway v. Bethlem Royal Hospital Governors* [1985] AC 871.
24. *Bolitho v. City and Hackney Health Authority* [1997] 4 All ER 771.
25. *Fv.R* (1983) 33 SASR 189.
26. *The Mental Capacity Act 2005*. London: The Stationery Office, 2005.
27. *Tarasoff v. Regents of the University of California* (1976)17Cal. 3d 425, 529P. 2d 334, 131Cal. Rptr. 14, 551P. 2d 334.
28. Dondershine HE, Cozzolino A, Greene JM, Novak B. Psychiatric malpractice: basic issues in evolving contexts. *Psychiatr Times* 2007; **24**: 5.
29. The Health and Social Care Information Centre. *Data on Written Complaints in the NHS 2009-10*. London: Health and Social Care Information Centre, 2010.
30. Ingram K, Roy L. Complaints against psychiatrists: a five year study. *Psychiatr Bull* 1995; **19**: 620–622.
31. Slawson PF, Guggenheim FG. Psychiatric malpractice: a review of the national loss experience. *Am J Psychiatry* 1984; **141**: 979–981.
32. Schwartz WB, Mendelson DN. Physicians who have lost their malpractice insurance. *JAMA* 1989; **262**: 1335–1341.
33. Taragin MI, Sonnenberg FA, Karns E *et al.* Does physician performance explain interspecialty differences in malpractice claim rates? *Med Care* 1994; **7**: 661–667.
34. Wikipedia. Bolam v Friern Hospital Management Committee. Wikimedia Foundation, 2011; http://en.wikipedia.org/wiki/Bolam_v_Friern_Hospital_Management_Committee [accessed 17 May 2011].
35. Knoll J, Gerbasi J. *J Am Acad Psychiatry Law* 2006; **34**: 215–223.
36. Wikipedia. Ignaz Semmelweis. Wikimedia Foundation, 2011; http://en.wikipedia.org/wiki/Ignaz_Semmelweis [accessed 17 May 2011].

37. MMWR. Achievements in Public Health, 1900–1999 Motor-Vehicle Safety: A 20th Century Public Health Achievement, *MMWR Weekly* 1999; **48**: 369–374.

38. Peters M. U.S. Secretary of Transportation Mary E. Peters announces new data showing record low highway fatalities; Americans safer than ever on the nation's roads, rails, and in the skies (http://web.docuticker.com/go/docubase/27795), 2008 [accessed 17 May 2011).

39. Graham N. Director, Air Navigation Bureau, International Civil Aviation Organization, video message, 2010.

40. Orkin FW. Patient monitoring during anesthesia as an exercise in technology assessment. In: Saidman LJ, Smith NT (eds) *Monitoring in Anesthesia*, 3rd edn. London: Butterworth-Heinemann, 1993; pp. 439–455.

41. Haynes AB, Weiser TG, Berry WR *et al*. A surgical safety checklist to reduce morbidity and mortality in a global population. *New Engl J Med* 2009; **360**: 491–499.

42. Royal College of Psychiatrists. *Good Psychiatric Practice*. London: Royal College of Psychiatrists, 2009.

CHAPTER 12

New ways of working: innovative cross-sector care in a competitive mental health environment

Kai C. Treichel[1,2] and Magdalena Peckskamp[3]
[1]Management Department, Medical Center Friedrichshain, Berlin, Germany
[2]Psychiatric Initiative Berlin-Brandenburg, Germany
[3]Department of Psychology, University of Vienna, Austria

Introduction

Hospital settings have long been the main location for treatment of psychiatric patients, and in many countries they are still the main workplace for psychiatrists. However, treatment of psychiatric patients in outpatient settings is constantly expanding due to political, clinical and economic reasons. Cross-sector psychiatric healthcare provision is delivered in different organizational forms.

One form is represented by community mental health services, which include a variety of healthcare providers such as nurses, social workers, physicians and other aiding healthcare professionals, and which are based in a community centre, sometimes attached to a hospital site.

Those teams are usually clinically led by consultant psychiatrists (i.e. senior psychiatrists with long experience in the treatment of psychiatric patients). These services are mostly present in countries where healthcare is funded by government agencies through taxes, the largest being the National Health Service (NHS) in England.

Another organizational form is (private) psychiatric outpatient care, provided by psychiatrists who run their own practices. This is mainly the case in countries where outpatient care is funded by healthcare insurance companies. In these care models the organizational structure is rather

How to Succeed in Psychiatry: A Guide to Training and Practice, First Edition.
Edited by Andrea Fiorillo, Iris Tatjana Calliess and Henning Sass.
© 2012 John Wiley & Sons, Ltd. Published 2012 by John Wiley & Sons, Ltd.

loose (i.e. psychiatrists see the patients in their practice, other services such as nursing or social workers may provide care but are usually not structurally linked into the process). Treatment pathways hardly exist and doctors work under their own management without any business structures in place.

In recent years another option – so-called *integrated healthcare provision* or *managed care* – has become an increasingly attractive way of providing care for psychiatric patients of various ICD diagnoses, from anxiety disorders to schizophrenia. Studies show that integrated, multidisciplinary, cross-sector healthcare provision including home treatment options can provide better clinical care and reduce costs through a lower probability of an exacerbation of psychiatric illness, i.e. reduced hospital admissions, reduced lengths of stay per admission and lower costs per unit of service.[1]

History of change

The shift from inpatient hospital treatment towards the outpatient public or private sector is mainly driven by political, economic and legislative changes. It is happening at different velocities and thus in some countries it is more visible than in others.

Historically, in countries such as the UK and Germany the ground for these changes and the opportunity for doctors in outpatient settings was set by legislative reforms – in the Mental Health Act in 1975 in Germany, and in 1983 in the UK. The reform demanded a radical change of paradigm in the treatment of psychiatric patients, stating that the hospital was to be a place for treatment only, not for keeping or custody of psychiatric patients.[2] As a result, the existing large asylums and hospital facilities were closed, smaller units or departments of psychiatry were established in or attached to general hospitals, and outpatient treatment facilities were established on a larger scale in the communities. Funding also shifted significantly into the outpatient sector. Most of this change demanded by the new laws was motivated politically and followed a controversial debate about the introduction of a so-called psychosocial model. This model claimed that environmental, educational and social factors were equally responsible for psychiatric disorders as were biological factors. Consequently, this view demanded a whole range of new treatment options. As a result, complementary services, such as supported community housing, sociotherapy or home treatment nursing, were first introduced in the 1970s and 1980s. Still the main driver of these developments was political will and a resulting shift in the funding of mental healthcare.

From the 1990s, change was mainly driven for economic reasons. By then, scientific data were available showing that inpatient treatment was disproportionately contributing to the direct healthcare costs of a patient. Expenditures by treatment and rehabilitation form an important part of psychiatric healthcare expenditures all over the world. Direct healthcare costs are calculated by multiplying the number of cases by medical care costs, i.e. the utilization of health service. Berto *et al.*[3] reviewed the costs of illness for depression in the USA, UK and Italy and found that the most important contributor to direct costs was hospitalization.

There are also data suggesting that outpatient treatment, if managed by a collaboration or network of psychiatrists and other healthcare professionals, including complementary services, could be far more cost effective and improve the quality of care for psychiatric patients at the same time.[1]

Psychiatric healthcare provision is still undergoing massive changes regarding funding, governance and the way doctors work. This is mainly due to a Europe-wide trend that government funding is decreasing, or at least stagnating, as budgets become tighter, not only since the recent global financial crisis. It can be expected that this trend will gain pace, in the future.

The system-wide reform agendas require organizations and psychiatrists to adopt new service delivery models if they are to succeed in the new market environment. In this situation, psychiatrists or mental health professionals who run medical centres have a significant need for management expertise in order to develop a strategy for their role within the changing healthcare environment. They must also develop a feasible strategy to reduce risk and to explore the opportunities of the change. In contrast to large hospital trusts, they do not normally have legal and business expertise in-house. This affects the way all providers and psychiatrists work together, the processes and the way the care is perceived.

Dehospitalization

The above developments explain why funding authorities – either governments or private health insurers – have a strong interest in reducing costs. Hence, the incentives increasingly favour outpatient treatment. This presents an opportunity for psychiatrists to participate in and benefit from this change of paradigm.

Most of the problems related to a mental disorder are not tackled by short-term inpatient treatment. Also, it is insufficient to treat chronic psychiatric disorders such as schizophrenia or bipolar disorder with only a medical approach. More and more it is understood that there needs to be a whole 'package' of interventions and treatments – inpatient, outpatient, medical, social and complementary. These interventions have to include not only the patients, but also their environment, such as families and the workplace. This psycho-social approach is improving results and reducing the (economic) burden of mental illnesses, and there is evidence that it will become increasingly important. However, in many countries there is currently no such system in place.

Healthcare insurers and government funding agencies want psychiatrists to facilitate stronger ties and more cooperation with other professions and complementary services that provide care to psychiatric patients. In a significant number of countries, these groups of service providers were or still are tending to work separately. Psychiatrists have to be aware of these developments and recognize the consequences of systemic change and current legislation. As quality aspects, process analysis and management skills grow in significance, it is important for psychiatrists to make decisions about the way they work, either independently or as part of a larger network. Thus, there is a need to take steps towards a more professional service model approach, whether psychiatric care is provided on a for-profit or non-profit basis.

It is crucial to develop new ways of working, to establish good clinical standards of patient care and a sound financial model in order to create value for patients, professionals and (if for-profit) for stakeholders. This can be delivered by a structured cooperative network of providers in outpatient psychiatric care or in the form of larger units, as ambulatory medical centres.

These changes may pose a threat especially to inpatient structures, as they might be forced to cut down on the length of stay of an admission or on the admission rate. This may lead to a reduction of beds and also a reduction in the number of psychiatrists working in hospitals. But these changes also bring new opportunities for psychiatrists.

From an economic point of view, large medical centres can help to improve entrepreneurship amongst doctors, and also allow junior psychiatrists to work in the ambulatory sector without carrying the financial risk that normally is included in running a private practice. Multidisciplinary and cross-sector cooperations are economically incentivized.

Managed care and integrated care provision

While federal initiatives were important forces in the healthcare industry, the major impetus to shift the focus from inpatient to outpatient care was actually the competition that occurred in the private sector, especially among the health insurance companies. They were the main driver to incentivize private and public sector initiatives that would deliver mental healthcare in an organized fashion, avoiding or reducing hospital admission, using clinical pathways, i.e. standardized clinical procedures, and shared documentation in order to manage the financial risk associated with the care of psychiatric patients. These programmes were started in the USA under the term *managed care* and are also being introduced in Europe as *integrated care provision*.

Managed care aims to reduce mental healthcare costs by using economic and quality incentives for psychiatrists, service providers and patients to choose an economically efficient form of care. This includes a variety of mechanisms, such as reducing inpatient hospital admission and minimizing lengths of stay, as well as implementing cost-sharing incentives for outpatient treatment. High-maintenance cases are managed through a quality control panel.

Contracts for the integrated provision of care are individual cross-sector contracts between a health insurance company and outpatient healthcare providers. The aim is to stimulate cooperation between traditionally separate sectors and to incentivize the use of medical pathways. These services are reimbursed additionally to the regular budget and thus mean potentially a new revenue stream for doctors.

Integrated or managed care may be provided in a variety of settings, such as health maintenance organizations (HMOs, mainly in the USA and Switzerland), large medical centres or integrated networks of psychiatric service providers. Contracting is mostly elective for insurers, providers and patients, which allows each party to opt out of the contract if not satisfied with the results.

Management of integrated care programmes

Historically, psychiatrists working in outpatient practices were guaranteed considerable autonomy in the way they carried out their work and related to colleagues and patients. Scientific evidence suggests that professional firms, such as medical practices and mental health service providers, traditionally have a very different code of working compared with other business environments. This is partly due to the professional peer ethos, but also the intrinsic conviction of many mental health professionals that they are not working within a business environment, but rather are providing a social service. This has been reinforced by the considerable suspicion traditionally shown towards managerial techniques of control.[4] The downside of this is that management expertise is often poor, with decisions being delayed, financial management being suboptimal and strategic opportunities being missed.

A change has come in response to the problems of managing greater size and complexity, and under pressure from health insurance companies. The old model, where a single psychiatrist was diagnosing the patient and chose treatments with no or minimal communication and interaction with other professionals, with no pathways in place, and no systematic control of clinical effectiveness and economic efficiency is not appropriate for the management of larger psychiatric networks or centers.

Evidence suggests that the introduction and implementation of professional management could not only help to improve operations, reduce costs and identify new opportunities, but also that it is fundamentally necessary as a *sine qua non* to achieve optimal results.[4]

In managing new integrated care or managed care contracts, psychiatric healthcare providers are faced with a higher level of morbidity risk, being paid by capitation or even as a global budget. This causes substantial uncertainty regarding future costs. Thus, financial and strategic planning of an integrated psychiatric healthcare delivery network needs to be more proactive in order to act systematically. A principal goal is to reduce the probability of financial loss and to remain successful in a competitive environment. Providers who focus exclusively on service delivery and good quality of services could face financial loss and ultimately extinction from the market. This is why it requires a professional management concept or, better, a management company that is capable of carrying out a thorough risk analysis and undertaking sound financial management in the framework of managed care contracts in the field of outpatient mental health.

The above does not mean that for-profit psychiatric service providers who operate managed care schemes can simply stint on service quality in order to gain financial stability, or even to generate profits. These negative developments have partly been seen in some instances in the USA, where psychiatric service providers have reduced costs through downsizing their workforce, or by minimizing contacts with the 'expensive' healthcare professionals, such as specialist psychiatrists or psychologists. Some critics have thus argued that managed care contracts with health insurance companies generally incentivize psychiatric health providers to reduce the quality of care in order to remain profitable.[5]

However, from both a customer (patient)-orientated and a management perspective, exactly the opposite can be argued: reducing the quality of care would be short-sighted as it would only pay in the short term, immediately after such measures were implemented. Ultimately, deterioration in the quality of care would not go undetected by patients, their families or carers. There is a risk that a substantial number of patients would opt out of such poorly managed contracts, and hence it is foreseeable that the financial damage of such strategy would be greater than any savings that the low-budget service had initially generated. A good and successful psychiatric service provider will therefore be anxious to meet both demands in order to remain competitive in the market: to implement professional management structures that ensure financial stability and to ensure long-term quality of care.

Good management also needs to negotiate contracts with manageable risks by implementing rigorous quality controls on all service providers party to the contract.

Service quality, customer processes and patient relationships

Client/patient-facing processes play an important part in larger psychiatric service operations. They are significant for contracts awarded by healthcare insurance companies to privately managed care organizations or networks of providers delivering outpatient care. Therefore, it is worth taking a closer look at these client processes.

Client/patient-facing processes have a significant influence on client behaviour and treatment progress. Perception of and interaction with psychiatrists or with the service can influence the outcome (success) of treatment and thus should be given strong emphasis. The perception of the service is crucial for any evaluation by patients. Unexpected waiting time due to overbooking, as happens often in psychiatric services, may have a negative impact and thus should be avoided in any new delivery structure. Involuntary waiting time potentially affects all patient-facing services, but can cause more problems in psychiatric patients due to the nature of their disorders.[6]

Circumstances very much influence the subjective view and thus have an important impact on how the patient feels and judges. In the specific case of mental health services, one can expect that many patients suffer from anxieties or are vulnerable. Some might have the expectation to be seen ad hoc. It is therefore a very demanding and responsible job for staff to act with empathy, but still keep control. In order to achieve this, training and support for staff is crucial. Feelings of boredom, injustice, stress, loneliness, uncertainty or anxiety can disturb the patients' relationship to service providers, and as a consquence may lead to poorer outcome of care and higher costs. Thus, it would be advisable for the service provider to offer a friendly, calm, reliable, respectful and supporting service besides maintaining a good professional standard.

Generally, improving service quality means improving patient satisfaction within the competitive environment of outpatient mental health services in times of choice and increased patient/client expectations. Because psychiatric patients often present with significant deterioration due to symptoms such as thought disturbances or hallucinations, they are traditionally not regarded as customers. But they have families and carers who often have very clear customer expectations towards the services.

Unfortunately, many medical practitioners still seem to have an attitude that their self-perceived service quality is good enough and that the patient will also acknowledge this. Research suggests that service-led and patient-facing organizations must be able to listen to the patient, to ask for his/her opinion via surveys and structured process mapping, and be prepared to change their service and processes according to the critique of the patients.

A negative service experience for customers not only forces existing customers to migrate to competitors, but also – due to the effect of negative word of mouth – results in fruitless efforts of the organization to attract new customers. Market research has shown that unsatisfied customers communicate their experience three or four times more often than satisfied customers.[7] Thus, for managed care organizations or integrated care contractors it can be essential to understand the patients' expectations in order to remain competitive, as patients can always opt out of the contract.

Improvement of the operations should be part of the quality management of any psychiatric healthcare provider independently of whether the services are run on a profit or non-profit model. Specifically, it is important to regularly ask patients directly about their perceptions and wishes.

It is important to train frontline staff in communication and client respect, but this needs to be embedded into a general corporate culture that not only respects but also values and empowers customers. Thus, it is important that this information is shared by the management with the employees in order to make sure that every single member of the company understands the clients' expectations. Here there is room for improvement. It is recommended that all professionals involved in the managed care process could receive communication training that includes both direct contacts and telephone and internet communication with patients and other clients.

Economic and financial management of integrated care contracts

As shown above, high-quality programmes for the provision of outpatient care for psychiatric patients pose a potential financial risk to providers within integrated care contracts. Risk can arise from different factors within managed care programmes. An initial risk is the changed form of payment, from direct payments for procedures to the payment of a lump sum or a capitation. The latter also implies a shift of the morbidity risk of the patients from the insurance company towards the service providers. Managed care contracts have therefore an increased need for administration and management systems that facilitate coordination and control of interdisciplinary and intersectoral clinical procedures.

The establishment of these structures also poses a risk to new entrants, as psychiatrists and other mental healthcare professionals usually lack the experience in operating management structures and negotiating contracts. This applies especially to contracts where budget responsibility is fully or partly handed over from the insurance company to the psychiatric care provider through prospective per capita payments (capitation). The transfer of medical and economic responsibility confronts the healthcare providers with an entrepreneurial risk that is a challenge to be dealt with. The real costs caused by patients may not equal the negotiated budget (set by the sum of the capitations). If expenses exceed the budgeted income the provider may face bankruptcy. However, if costs can be kept under the negotiated capitation budget while maintaining a good standard of service to the patient (i.e. by reducing relapses that cause hospital admission) the gain can be shared between the psychiatric service providers and the contracting insurance company according to a negotiable ratio. In order to minimize financial risk, control becomes essential and it is strategically important to implement (contractually binding) professional management.

Implementation of professional management

Healthcare providers often do not implement professional structures compared to other businesses. The aim of integrated provision networks for mental health is to provide integrated managed care to a certain population of mental health patients. These networks have to form interdisciplinary and contract-binding collaborations. They promise some major advantages for insurers and patients, compared with the traditionally highly segmented care models. Successful managed care and integrated provision networks offer: (i) regional clusters of linked multidisciplinary providers through assignment concepts; (ii) implementation of cross-sector elements of care; (iii) improvement of patient bonds and services; (iv) interdisciplinary communication and control via shared IT; (v) improved economic efficiency; (vi) gathering of treatment data and health service research.

Members of the networks can be independent psychiatric practices, psychologists, providers of socio-therapy, home treatment teams, nursing homes and potentially any complementary service that provides treatment of mental disorders. Clinical leadership by psychiatrists is advisable, although some health insurers and non-medical professionals are questioning the traditional leadership of psychiatrists in the treatment of psychiatric patients.

The goals of successful operations in the provision of integrated mental healthcare under psychiatric leadership are the improvement of quality and efficiency of care while having a competitive advantage. One main goal is therefore the development of sustainable structures and procedures by guaranteeing reliable access to the expertise of cooperating partners and mental health professionals within the network, if possible across the sectors. This will enhance the spectrum of procedures offered to the patient and will also increase the perceived quality of care and improve patient satisfaction.

In order to achieve these goals, successful providers of outpatient managed care will need to professionalize both internally and externally. This includes strategic planning of the service model towards the competitive market, especially regarding the negotiation of contracts with healthcare insurance companies.

Management of innovations and processes includes the definition and implementation of standards and procedures (clinical pathways) and cross-sector models for care delivery. Management will have to be able to coordinate human resources and exercise sound financial control, especially when capitation or quality- and efficiency-based reimbursement systems are negotiated. It should retain the capacity to integrate new financial and economic models (e.g. public-private partnerships, investors, etc.) while maintaining leadership over the enterprise.

Last, but not least, it is also advisable to integrate functioning quality management and scientific research projects that monitor the outcome of provided care.

Many health insurance companies only enter into contracts with providers that have a professional management team in place. Contracts are usually negotiated between the leadership of the managed care network and high-ranking officers of insurance companies. For legal and liability reasons, it is advisable for providers who seek to negotiate an integrated or managed care contract to establish a management company in the form of a limited company or a similar legal form, and to implement professional management structures that can manage for-profit companies. In this way the liability and financial risk of the individual service provider to the programme is reduced.

Possible areas of action for a management company of a managed care network include the following:

- Design and delivery of innovative service concepts.
- Development and facilitation of cooperative and joint ventures.

- Purchase management.
- Implementation of an internet technology communication platform for service providers and users.
- Control of service delivery.
- Quality management.
- Financial management of contracts with insuring companies/funding authorities.
- Data management.

Information technology (IT) infrastructure: optimizing transfer of information

Internet technology (IT) plays an increasingly important role in achieving successful positioning of psychiatric care in the changing healthcare environment. Psychiatric practices have often been backward when it comes to implementing technological innovations. This is partly due to the nature of the field, where traditionally diagnosis does not primarily rely on technological devices but is performed through direct patient contact, exploration, psychiatric interviews and questionnaires. Even so, in hospital settings it has become more common to install IT systems that gather the results of most procedures and tests within an electronic patient file.

However, outpatient care providers have been rather reluctant to implement such systems. In particular, electronic patient files in psychiatric practices are often used reluctantly and with limited functionality. It is very rare that other service providers such as hospitals, nursing companies, other psychiatrists or funding organizations can access digital information about a patient. The main reason for this is not a technological gap, but the fear that patient confidentiality could be breached.

The management of psychiatric health services within the integrated healthcare delivery system has to be capable to monitor quality and quantity of services provided, to control financial budgets and provide information to ensure the compliance of psychiatric care providers with negotiated contract arrangements. A means of ensuring both quality and financial control is a netwide IT infrastructure that is designed to link all service providers and simultaneously allow the net or central management to access real-time information. Through this tool, analysis of the care delivered and control of the costs incurred by psychiatrists and other healthcare providers can be monitored. In the management of full-budget capitation contracts especially, it is vital that the IT infrastructure also includes any cooperating inpatient facilities. Only if the duration and costs of (expensive) inpatient treatments are checked closely can outpatient service management estimate whether they will meet their negotiated target budget.

Voluntary inscription and data protection

In community mental health services, patients depend on the care offered by a mental health trust in their catchment area, with only limited choices. With for-profit integrated managed care, programmes involving an outpatient psychiatric service provider and health insurance companies rely on the voluntary and active subsription of psychiatric patients into the contract. Because of their voluntary participation, patients need to actively agree to the monitoring, analysis and exchange of their clinical data. In order to avoid (legal) conflicts, service providers should ensure explicit transparency and open communication about clinical data records. In this respect, a private contract gives more rights to psychiatric patients, who normally have only limited access to their inpatient treatment files. Initially this can be seen as an additional administrative burden for the management of integrated care organizations, but it is also an opportunity for those providers to explain the advantages of an integrated care model to the patients. The greater transparency of the structured care and cooperation provided by the aligned professionals can motivate ambivalent patients to subscribe to the integrated care programmes available in their region.

Innovation management in future psychiatric outpatient care models

Entrepreneurs in changing economic environments and emerging markets routinely face more challenges then in mature markets. Thus alliances are important to establish a new model of service delivery. Networking strategies should include collaboration with competitors.[8] Core competencies that providers of integrated care models should develop are competitor differentiation, customer value and extendibility of the business model.

New entrants and entrepreneurs have to adopt to constant change in the current healthcare market. The traditional form of delivering mental healthcare is eroding and new models are facing increased competition and financial risk. In this environment creating tangible delivery structures will be essential but it remains important to accept asymmetries and competing visions. This is a challenge for the leadership qualities of psychiatrists as entrepreneurs. Within the network of contracted providers of a mental health programme it is helpful if the participants share the same culture, i.e. to build and stimulate an interdisciplinary corporate identity where the continuous changes that are inevitable are seen as stimulating challenges rather than threats. The demand for psychosocial treatment in outpatient settings is on the rise. This is because hospitals face the dilemma that even if they identify this demand, their cost-ridden structures and processes cannot integrate these lengthy processes

efficiently and effectively. That is why they increasingly rely on cooperation with medical and non-medical providers of outpatient care plans.

Outpatient psychiatric competence centres, which bring together
different professions and multidisciplinary teams, including professional
management, clearly have a competitive advantage as partners of health
insurance funds. Integrated provision of care is currently only starting
to be established. Traditional boundaries and rivalries must be overcome
in a cooperative manner that leaves both sides feeling they are part
of a win-win situation. Here, clearly, there is still a lot of room for
improvement, and leadership of management is essential to build trust
between the sectors.

Increasingly, investment capital can be generated for innovative
partnerships in the healthcare market. Investors range from hospitals to
insurance companies to business angels and pharmaceutical companies.
However, investors are nowadays more selective. If the for-profit
providers of integrated managed care in mental health are seeking to
raise venture capital they have to be well-researched, offer innovative
propositions with some capital already in place, have the potential to
take a leading position in their local healthcare market, and have an
experienced clinical and management team. Ideally, they should also
have innovative concepts, a reliable and sophisticated IT infrastructure,
and partners who have started successful businesses before – to provide
contracts, commercial knowledge and high standards of corporate governance. It is the current transition period in this market environment,
with power shifting away from traditional incumbents (doctors) towards
new entrants in the outpatient treatment market (healthcare insurers,
hospitals), that makes a proactive strategy so important.

An outlook for early career psychiatrists

Psychiatrists with the desire to lead and make a positive impact on managed outpatient psychiatric healthcare must consider leaving the 'front
line' of clinical psychiatry and consider an alternative way forward. There
are many options, from working as a consultant developing innovative
changes in psychiatric healthcare strategy, to working in management
firms that provide healthcare in outpatient settings or organize patient
flow and treatment operating as a link between the hospitals and the
ambulatory sector. This may involve playing a part in the restructuring of
entire health authorities.

Within Europe and globally, there are insufficient numbers of psychiatrists in these positions, while the demand for these services is growing.
Especially in developed countries, the downsizing of hospital capacity is
not necessarily a threat to future psychiatrists, but rather an opportunity

to make a significant impact on the development of new ways of treating patients in psychiatry.

As regards training in psychiatry, economic understanding and leadership skills should form part of postgraduate psychiatric training curricula. Training schemes should include basic knowledge of the evaluation of key economic data and practical experience in the management of projects and teams as well as the management of quality and processes.

Tasks for more experienced and senior psychiatrists within the management of an outpatient centre or a managed care network involve leadership, and the acquisition and management of projects and contracts, including clinical and financial analysis as well as liaison with partners. Psychiatrists seeking a leadership role in this domain will need to provide evidence of the following key skills and attributes:

- ability to work in a team;
- interpersonal and communication skills;
- problem-solving attitude;
- analytical skills;
- sound economic and financial knowledge;
- flexibility;
- adaptation to fast-changing market environments;
- drive for innovation;
- ability to cope with imperfect markets and resulting challenges.

There are tendencies to grant contracts to providers who mainly work with employed non-medical staff and only give medical psychiatric treatment in times of crisis, one of the reasons being that it is cost-saving. Whether it is cost-effective in the long run must be doubted, apart from concerns that patients do not receive the care of the health professionals with the longest training.

Conclusions

Implementation of new ways of working in large managed care networks and outpatient medical care enters offer a wide range of new roles and tasks for future psychiatrists. In the future it will however be a challenge for the psychiatric profession to maintain its clinical leadership role in outpatient managed care models. This will require mutlidisiciplinary and crossector cooperations as well as additional skills for the management of patients, processes and budgets. In order to prepare early career psychiatrists to be succesfull in their field, training in psychiatry has to provide the opportunity to develop management skills and interdisciplinary competencies additional to sound specialist psychiatric knowledge.

References

1. Goldman W, McCulloch J, Sturm R. Costs and use of mental health services before and after managed care. *Health Affairs* 1998; **17**: 40–52.
2. Department of Health. *Mental Health Act 1983*. London: Department of Health, 1983.
3. Berto P, D'Ilario D, Ruffo P *et al.* Depression: cost of illness studies in the international literature: a review. *J Ment Health Policy* 2000; **3**: 3–10.
4. Maister DH. *Managing the Professional Service Firm.* New York: Simon & Schuster, 1993.
5. Daniels N, Sabin J. The ethics of accountability in managed care reform. *Health Affairs* 1998; **17**: 50–64.
6. Van Dijk NM. Why queuing never vanishes. *Eur J Oper Res* 1997; **99**: 463–476.
7. Mitchell M, Tseng MQ, Chuan-Jun S. Mapping customers' service experience for operations improvement. *Bus Process Manag J* 1999; **5**: 50–64.
8. Hamel G, Doz YL, Prahalad CK. Collaborate with your competitors – and win. *Harvard Bus Rev* 1989; **67**: 133–139.

CHAPTER 13

Choosing a career in psychiatry and setting priorities

Joshua Blum[1] and Andrea Fiorillo[2]
[1]Department of Psychiatry, University of Massachusetts Medical School, Worcester, MA, USA
[2]Department of Psychiatry, University of Naples SUN, Naples, Italy

Introduction

The process of figuring out how best to spend one's own life is not an easy task. Part of the reason why it is hard is that it requires first to have at least some idea of who you are, and that's hard enough. It also requires having some idea of what you want out of life. And that means *you*. Not your friends, not your parents, not your significant other, not your children. They may all want things for you, but in the end, it is up to you to determine if what they want allies with what you envision for yourself. And frankly, most people have a hard enough time telling you what they want for dinner, let alone what they want out of life.

Professor Norman Sartorius, during his courses on leadership skills for young psychiatrists, provides lectures and materials on 'How to decide on priorities'. It is always difficult to set priorities, in particular when priorities for different areas of your life do not coincide. At different stages of life, we have to choose between our family, our professional career or our own life. And this is hard for everyone. Even within each of these domains, there are some choices to be made. For example, if you decide to dedicate your life to medicine, then the choice can be between public health, research, clinical activities or academic life. So, how can someone select the appropriate priority when he/she does not have the relevant basic knowledge to choose? In this chapter, we will provide some suggestions on how to choose a career in psychiatry and how to

How to Succeed in Psychiatry: A Guide to Training and Practice, First Edition.
Edited by Andrea Fiorillo, Iris Tatjana Calliess and Henning Sass.
© 2012 John Wiley & Sons, Ltd. Published 2012 by John Wiley & Sons, Ltd.

set priorities, reporting – at the end of the chapter – on the importance of leisure activities in order to prevent work stress and burnout. The role of exercise will be emphasized, but it can be considered an example of any other hobby or leisure activity.

Choosing medicine

One of the most difficult decisions is already behind you – deciding to go into medicine. Many of you reading this may have gone a step further and narrowed your career focus to the specialty of psychiatry. Congratulations on making it this far! It is easy in the midst of your day-to-day activities to forget what attracted you to your choice of specialties to begin with.

Although you may spend your days hearing about the stories of others, this is the time to concentrate on your own story. So often in medicine, we forget to look after ourselves, and although it may have become a cliché to view doctors as making bad patients and being the last to take care of themselves, clichés sometimes have a bit of truth to them. Let's begin.

Personal assessment

In order to get pleasure out of your career, it is important to have a good idea of who you are. We often don't put in the time or effort to do it properly, and as a result, we may feel unsatisfied with the results. There is more to a job than a paycheck, but it may not be within many people's reality to ask for more.[1]

This first step is the most important, because it is where you define what you want. If you don't know what you want, how can you know when you have achieved it? Those of you who have done cognitive behavioural therapy with patients will recognize this process.

Box 13.1 contains a list of questions to consider in order to better define goals. We will first consider work, then non-work activities. In order to best encapsulate your reasoning, try to distill your answer down to the bare minimum (e.g. if your answer to the question 'Why medicine?' is that you like the ability to move around geographically and still be able to find a job, ask yourself which adjective would best fit that aspect – independence? autonomy?).

Note: Self-honesty is particularly important here, even if it isn't what others around you may want. Have the courage to put down what you really think, without worrying about what other people might think or say.

When answering questions 3–6, keep in mind the following qualifiers, some of which are paraphrased from the article, 'How to love your job' by Andrew Harrison.[1]

- Do you want to be a solo practitioner?
- Would you rather be part of a group practice?

- What type of patient demographic do you want to see? Think ethnicity, race, socioeconomic status, age...This is not a time to exercise self-judgment. Be honest! It is OK to like what you like.
- Along these lines, is there a specific population that you would like to treat? While it may not be necessary to seek out additional training, there may be subspecialty programmes you may be interested in that are available depending on your location, e.g. child and adolescent psychiatry, transitional age youth, geriatrics, consultation-liaison work, addictions, pain medicine, sleep medicine, forensics, and neuropsychiatry.
- Do you want to see lots of patients in short bursts? Less patients in more depth for longer?
- Do you gravitate towards inpatient, partial hospitalization or outpatient settings? What do you like or dislike about each?
- Do you want to have a practice that includes therapy, medication management or both?
- Do you like consultation on medical floors or outpatient medical offices?
- How much direct medical care do you want to provide? Research, writing, teaching, and administration are options that do not directly involve patient care.
- Do you want to incorporate research in your career?
- Do you want an academic setting with built-in teaching of medical students and residents?

Box 13.1 Internal Assessment Questionnaire – work life

1. Why medicine?

2. Why psychiatry?

3. Which parts of psychiatry do you like best?

4. Which parts of psychiatry do you dislike most?

(Continued)

Box 13.1 (Continued)

5. Which parts of psychiatry are most meaningful to you?

6. If you could pick and choose the most enjoyable and/or most meaningful parts of psychiatry to make the ideal career, what would you include?

7. What would you exclude?

8. What do you want to accomplish in your career?

9. From time to time, it pays to step out of the ivory tower and reality test. Does your vision of the ideal career allow you to accomplish these goals?

10. Reality testing: being mindful that there are no ideal careers, it's helpful to consider what parts of your 'dislike' list you would tolerate and which are absolute 'no-nos':

Setting priorities in psychiatry

Psychiatry is a medical discipline with very different and complex domains. One can decide to work in clinical psychiatry, social psychiatry, biological psychiatry or forensic psychiatry. One can decide to work as a clinician, as a researcher or as an academic. It is possible to work with children (child and adolescent psychiatry), with the elderly people (geriatric psychiatry), with adolescents (early intervention in psychiatry), in collaboration with other medical specialties (consultation and liaison psychiatry), in jails or with detained patients (forensic psychiatry), and so on. There may be different priorities for doctors working in private settings, in hospital wards or in community services (for this, we suggest you go to the relevant chapters of this book). It would probably be impossible to set a rule of priorities in this sense (and also beyond the scope of this chapter), although very interesting.

It is essential, however, that early career psychiatrists decide as soon as possible what kind of career they want. Curricular needs may be different if for example, you want to work in an academic institution or in a community service. For the former, publications in peer-reviewed and high-impact journals are strongly needed; also, it is important to attend national and international conferences, to develop teaching and presentation skills, and to read the existing literature in your field of interest. Yes, choose your field of interest: the sooner the better. The complex structure of the mind is reflected by the complex structure of psychiatry – a branch of medicine that spans neuroscience, public health, social medicine, internal medicine, psychoanalysis and philosophy.[2,3] Before choosing their field of expertise, young psychiatrists should at least know the basics of each of these domains of the discipline and rely upon a mentor or leader.

If you decide to go for clinical work, other professional aspects are demanded. You should learn how to deal with difficult patients, how to perform night shifts, how to negotiate with nurses and other non-medical professionals, how to work in a team; in this case you should identify senior colleagues who are already experienced in working in clinical settings. Ask them for help and advice: you may find yourself having to decide which therapy is best for that given patient in that particular moment. You can rely only upon yourself. When you start working as a doctor, you have full responsibility for your patients – no matter how old or experienced you are. See Chapter 16 for more about professional responsibility. Again, the choice is not an easy task, but choosing is essential.

Setting priorities in own life

Now that you have a better idea of what you want in your professional career, it's time to consider the rest of your life. Your profession is one of only many ways to define yourself. Like many jobs that require significant time, effort and personal sacrifice, medicine can be all-encompassing, so don't be surprised if you find that your personal life seems more amorphous and less goal-directed than your professional life. Yet, chances are, you want some things out of your non-work life, too. We have just spent some time considering the goals of your work life. Let's do the same with your non-work life.

When considering your life, please take into account all the aspects of your personal life and rate them. In particular, what about your partner? Do you have a partner? Do you spend enough time with him/her? Is he/she satisfied about your relationship? Are you satisfied? In a recent survey of Italian young psychiatrists, although 90 % stated they had a stable relationship, only half of them reported they were satisfied with it.[4] This is something we should take care of!

And, do you have (or do you want) children? If yes, how many? Is the house where you live large enough? Is your salary of a young doctor sufficient for a new family? Do you have enough time off work to spend with your children?

What about other family members, for example your parents? How often do you go to visit them? Do you have (or did you have) hobbies? Do you have enough time to pursue your hobbies? Do you like your house or do you want to change it, sooner or later? And, we have not included in this question list your friends and mates! We already know you don't have time for them. Friends seem to be a privilege for young people: when did you spent quality time with your friends last time?

All these questions relate to setting priorities in your life, so that you cannot one day say 'Oh, what happened to my life?' So, please fill in the questionnaire in Box 13.2. Again, be honest!

Box 13.2 Internal Assessment Questionnaire – personal life

1. Ideally, what would you like to accomplish in your non-work life?
   Think non-work interests, hobbies, travel, etc.

2. In your life right now, how big a role do these things play?

3. Is that enough?

4. Is that by choice?

(*Continued*)

Box 13.2 (Continued)

5. Ideally, how will family (e.g. spouse, significant others, children, parents, siblings) and friends fit in?

6. In your current life, how big a role do these people play in your non-work life?

7. Is that enough?

8. Is that by choice?

9. Where do you want to live (e.g. urban vs suburban vs rural)?

10. Does your ideal geographic location allow you to pursue your interests?

11. Does your ideal geographic location allow you to pursue your work goals?

12. Reality testing: which is more important, your work location or your home location? In other words, would you, for example, be willing to do a longer commute if you could live in a better location?

When setting priorities, it is important to consider own limitations. For example, if you have some (even mild) disorders that prevent you from driving, you must take this limitation into account when choosing the house and the place where you want to live. Other limitations may apply to the area where you live or work (e.g. is there public transport?), to the discipline you have chosen (e.g. do you feel adequate to treat persons with mental disorders?) or to the subspecialty you may undertake (e.g. do you have enough empathy if you wish to pursue a psychoanalytic career?).

Balance between work and life

Once you have completed the sections assessing your ideal and current assessments of your work and non-work lives, it is time to put them together. Yes, *time*. Time is an interesting concept. You may have heard patients telling you that they have too much time. In the absence of an external structure, the mind may find ways to fill the time, leading to rumination and self-doubt. Yet, if time is lacking (and for sure you have experienced this at some point during your career), non-urgent matters get pushed to the side to make room for priority goals.[5] The end result is stress, which may lead to depressive symptoms. Being able to manage time allows the opportunity to balance work and non-work activities. However, 'balance' does not necessarily mean 50/50. It is for you to determine what your 'balance' is.

It can be an interesting exercise to see just how much time you actually have. There are 24 hours in a day, 7 days in a week. That is $24 \times 7 = 168$ total hours/week. In the UK and other parts of Europe, there is currently a 48-hour/week limit on work hours according to the EU Working Time Directive, which also applies to medical trainees.[6] According to the American Medical Association 2000–2002 data from *Physician Socioeconomic Statistics*, the general psychiatrist worked an average of 48 hours per week. The average for all US specialties was 53.9.[7] In 2008, according to the US Bureau of Labor Statistics, 43 % of all US physicians worked more than 50 hours/week,[8] but since it's just an estimate anyway, let's just say 48 hours work/week for the sake of this argument.

So, in an average week, 168 hours total − 48 hours of work = 120 hours/ week left for non-work. How does that time get spent? According to the US Bureau of Labor Statistics, the average American spends 8.67 hours/day sleeping and 1.22 hours/day eating and drinking.[8] Just to make the arithmetic easier, let's do a little rounding off. Let's say you spend 8.5 hours/day sleeping $\times 7 = 59.5$ hours/week sleeping. Let's also say you spend 1.25 hours/day eating × 7 = 8.75 hours/week. That's 59.5 + 8.75 = 68.25 hours/week eating, drinking and sleeping.

So, this means that 120 hours/week not spent working −68.25 hours/week on eating, drinking and sleeping = 51.75 hours/week left over for activities like hobbies, personal care, chores, socializing, etc. This begs the question, how do *you* want to spend your 51.75 free hours?

Therefore, the next time you find yourself saying, 'I don't have enough time', ask yourself if that is really true. We all work within the confines of a 24-hour day. Could you use your time more efficiently? Be mindful of resistance, just like you would when doing psychodynamic psychotherapy. Our words and actions are an expression of what we think, even if those thoughts are unconscious.[9] So, by saying you don't have time and then procrastinating, what are you really saying? People avoid things for many different kinds of reasons. Perhaps the task you did not do was something you considered unimportant. Perhaps it is something you dislike or are afraid of.

Keep in mind, too, that resistance comes in a number of forms. You may have noticed some self-struggle when filling out the Internal Assessment Questionnaire. There is always the temptation to put down something to make yourself look good or fulfil some other needs. If you found yourself doing this, stop reading now! Go back and, as honestly as possible, redo the questions that gave you conflict. The purpose of doing this exercise is not to look good. The purpose is to make your life better, and that may involve change. The natural inertia of matter applies to human change as well. Expect resistance to come whenever you are about to make a change. Instead of viewing it as a roadblock, view it as a sign that you are on the right track.

Job satisfaction and prevention of burnout

Job satisfaction depends on a number of factors, but interestingly, the feeling of making a difference seems to rank above money.[1] Being involved in direct medical care means that there are opportunities to help others, though that may not necessarily translate into the feeling that one is making a difference. Bureaucracy, excessive paperwork, frustration when dealing with the government, insurance companies, and other aspects of health-care systems, lack of patient improvement, and financial debt from your own schooling are only some of the reasons why doctors become disillusioned with their practice.[1] Therefore, when answering the self-assessment questions above it is critical that you pay attention to what you find most fulfilling and make that a priority when you decide where to go and what you want to do.

What happens when you ignore, forget or simply lose touch with what gives your career fulfillment? Burnout.[10] In this book a whole chapter (Chapter 19) is dedicated to burnout and the mental health of early career psychiatrists, and therefore we will not go into detail here. What we want to stress in this chapter is that it is, of course, much easier to prevent burnout than to deal with it once it exists. It is easy to say, 'take care of yourself'. It is something we may have even said to our patients without a clear idea how to break it down. It is an entirely different thing to be able to do this ourselves. Here are some practical ways to think about this challenge.

Just as we carry on a biopsychosocial assessment of our patients, we can think of biopsychosocial aspects of taking care of ourselves. You can think of yourself as a wheel. The bio, psycho and social parts make up spokes of the wheel. In order for the wheel to roll smoothly, the spokes must be of equal length. Given that we are human beings and are not perfect, our spokes are not of exactly equal length. That's OK. But it doesn't mean that we are stuck with an uneven wheel for life. If you recognize an area that needs work – a spoke that is shorter than the rest – it is an area that can potentially be improved with some work or attention. Also remember that because we're taking a holistic view of health, there are multiple parts to consider. As much as we may try, human beings do a very poor job of multi-tasking.[5] That means that when you make time for one aspect of your life, something else must get less. Therefore, the trick is not so much trying to cram in more, it is trying to balance better. If that means putting off or taking shortcuts sometimes, so be it (Table 13.1).

Exercise

Does the very thought of exercise seem onerous? Do you hate the idea of going to the gym? Certainly you are not alone. 'Exercise' is simply part of the day. Pretty much all aspects of life, involve muscular effort and energy. You don't need a mastodon chasing you down to find ways to incorporate exercise in your daily life. Table 13.2 gives some suggestions that involve minimal equipment and little, if any, money. Many of these exercises take up very little room and can easily be done inside, in your hotel, living room, kitchen, basement or, if you are feeling particularly energetic, in the confines of a small hospital on-call room, which typically contains nothing more than a bed, a chair and a desk. We could call some of the exercises below 'The Call Room Workout'. The exercises have been broken

Table 13.1 Biopsychosocial self-care formulation.[11]

Bio	Psycho	Social
Tending to biological needs:	Cultivate good coping skills, e.g.:	Tending to your relationships:
• Adequate: • Sleep • Rest • Food • Exercise • Sex*	• Exercise • Relaxation • Progressive muscle relaxation • Guided imagery • Deep breathing/meditation • *Chi kung* or *tai chi chuan*[†] • Supervision with peers or a mentor • Confiding in peers or friends • Your own therapy • Sublimation (directing potentially negative emotions and energy into more positive experiences) • Humour	• Family • Friends • Significant others* • Children • Pets Do you have a mentor?
Addressing adequate preventive health measures • Going to your primary care doctor, dentist, eye doctor, psychiatrist... • Taking medications/vitamins • Proper nutrition		Tending your personal comfort in places you inhabit most, e.g.: • Your home • Your work space • Your mode of transport (car, bike, etc.) Do you have adequate control over your finances?
Making adjustments to reduce work hours or stay home when physically or mentally ill	Reflecting on your own imperfect defenses (you are a human being, after all), through, e.g.: • Journalling • Therapy • Meditation	Making time for religion or spirituality Do you have legal obligations that need to be fulfilled? Anything legal tends to involve a lot of time
Minimizing or controlling substance use		Vacation Hobbies

*As with other physical needs, the gratification of sexuality is complex.[11] It is, of course, not necessary to be in an intimate relationship to be sexual, but there has been a fair amount of literature that supports the idea that those who enjoy loving relationships that are emotionally and sexually fulfilling are likely to experience better physical and mental health.[1]

[†]A word on two Chinese martial arts (*chi kung* and *tai chi chuan*) that do not fit neatly into the above categories. They have been placed along with other relaxation-based exercises since deep breathing and slow, gentle movement form the core of these exercises. Although they are martial arts in their own right, they can easily be practised for health benefits.

Table 13.2 The Call Room Workout.

Body weight, strength and flexibility	Cardiovascular
Upper body • Push-ups • Triceps dips • Advanced: pull-ups • Advanced: handstands against a wall (handstand push-ups can also be done ... prerequisite: the ability to support your bodyweight entirely on your hands; don't attempt unless you are comfortable standing on your hands already)	Walking laps around the hospital (can also be done in any indoor setting, like a mall) Walking or jogging up and down the stairs Advanced: jumping rope Shadowboxing (prerequisite: knowledge of boxing, kickboxing or other martial arts as well as adequate flexibility to perform them safely) Jogging in place
Lower body • Squats • Lunges • Calf raises (either on the ground or a raised platform, like the stairs)	
Core • Sit-ups/crunches (to the front to work the *rectus abdominis*, side to side for oblique muscles) • Advanced: leg lifts	
Flexibility • Stretching muscle groups and loosening up the joints • Yoga (consider doing it along with a video)	

As always, the usual disclaimer: please take measures to evaluate your own health if you are not currently physically active. Consider it part of taking care of yourself. Talk to your primary care physician (if you don't have one, a good first step would be to get one) before starting a new exercise programme, and start slow and with exercises you definitely know how to do and proceed at your own pace. It is always helpful to loosen up the joints prior to doing any exercise. This is not meant to be a treatise on how to exercise. It is merely meant to provide interested parties with some ideas on how to do it cheaply with common household items.

into two artificial categories. Of course, many of the exercises contain aspects of both, and almost anything can become a cardiovascular exercise if done long enough.

Conclusions

This chapter can be summed up in a single word: change! If you are unhappy with where you are now or are simply looking for a more fully actualized career and/or personal life, take heart. There is always potential for improvement if you know who you are and what you want. If you don't know those things, you can learn. The purpose in doing the above self-assessment is to help you narrow down a career that will not only allow you to do what you want, but in a way that is personally fulfilling. If you love what you do, not only are you more likely to make a difference in the world, but life is better not only for you and your family, but also for your patients.[1] If some of the advice given above seemed like what you might give in therapy to your patients, that's because it is. We are not immune to the same stresses and problems our patients face, but our patients can rely on us. Who will we turn to? It is important to remember that we must all have teachers and mentors: we cannot shoulder the burden alone. Use the experience and expertise of those who have come before you. Generally, all you have to do is ask. Most people are more than happy to talk about themselves.[1]

One of the saddest things is lost potential. After having invested so much time and energy to get to where we are, we deserve to feel that it was worth it. If that involves making changes in our lives that can create temporary discomfort, such as moving to a new home, reducing time for personal psychotherapy, or changing jobs in order to get longer-term quality of life, it might be worth the gamble. In the end, be kind to yourself. It isn't a bad way of taking care of yourself, either.

References

1. Harrison A. How to love your job. *Practice Link* 2011; **21**: 69–71.
2. McHugh PR, Slavney PR. *The Perspectives of Psychiatry*, 2nd edn. Baltimore, MD: Johns Hopkins University Press, 1998.
3. Kandel ER. A new intellectual framework for psychiatry. *Am J Psychiatry* 1998; **155**: 457–469.
4. Giacco D, Luciano M, Volpe U, Fiorillo A. Opinions of Italian residents in psychiatry on their training course. *Eur Psychiatry* 2010; **25**(S1): 3–170.
5. Ferriss T. *The Four Hour Workweek*, New York, NY: Crown Publishers, 2007.
6. British Medical Association. European working time directive. Available at: www.bma.org.uk/employmentandcontracts/working_arrangements/hours/index.jsp.

7. Dorsey ER, Jarjoura D, Rutecki GW. Influence of controllable lifestyle on recent trends in specialty choice by US medical students. *JAMA* 2003; **290**: 1173–1178.

8. US Bureau of Labor Statistics. American Time Use Statistics – 2009 Results. BLS, 2010. Available at: www.bls.gov/news.release/pdf/atus.pdf.

9. Livingston G. *Too Soon Old, Too Late Smart*. New York, NY. Marlowe & Co., 2004.

10. Kumar S. Burnout in psychiatrists. *World Psychiatry* 2007; **6**: 186–189.

11. Baker E. *Caring for Ourselves: a Therapist's Guide to Personal and Professional Well-being*. Washington, DC: The American Psychological Association, 2003.

CHAPTER 14

How to collaborate with other specialties

Silvia Ferrari,[1] Joshua Blum[2] and Patrick Kelly[3]

[1]Department of Mental Health, University of Modena and Reggio Emilia, Policlinico di Modena, Italy
[2]Department of Psychiatry, University of Massachusetts Medical School, Worcester, MA, USA
[3]Division of Child and Adolescent Psychiatry, Department of Psychiatry and Behavioral Sciences, Division of Child and Adolescent Psychiatry, The Johns Hopkins Hospital, Baltimore, MD, USA

Introduction

The Western tradition of medicine has conventionally divided the mind and the body. In the nineteenth and twentieth centuries, however, due to increased knowledge about biology and physiology, the split between mind and body began to lessen.[1,2] Sigmund Freud brought the idea of the somatic conversion reactions into the scope of medicine, and increasing knowledge about endocrine hormones, emotional stress and social factors helped to produce a more holistic approach to medicine.[1] However, despite this more modern view, there is still stigma and confusion when it comes to mental illness. The famous work by George Engel opened the way to discuss the faults and limitations of contemporary biomedicine, along with those of psychiatry: 'All medicine is in crisis and, further, that medicine's crisis derives from the same basic fault as psychiatry's, namely, adherence to a model of disease no longer adequate for the scientific tasks and social responsibilities of either medicine and psychiatry. [...] The dominant model of disease today is biomedical, and it leaves no room within its framework for the social, psychological, and behavioral dimensions of illness. A biopsychosocial model is proposed that provides a blueprint for research, a framework for teaching, and a design for action in the real world of health care'.[3] Ever since, his biopsychosocial paradigm of human disease has gained a general and undisputed consensus, but it might still lack effective translation into practice and culture.[4]

How to Succeed in Psychiatry: A Guide to Training and Practice, First Edition.
Edited by Andrea Fiorillo, Iris Tatjana Calliess and Henning Sass.
© 2012 John Wiley & Sons, Ltd. Published 2012 by John Wiley & Sons, Ltd.

In most Western countries, medical students are typically exposed to a certain amount of preclinical didactics in psychiatric diagnosis, interviewing and treatment, as well as 1–2 months of psychiatry in their medical school clinical rotations.[5] Psychiatry is part of the US national board testing system (USMLE Steps 1, 2 and 3), generally included among ethics and statistics. Therefore, all graduates of medical schools and residencies should know a certain amount of psychiatry, but aside from these formal requirements, it may be the last time trainees are exposed to a concentrated dose of the field.[5]

Residents in psychiatry find that their colleagues in other specialties often have the same prejudices and misconceptions that the general public does.[5] Unfortunately, the media often do very little to correct those perceptions. It's no wonder that psychiatry is on the 'bottom of the totem pole' in many hospitals. An example of this are the caricatures of psychiatrists portrayed in popular medical TV series, such as *ER, Scrubs* or *Grey's Anatomy*. The World Psychiatric Association (WPA) expressed concern about the shortage of psychiatrists, particularly in some countries, supporting a survey (the ISoCCiP study, currently ongoing) among final-year medical students about their preferences in choosing a medical career and reasons affecting this choice.

The general public is often still confused about the difference between psychiatry and psychology. In the end, the difference is simple: psychiatrists are, first and foremost, medical doctors. They go through several years of medical school, and much of their training is spent on biochemistry, physiology, pathology, the divisions of internal medicine, and aspects of surgery. As mentioned, the pathology and treatment of mental disorders forms a relatively small part of this curriculum. It is only after graduation from medical school (where everyone – future gynaecologists, family doctors, psychiatrists and surgeons alike – are educated with the same basic curriculum) that future psychiatrists enter residency, the apprenticeship where they actually learn their trade.

In this chapter, pitfalls and opportunities in the interaction between psychiatry and the rest of medicine will be described, hopefully providing early career psychiatrists with practical suggestions and possible improvements of their working situations.

Main reasons and examples of collaboration

Despite the controversial relationship between psychiatry and the rest of medicine, which parallels that between mental health professionals and professionals from other branches of health care, there are many good reasons for establishing effective collaborations, and some good examples of how to do this. Consultation-liaison psychiatry (CLP) and psychosomatic medicine (PM) developed progressively through the second half of the twentieth century as the conceptual and clinical area of psychiatry dedicated to operationalize the dialogue between psychiatry and the rest of medicine.

CLP is often considered an inpatient hospital service, but in actuality the ideal consultation from any specialist, inpatient or outpatient, psychiatric or not, has elements of both consultation and liaison. The consultation part comes from the primary doctor asking a colleague to help answer a particular diagnostic or treatment question. The liaison part refers to collaboration. 'Liaison' comes from French and refers to 'binding' or 'joining'.[2] In an ideal situation, consultants are able not only to provide some kind of clinical service, but also to educate and promote awareness to their colleagues, thereby imparting some of their knowledge, helping their colleagues to become more aware of some particular aspect of patient care so that in the future the consult may not be needed. Like a good therapist, a good consultant wants to render his or her services obsolete. Therefore, given that psychiatry is a specialty, psychiatrists are, in a way, automatically consult-liaison doctors to the rest of medicine whether they choose to be or not.

This is the reason why CLP has been included as mandatory in the specialization training curricula of most psychiatric schools. In Italy, for example, residents in psychiatry and child-adolescent neuropsychiatry are requested to deal with at least 20 clinical interventions of CLP. At the Modena University School of Specialization in Psychiatry, all residents in their second/third year perform a 6-month rotation at the CLP Service. In Europe, standards for postgraduate training in CLP have been formulated by the European Association for Consultation-Liaison Psychiatry and Psychosomatics (EACLPP) and can be found on the website of the Association (www.eaclpp.org). In the USA, PM is a recognized subspecialty of psychiatry by the American Board of Psychiatry and Neurology. As such, most professionals in this field have taken additional training above and beyond that offered in a general psychiatry residency. According to the Accreditation Council for Graduate Medical Education (ACGME), fellowships must consist of 1 year of 'advanced training'. Specific requirements can be found at www.acgme.org, and each programme does vary slightly in its offerings. At the end of that year, practitioners are eligible to sit for a subspecialty examination after which they will be certified to practise PM by the Board.

In the following paragraphs, examples of effective collaborations will be provided, described and discussed; these are logically organized into three different perspectives: (i) according to the clinical setting; (ii) according to type of activity (clinical, training, research, organization of service); (iii) according to specific clinical issues and psychiatric conditions.

Collaboration related to the clinical setting

Segregation of the mentally ill from the physically ill, mainly represented by the institution of the mental hospital, is a relatively recent historical phenomenon, since in medieval hospitals no such division was observable and the management of mental illness had a 'legitimate place' in medical care as a whole.[6,7] The institution of special, separate asylums for 'lunatics' dates back to the eighteenth and nineteenth centuries and was the starting point for a segregation of psychiatry, which, from being physical and geographical, ended up being also cultural and scientific. It was only at the beginning of the twentieth century that psychiatry started regaining both a clinical and educational role within the rest of medicine: this was evidenced by the gradual establishment of acute psychiatry wards in many general hospitals both in the USA and in Europe, an event that is officially considered as the symbolic birth of CLP.

With psychiatry wards and psychiatrists back in the general hospital, many new opportunities for encounter and exchange were available, more or less satisfactory for both psychiatrists and specialists from other disciplines, the first and most typical being consultation referrals in the wards and in the emergency departments. So, internal medicine physicians, surgeons or dermatologists started being called for related comorbidities in patients admitted to the psychiatric ward, and came face to face with the rather strange and sometimes scary aspects that even now mark the differences: some of these real (i.e. the locked door, the totally non-compliant patient, physical restraints, the smoking room), some more related to ideology or stigma. The medical health of the mentally ill has been, and still is, greatly neglected, partly as a consequence of difficult relationships and different perspectives on illness between medical doctors.

Psychiatrists do not feel 'at ease' when their medical or surgical skills are required, no matter how basic, rather as non-psychiatrists feel when they have to recall their well-forgotten memories of psychiatric disorders or therapies. Psychiatry is by no means unique in that once training became increasingly specialized, many basic medical skills – things like physical exams and management of basic medical complaints – were not handled by psychiatrists any more but delegated to medical colleagues as consultations.[8] Of course, we should be able to trust our colleagues and their judgment, which is one argument for consulting. However, the culture of consulting does seem to have had the adverse effect of making clinicians less self-confident. In fact, due to concerns about liability and 'practising outside of one's field', some psychiatrists may simply prefer to have an internist or family doctor managing all non-psychiatric issues. Unfortunately, lack of exposure leads to less practice, which ultimately becomes a feed-forward cycle resulting in less confidence.

Psychiatric assessment tends to rely heavily on the clinical interview, and with a lack of practice, confidence in skills such as physical exams wanes. And, even if residents do perform these skills while in training, there is often not the need to continue after graduation, when they can be performed by someone else. There is always the excuse that a trainee is 'closer to his or her medical training' than an attending physician, so is therefore more competent to perform these skills. In addition, in many settings, particularly outpatient offices, the constraints of time and the lack of adequate exam rooms, tools and chaperones make basic medical exams and studies difficult to perform. In addition, the issue of who provides the medical treatment for a patient becomes complicated in psychotherapy, leading to concerns about changing roles, boundary violations and transferential issues. Moreover, on a purely logistical level, in many psychiatric hospitals (which are often free standing), basic medical treatment as one would find on a typical inpatient internal medicine ward (with access to medical paraphernalia such as oxygen, intravenous access and telemetry) is unavailable. When psychiatric units are located in the same hospital, they are often locked. Not only does this lead to the isolation of psychiatry from the rest of medicine, but it keeps the rest of medicine from knowing exactly what psychiatrists do. In some hospitals, the separation goes beyond geography and extends to the medical records as well, where psychiatric records are kept separate from the general medical charts.

At the same time, with the return of psychiatric wards to the general hospital, psychiatrists started being called into medical wards or in the ER, and had to update their terminology, practices and attitudes as well. Box 14.1 gives a classification of the most common reasons for psychiatric referral.

Box 14.1 Reasons for psychiatric referral

1. Generic, unspecified referral, one among all the other referrals of the diagnostic pathway.
2. 'Magical' referral, at the end of a long, complex diagnostic pathway that has not revealed the presence of a medical disease: psychiatric referral as the 'last resort'.

(Continued)

Box 14.1 (Continued)

3. Referral for custody-control reasons, for 'difficult' patients (behavioural problems, not necessarily of psychiatric pertinence).
4. Specified referral, if the presence of a psychiatric disorder has been suspected by the ward physician.

This divide between psychiatry and internal medicine is based on many aspects, both big and small, such as managing medically/surgically unstable or suicidal patients in wards that do not guarantee protection for the patient. The insistence of psychiatrists on announcing their consultations properly to the patient or on conducting them in a private, quiet and dedicated room has sometimes been seen as an incomprehensible and pointless quirk of doctors known to be 'stranger than their patients'. Some degree of inferiority complex on the account of psychiatrists is involved, pairing suspicions and ideology from other specialists, and leading to daily 'skirmishes', which nevertheless also had the effect of increasing awareness and reciprocal respect.

The general hospital is ideally the place where all medical disciplines and specialties meet and complement each other, not only as an academic concept but also as a concrete opportunity, for example in discussing a case with a colleague at the coffee shop, or while conducting a difficult differential diagnosis, since exchange of views is more feasible than in other more dispersed clinical settings. Nevertheless, the expense of the hospital setting has in recent years led to a shift to primary and community care, for both psychiatry and other medical disciplines. However, many examples of collaboration between psychiatry and the rest of medicine have been accumulating in primary care as well.[9]

Collaboration related to type of activity

The clinical, research and education-training activities performed by psychiatrists are closely linked. CL psychiatrists act in an area (also from the spatial point of view) that is especially conducive to the development of working processes dependent on cooperation among very widely divergent professional figures as regards their roles, functions and professional and cultural identities. Therefore, collaboration takes place not only while dealing with patients in everyday clinical practice, but also in training, research and organizational activities.

As to training, psychiatry was included many decades ago in the undergraduate and postgraduate educational curricula of most medical and social professions (not only medical doctors, but also nurses, social workers, educators, physical therapists, midwives, etc.). Moreover, many local, national or international training initiatives focus on development of theoretical and practical skills at the boundaries between psychiatry and the rest of medicine, such as programmes dedicated to dealing with specific disorders (see below) and on more general issues. Specific programmes of CLP exist within most medical schools and have an increasing role in supporting and implementing the biopsychosocial paradigm.[10] More and more, the initiative for organizing training events is taken by non-psychiatrists, particularly primary care physicians, on the basis of real-world educational needs and methodologically inspired by Balint groups as the most effective and respectable predecessor.

Collaborations between psychiatry and other areas of medicine have been particularly significant in research. On the one hand, there has been the need to verify and quantify the epidemiological impact of medical-psychiatric comorbidities, which has generated a massive amount of literature.[11-15] On the other hand, research on the biopsychosocial correlates of human illness has been exploding, with many promising insights, involving specialists from virtually all the branches of medicine and basic sciences. One of the most advanced areas is arguably the study of the correlates between depression and cardiovascular disorders, the prototype of a 'new', contemporary concept of a complex multi-morbidity disorder;[16-20] another well-known expanding field is that of neuro-psycho-immuno-endocrinology. Advances in the fields of physiology and pathophysiology suggest that it is useless, limiting and even misleading to refer to human illness as single disorders of separate organs and systems, diagnosed and treated by separated consultants, and that we should move to a more articulated and 'circular' idea of aetiology and treatment: this is not just a beautiful paradigm of abstract medical epistemology with few practical implications, but should also be the source for more specific and effective care interventions.

Inputs from clinical practice, training and research should be channelled into the organization of services, with all structures, strategies and procedures improving collaboration. The main example is in itself the establishment and maintenance of a CLP service in a general hospital or in the community: different experiences and original solutions to problems have been developed in many Western countries. CL psychiatrists have to face a paradoxical negative rebound effect of their own efforts in convincing colleagues of the relevance of psychosocial issues in medicine, with referrals to psychiatric consultations dramatically increasing in all settings of care and rapidly overwhelming available resources. Many authors have criticized the obsolete model of CLP and called for original models of collaboration, accounting for the contemporary conceptualization of complex illness.[17,20,21]

Collaboration related to specific psychiatric conditions

The most frequent and/or most severe clinical conditions involving specialists from both mental health and other disciplines are related to specific examples of collaboration, among which the following should be mentioned:

- The model by Katon for the care of depression.[22]
- The experiences of medical psychiatric units in the USA[21,23] and in Europe.[24]
- The model for delirium, based upon the work by Trzepacz[25] and Inouye.[26,27]

Medical complications of psychotropic treatments, as well as psychiatric complications of medical treatments are also very common clinical reasons for collaboration. Examples of the former are the long QTc syndrome and the metabolic syndrome for patients treated with first- and second-generation antipsychotics. Routine monitoring of basic physical parameters such as ECG, blood pressure, weight and metabolic indicators are now mandatory in clinical psychiatry practice, and examples of managing strategies also exist.[28] Examples of psychiatric illness due to medical treatments include drug-related delirium and psychiatric side effects of interferon therapy. Routine psychiatric assessment and follow-up before and during interferon therapy has been successfully introduced, reducing rates of drop-out and complications.[29]

Medically unexplained physical symptoms (MUPS) are another common and clinically relevant issue requiring strong collaboration between psychiatrists and other clinical doctors, and these are dealt with below.

Medically unexplained physical symptoms (MUPS)

The fragility of the biomedical model

Psychiatry and psychiatric disorders are a real thorn in the side of biomedicine, due to their uncertain aetiology, complexity, arbitrary classification and overall unpredictability, explaining why they often tend to be sidelined or ignored by biomedical specialists. But also well-certified and unquestionably somatic disorders, such as diabetes, coronary heart disease and cancer, share some of these features.[19] On the other hand, research on the biological correlates of psychiatric disorders, such as depression or schizophrenia, has shown that these disorders share many pathophysiological mechanisms with primarily organic disorders.[16,20] A model based on reductionism and linear causality is too simple and limiting to be of any use in everyday clinical practice, since explanations and solutions of one side of the problem would inevitably and continually generate other problems.

Primary care physicians and other 'first-line' medical doctors especially are used to a pragmatic clinical approximation, which is nothing less than a very complex, circular integration of notions and scientific facts to less physical, immeasurable evidence: this is because human illness, i.e. the phenomenon of 'illness' affecting a human being, is a matter of complexity, as beautifully remarked by Graeme Smith:[17] 'Complex means intricate, not easily analyzed and disentangled. [...] the patterns that emerge through the interaction of multiple agents ... can be perceived but not predicted, because the number of agents and the number of relationships defy categorization or statistical analytic techniques'; he evidently refers to the theory of systems.

MUPS features

Patients presenting with MUPS are dramatically common; they have a prevalence of up to 50 % in both clinical and non-clinical settings,[24] and are typically dealt with by primary care physicians. Only for a very small proportion of common complaints can a well-defined organic cause be defined with certainty. Of the many physical symptoms that each of us experience every day, the vast majority remains unexplained, without much concern and consequences due to self-limitation or trivial importance. In some cases, the problem persists, usually via reinforcing cognitive mechanisms such as sensory amplification, leading to MUPS. Interestingly, a recent study provided evidence that quality of life in patients with multiple somatic symptoms is more affected by the number of symptoms and comorbid anxiety/depression than by an existing sound explanation of the origin of symptoms.[30] Chronicity, disability, high comorbidity with anxiety and depression, and excessive and inadequate use of health-care resources are typical features of MUPS,[31] which represents an epidemic with important consequences for health care organization and budgets. Dysfunctional and disrupted practitioner-patient relationships are also very common, these patients usually being much disliked by doctors for their oppressive and sometimes manipulative and aggressive attitudes. The doctor-patient relationship is described as unsatisfactory by both doctors and MUPS patients, although the latter admit they prefer their GP to other specialists. Many recent studies have delved into the features of such relationships, both as cause and consequence of MUPS and frequent attendance, for example those from olde Hartman *et al.*[32,33] Results from qualitative studies should guide training of medical doctors aimed at improving self-awareness of how their communication styles and behavioural idiosyncrasies might affect their relationships with patients and, ultimately, the effectiveness of their clinical practice. MUPS patients contribute strongly to the development of burnout syndrome in their physicians, and this issue is often a lively subject of discussion during Balint groups. The phenomenon has received attention in the media, where it has been often quite funnily portrayed (see, e.g., the Nick Hornby novel *How to be good*).

Each medical specialty has its own 'functional' disorder

All medical specialties have their own 'functional' syndrome: there is irritable bowel syndrome for gastroenterology, fibromyalgia for rheumatology, non-cardiac thoracic pain for cardiology, chronic fatigue syndrome for infectious diseases, and so on, down a list getting longer each day. The increasing need for somatic doctors to invoke functionality is direct evidence of the shortcomings of the biomedical model.

These syndromes all share common features, such as poorly defined pathophysiology, uncertain results at diagnostic examinations, chronicity, and high levels of comorbidity with anxiety and depression. Kanaan et al.[34] discuss whether it is more useful – also for clinical aims – to focus on these common features rather than on specificities. In other words, would it be better – and feasible – if in a general hospital there existed a 'MUPS ward' rather than the many overlapping specialist clinics? Medical psychiatric units and outpatient clinics were conceived to address this need. In Europe, the model of the German psychosomatic medicine service is paramount;[35] a recent and promising experience in Europe is described by Leue and colleagues,[24] who conducted an amazingly accurate analysis of cost-effectiveness of the intervention.

These patients never go to 'the shrink'

How come the incidence/prevalence of somatoform disorders is so low in clinical and non-clinical populations, in the face of such a widespread and commonly accepted view that MUPS are very frequent? The diagnosis of somatization is a very poor clinical tool, and therefore unpopular among physicians, patients and psychiatrists: it seems that everyone considers, but cannot formalize the condition, due to fear of missing a somatic diagnosis and of being sued for this. Moreover, even if one correctly and appropriately diagnoses somatization, very often one is left with only a sense of impotence and frustration for not being able to do anything helpful. Some of the excesses and perversions of contemporary medicine are possibly just defence mechanisms against such feelings.

Mental health professionals rarely see these patients, who often refuse and resist psychiatric referrals. About this, Stone et al.[36] discussed the disappearance of the 'hysteria' syndrome according to psychiatrists. Secondly, psychiatrists, as well as other clinicians, tend to stick to their own, more familiar diagnostic categories of anxiety, depression, and may be sometimes invoking personality traits or disorders, for which they feel they have some kind of intervention available, either pharmaceutical or psychotherapeutic, whereas they feel they lack effective and/or feasible therapeutic options for MUPS.

Physicians need effective clinical solutions for these patients

A diagnosis of 'somatization' is usually perceived as inappropriate and stigmatizing by patients with MUPS, and may lead to interruption of communication between patient and doctor, or 'doctor-shopping' behaviour. Psychologization of somatic symptoms is felt by both doctors and patients to be a vague and unsatisfactory 'dress for all seasons': if 'stress' is the reason for everything, then it is the explanation of none.

Controversies and reciprocal misunderstanding often occur between physicians and psychiatrists when MUPS patients are concerned, even once the patient has somehow agreed to the psychiatric consultation, with frequent and annoying 'passing of the buck'. Psychiatrists blame their consultees for impossible, last-resort requests, while physicians blame the absence of pragmatism and substance in psychiatrists' clinical reports. Interventions for MUPS patients are few and poorly studied. Recently, evidence in favour of cognitive behavioural approaches has been discussed.[37] Many recent studies have been accumulating evidence favouring reattribution techniques.[38]

Practical suggestions for improving collaboration

Improving cooperation has many obvious consequences, not only improved quality of patient care but also greater satisfaction with one's professional situation (leading to proactive attitudes, long-term investments, less burnout, etc.). In Table 14.1 we list some of the most common obstacles to collaboration, leading to conflicts or misunderstandings, and possible indications of how to better cooperate with specialists from different branches of medicine.

While discussing the subject of conflicts between consultants from different specialties, Caplan et al.[39] outline three main responses to conflict: (i) avoidance – by far the most common among medical doctors – i.e. refusal to acknowledge the presence of conflict or tension and therefore having to deal with it; (ii) 'forcing' – when a more powerful party tramples on the other without much consideration; (iii) negotiation, the most effective and least utilized strategy. The authors also list some practical advice for confronting conflicts and improving collaboration by promoting negotiation and discouraging avoidance or forcing.

Table 14.1 Obstacles and indications for improving cooperation.

Obstacle	Actions/solutions
Stigma and prejudices	• Organize dedicated seminars or round-table sessions at local institutions • Take some time at the end of the referral to explain to doctors and nurses who the patient is, and who the person is behind the patient • Provide gentle reproach for stigmatizing attitudes of colleagues, to help increasing self-awareness • Be aware of your own stigmatizing attitudes
Language	• Avoid expressions that are too technical or abstract in favour of more user-friendly terms, but without sacrificing completeness and the need to convey the sense of complexity
Lack of/fear of basic clinical notions in reciprocal fields of competence	• Keep updated, be curious, ask about what you are not familiar with (usually colleagues are happy to give you a little lecture!)
Lack of familiarity (with persons, procedures, etc.)	• Let your colleagues know you, provide indications on how to find you (within the terms of your professional availability) • Take some time to explain the appropriate procedures of referral to doctors and nurses • Do not change procedures too often and clearly advertise any change
Excessive turnover of professionals	• Establish a standardized procedure for transmission of information when colleagues move away and new ones come
Previous negative experiences (during and after training)	• Be aware that there might be a prejudice affecting your judgment, and give new people and new situations a chance • Express as openly as possible your concerns and make simple and clear requests to prevent bad things from happening again
Pressure in clinical practice due to shortness of time and resources	• Try and assume your colleagues' point of view, and ask them to do the same • Be creative!
Fear of reciprocal manipulation (i.e. faking of severity to get urgent referrals)	• Openly address your concern • Do not manipulate yourself • Take some time in 'educating' your colleagues to respect you
Shortened time for face-to-face discussions on problems	• Do not postpone discussions, as they often prevent time wasting in the future

Part of finding your place as a psychiatrist in the wide world of medicine is figuring out how you want to interact with your medical colleagues.[2,8] What follows may seem a bit like cognitive behavioural therapy, and in a way, it is. We learn by modelling, even if the model is virtual. If you don't know what it is you are trying to become, you'll never know when you've got there. Take a few moments and think about some situations that you've encountered where you felt that collaboration between psychiatry and a non-psychiatric service worked particularly well. How did those involve interact with each other? How did they communicate? How did they carry themselves? Ask yourself – is this something that I would realistically be able to do on a regular basis? Now think of the opposite situation, where collaboration was handled poorly, or where there was none at all where there should have been. Or consider situations where you felt insulted, talked down to, or just ignored by a colleague for the question you had. Why was there poor collaboration? We all work under the constraints of time, money and large caseloads. Was there another reason? How could things have been improved? Now ask yourself – are there times when I have acted this way to others when they have asked for help? Also ask yourself if there were times when you could have educated yourself more prior to asking for help. Table 14.2 offers a few examples of general medical conditions that psychiatrists often see in consulting services or in their own patients.

This is by no means a proposal that we get in over our heads. Part of providing good care is knowing when to ask for help and doing so. But, the answer to our initial question is probably always 'yes'; we can always educate ourselves more. However, if you ask a colleague to help with something you feel is 'beneath' you or something you have no interest in, it does beg the question why you are asking the question in the first place. Is it just for the purposes of documentation? Or, as mentioned in *The House of God*, 'buffing the chart'?[40] Do you have vague concerns that something is wrong but are unable to formulate a question? Would that be something that you could share with the consulting service? Perhaps you could jointly create a question to answer. Remember, everyone wants to have their services valued. We all want to feel that what we worked for was worth it in the end. A little self-education prior to calling for help may not always be realistic, but if you share what you tried to figure out before calling for help, it can be a good way to show not only that you are concerned enough to investigate it on your own, but also that you are interested in the subject matter. This, may, in turn, make for a more high-yield consultation. We are usually more likely to want to teach and help those who seem interested.

Table 14.2 Examples of psychiatric/general medical overlap.[54]

In the event of . . .	. . .consider:
Dysmorphic features	Developmental disabilities (consult a reference such as *Smith's Recognizable Patterns of Human Malformation*[55])
Overly thin body habitus	Eating disorders, malnutrition, alcoholism (especially if signs of liver failure are present – e.g. scleral icterus, ascites, jaundice), opioid dependence
Central obesity	Cushing's syndrome (especially if with other features, such as violaceous striae and moon facies), metabolic syndrome (many causes, not the least of which are atypical antipsychotic medications)
Repetitive perioral/lingual movements	Extrapyramidal symptoms or tardive dyskinesia secondary to antipsychotic use
Lid retraction, widened palpebral fissures	Psychosis, hyperthyroidism
Puffy, non-pitting oedema around face and extremities	Myxoedema secondary to hypothyroidism
Bumps under the skin	Lipomas, cysts, abscesses, neurofibromatosis type 1 (especially if seen with other features such as café-au-lait spots)
Resting tremors	Parkinson's disease, Parkinson's plus syndromes (e.g. Lewy body dementia, multi-system atrophy)
Tics	Tourette's syndrome, obsessive-compulsive disorder (OCD)
Dysarthric speech	Alcohol or substance intoxication, traumatic brain injury, mental retardation, delirium
Word-finding difficulties, aphasia	Dementias, stroke, transient ischaemic attack (TIA)
Shortness of breath, chest pain, tachypnoea, tachycardia	Wide differential! myocardial infarction (MI), pulmonary embolus, aortic dissection, panic attack, gastro-oesophageal reflux disease (GERD), asthma exacerbation, pneumonia, etc. (psychiatric patients get all these, too)
Disorientation (both with agitation or excessive quietness)	Sundowning, excitatory catatonia, various and many causes of delirium – e.g. sleep deprivation, hypoxia, hypercapnia, alcohol intoxication/withdrawal, substance intoxication/withdrawal, hepatic/metabolic encephalopathies, and many others
Frequent falls	Peripheral neuropathy, alcoholic neuropathy, cerebellar atrophy, seizures, syncopal and presyncopal events due to hypovolaemia, vasovagal episodes, autonomic instability, etc.

Two examples of collaboration

The interface between child and adolescent psychiatry and paediatrics

As a discipline, child and adolescent psychiatry (CAP) is relatively young. It was not until the late 1800s that children were recognized as individuals who may suffer from psychiatric illnesses, at times similar to those seen in adults. Prior to this distinction, children were expected to either be developmentally/neurologically disabled (with accompanying psychiatric symptoms) or 'normal'. It was only through the accumulation of harmful life experiences that children developed psychiatric illnesses, and therefore it was difficult for children to be so damaged as to express symptoms worthy of treatment at such a young age. It is true that historical figures such as Anna Freud and Melanie Klein began to study and understand child development, but it was particularly focused on what can go wrong in this development and how it influenced adult psychopathology, rather than treating children as such. In many areas of the world, CAP began to emerge as a field around 1930. In the USA, Adolf Meyer, then the director of psychiatry at the Johns Hopkins Hospital, recognized a need for specialized treatment of children and adolescents. This was primarily driven by the paediatrics department, who felt somewhat neglected in the area of psychosocial support for what were obviously suffering children and families. Leo Kanner was then recruited to chair the first division of CAP in the world. Kanner used his experience to gather information for his book, *Child Psychiatry*, published in 1935.[41] At around the same time in Switzerland, Moritz Tramer created the first *Journal of Child Psychiatry* in 1934.

Given that paediatricians were among the primary proponents of bringing psychiatry into the realm of childhood, one would think that relationships between paediatrics and CAP would in some way be smoother than the one between medicine and adult psychiatry. In fact, some paediatricians felt that psychiatrists had no business in childhood. In 1931, the Chicago paediatrician Joseph Brenneman wrote, 'there is a menace in psychologizing the school child, psychiatrizing his behavior and over organizing his habits and his play'. He attacked the psychologists of the day for interfering with the innocence of childhood and trying to pathologize the developmental process. Despite this controversy, one would think that the department of paediatrics at Johns Hopkins at least would have an easier time relating to the division that it helped found (CAP). Unfortunately, a short decade later, Leo Kanner, who had already pioneered a joint paediatrics clinic, noted that there was 'a tendency to ridicule and resent any psychiatric offerings' among paediatricians in his own hospital.[42] One could speculate as to the reasons for this observation, but it is likely due to the same reasons why such attitudes to psychiatry exist in other areas of medicine.

Child and adolescent psychiatrists are likely to be asked for assistance in two clinical settings, inpatient and outpatient. In the inpatient setting, the reasons for consulting psychiatry can be as varied as in adult services. However, paediatricians tend to be less likely to consult the team in order to have the patient removed from their service. A common reason for involving psychiatry in the adult population involves a subsection of patients who are seen as 'inappropriate' for the adult inpatient service (whether they are behaviourally difficult, malingering, primary substance abusers, etc.). The consultation, veiled in technical terms and innuendos, is essentially to request 'please take this patient away from us'. This is far more unusual in the paediatric realm, but does occasionally occur. Most often, paediatricians consult because they have already identified that something is going on that makes them feel out of their element, even though they may not be able to describe the exact problem. Often they get a vague sense that something psychiatric is impeding the patient's development or ability to maintain their medical health, but have no idea how to address these concerns. In a recent survey, only 54 % of paediatricians said that they were comfortable in their own skills at identifying psychiatric illness and depression in children, and only 10 % felt comfortable caring for these patients. When asked what led to these determinations, 68 % stated that they did not have time to do a complete assessment, and 54 % cited a lack of adequate training.[43]

Despite wanting to treat their patients, involving psychiatry can be seen as a double-edged sword. In one survey, the most important aspect of any consultation was not the accuracy of the diagnosis or the quality of the treatment provided; it was the timeliness of the response by the psychiatric team.[44] In fact, the primary limiting factor to involving psychiatry was the concern that the consultation would lengthen the inpatient stay and/or create more work for the primary team (in finding outpatient referrals, etc.). This concern is to some extent true – CAP and paediatrics do operate on something of a different timescale. Whereas the average length of stay on many US inpatient CAP units is 7–10 days, the average time on a paediatrics unit is significantly shorter. Psychiatry comes to diagnostic conclusions usually by gathering historical data, interviewing the patient, the family, the school, the outpatient mental health provider (if any), previous records, etc. Serial mental status examinations are also critical to accurately formulating the diagnosis. All of this takes great amounts of time, but is critical for putting together an appropriate treatment plan. Though paediatricians of course want the best for their patients, they have a difficult time justifying continued inpatient treatment once the medical condition is addressed – hence feedback from psychiatry that the workup is not complete is typically met with frustration. Even simple questions, such as 'is this patient truly at risk to hurt themselves and can they safely go home?' can take days to determine, but from the paediatrician's standpoint the answer may determine whether or not they discharge the patient.

The outpatient experience is quite different. Typically, outpatient paediatricians involve child psychiatrists by referring their patients for an evaluation, rather than having them seen in the office. This is despite the fact that many paediatricians frequently see psychiatric problems in their own outpatient clinics. About 75 % of children with psychiatric disorders are seen only in primary care settings, and about half of all paediatric office visits involve behavioural, psychosocial and/or educational concerns.[45] So, why do paediatricians refer? The majority of paediatricians and child and adolescent psychiatrists agree that paediatricians should be responsible for identifying and referring, but not treating, child mental health conditions, except attention deficit hyperactivity disorder (ADHD).[46]

Unfortunately, this model has its own difficulties. The primary issue seems to involve communication between the child psychiatrist and paediatrician, and both practitioners seem equally at fault. In one study, only 25 % of paediatricians communicate with a child psychiatrist when referring their patients. Interestingly, 66 % thought that prior communication would result in improved patient outcomes after the consultation. On the other side of the equation, only 14 % receive information back from the psychiatrist after their patient is seen. More than 90 % of paediatricians reported that they are more likely to get communication from surgeons and other medical subspecialists than psychiatrists. Most paediatricians (88 %) reported that the family is the primary source of information about the content of the psychiatric consultation, while only 14 % of the paediatricians thought the family was a dependable source of information.[47]

With regard to clinical activity, the major area that seems to be starved of child psychiatric input is training. When paediatricians were asked about mental health, most (89 %) did not feel adequately trained in psychiatric care and thought more training should be included in residency (92 %) and continuing medical education (95 %).[47] In fact, lack of knowledge was cited as the primary reason that paediatricians did not prescribe selective serotonin reuptake inhibitor (SSRI) medications for depression to children and adolescents – not the black box warning, nor concerns about time.

The interface between neurology and psychiatry

Another example where there is ripe opportunity for collaboration is the area where psychiatry, neurology and neuropsychology intersect, not only because of the inherent similarity between these fields, but also because so many psychiatric disorders result from 'faulty wiring' in some way, and the more we learn about the pathology behind psychiatric disorders, the more and more outdated the terms 'organic' and 'non-organic' illness become. Although psychiatrists may not be responsible now for treating illnesses that were once considered psychiatric (such as epilepsy), there is enough literature to support minor neurological exam findings in many of their patients.[48–50] What follows is a brief discussion of selected common psychiatric conditions and some of the neurological components of how these conditions present. Although it is an area that is relatively underdeveloped in relation to the rest of neurology and psychiatry, increased knowledge about this area of crossover is not only a potential goldmine for future research, but also one that has built-in potential for collaboration between these fields.

In psychiatry, the doctor's primary objective tool is the mental status exam, which comments on the patient's appearance, behaviour, cooperation, speech, thought process and content, affect, insight and cognition. The latter may include testing of some aspects of memory, attention and executive function.[1] The goal is to screen for mood, thought, cognitive and anxiety disorders. Because many of those disorders involve verbal expression of subjective internal states, the exam is also largely verbally driven. A disadvantage is that patients unable to express themselves may be misunderstood and misdiagnosed (one example is patients being misdiagnosed as schizophrenic because they describe hearing 'voices'). Because of this risk, the importance of collateral information from family, friends and others who know a patient becomes more important (whereas, in other parts of medicine, it is not stressed nearly as much).[1,2] And, while laboratory studies may show abnormalities that can hint at reasons for psychiatric diagnoses, there are as yet no laboratory markers for most psychiatric illnesses.[51]

In neurology, the doctor's primary objective tool is the physical exam – examination of the general appearance and state of the patient, his or her mental status and, potentially, many of the same aspects of the psychiatric cognitive exam. In addition, there is testing of the cranial nerves, strength, reflexes, coordination, gait, and cardiovascular system to pick up major neurological signs, such as an upgoing toe or clonus.[50] Afterwards, a wide range of laboratory and radiological tests can be employed to screen for signs not readily seen on the physical exam. Unlike psychiatry, which still relies mainly on clinical judgment, neurology is now at the point where many diagnoses can be made in large part using these tests (e.g. EEGs, CT scans, MRIs).

The neuropsychiatric exam takes the mental status exam of psychiatry and combines it with the physical exam of neurology. Psychiatrists may already employ some of these techniques in examining for extrapyramidal symptoms from antipsychotics, for instance with the Abnormal Involuntary Movement Scale, which already examines for the presence of abnormal gait, dysdiadochokinesis, motor impersistence, muscle tone, mirror and overflow movements, tremors and choreoathetosis.[50,52] In essence, as stated by Sanders and Keshaven,[50] 'the objective of the psychiatric neurological exam...[is] evaluating performance decrements in psychiatric patients without identifiable neurological disorders...Such assessments may be described in terms of degree of performance decrements rather than by the presence or absence of abnormality.' These minor neurological abnormalities described above are often called 'soft signs' or 'neurodevelopmental signs', as they are often seen in immature or elderly nervous systems.[52] They are not easily localized, which makes them distinct from so-called 'hard' (reliable/reproducible) signs, such as asymmetric reflexes. Soft signs are seen in a variety of psychiatric disorders and can be broken down into three main areas, as shown in Box 14.2.

In the dementias there are a number of these minor neurological signs. Primitive reflexes, olfactory deficits, and pyramidal and extrapyramidal signs are correlated with disease severity.[50] One question that often comes up is whether the so-called 'dementia' is actually depression ('pseudodementia'), and the presence of these neurological signs can help distinguish between the two. In Alzheimer's dementia, astereognosis, agraphesthesia, olfactory deficits, hyperreflexia, upgoing toes, extrapyramidal choreoathetosis and cerebellar signs such as dysmetria have all been described. Lewy body dementia, in particular, is characterized by the presence of early parkinsonian extrapyramidal signs.[50]

Schizophrenia has a long history of abnormal movements, even before the neuroleptic era. Hollander *et al.*[52] estimate that there are minor neurological abnormalities present in 50–65% of schizophrenics (vs around 5% for healthy controls). All of the abnormalities present in Box 14.2 have been described in schizophrenics. Interestingly, some of these same soft signs have been seen in schizophrenics who have not been exposed to antipsychotics.[52]

Compared with thought disorders, there has been much less work done on the presence of soft signs in mood disorders, and what has been done suggests that patients with mood disorders have milder or less visible neurological abnormalities than their counterparts with psychosis. In addition, although there does not seem to be a clear difference in

> **Box 14.2** Examples of 'soft' neurological signs and ways they might present on testing[50]
>
> *Integrative sensory dysfunction*
> - Agraphesthesia (e.g. difficulty recognizing numbers drawn on one's hand)
> - Astereognosis (e.g. difficulty recognizing objects placed in one's hand)
> - Right/left confusion (e.g. difficulty identifying one's own right and left or those of the examiner)
> - Impaired auditory/visual integration (e.g. difficulty with figure copying or cube drawing)
>
> *Motor incoordination*
> - Dysarthria (e.g. difficulty enunciating or speaking)
> - Gait ataxia (e.g. difficulty keeping one's balance when walking)
> - Dysmetria (e.g. difficulty with finger to nose testing)
> - Dysdiadochokinesia (e.g. difficulty with rapid alternating movements)

neurological presentation between bipolar and unipolar depression, frontal and parietal lobe deficits (motor sequencing difficulty, astereognosis and agraphesthesia) have been described in bipolar patients.[50,52]

Interestingly, there is a fair amount of literature dealing with primary anxiety disorders and the presence of soft signs. In obsessive-compulsive disorder (OCD), the right hemisphere may play a role in the disease, and a number of studies have looked at right caudate volume/metabolism as well as right orbitofrontal metabolism and their correlates to OCD severity and response to treatment. In a 12-week, double-blind, randomized controlled trial by Hollander *et al.*,[52] in which 117 patients with OCD were treated with either fluvoxamine (100–300 mg daily) or placebo, treatment non-responders had more left-sided visuospatial difficulties (difficulties with cube drawing, left > right asymmetry on left/right differentiation testing) and more left-sided sensory problems (astereognosis, agraphesthesia), which the authors correlated with potential problems in the right (generally non-dominant) parietal lobe. In a study looking at male and female patients with post-traumatic stress disorder (PTSD), there seemed to be more soft signs (decreased motor sequencing, more cube drawing difficulties) among those who developed PTSD than those who did not.[53]

The value in looking for these signs is not that their presence will necessarily change your management. However, they are tangible evidence of minor neurological lesions and may become more significant in the future when we understand more about the biological basis of psychiatric illnesses. Testing for neurological soft signs requires relatively little time and can be easily incorporated into a standard mental status exam. In settings that are more psychoanalytically inclined, or situations where laying hands on a patient may be harmful (e.g. for someone with a history of sexual abuse), many of these tests can be done without any physical contact. Lastly, being able to perform a competent exam of a patient not only maintains skills developed during training, but can give ammunition when working with other services, who may not expect psychiatrists to perform their own physical exams.[5,48,49]

Conclusions

It seems sometimes that psychiatric issues have the power to elicit contrasting reactions among colleagues from other specialties: some would idealize psychiatry or are fascinated with it; others despise or ridicule it. Both attitudes are recognizable in consultants coming to the psychiatric ward or referring their patients to psychiatry, and have many effects on the care of patients. But there is a twist in all this, as well as an element of personal responsibility. While psychiatrists may complain about how they and their patients are viewed, it does mean that they have the opportunity to practise their craft out of love for the subject. And, as stated in *The House of God*,[40] though psychiatrists may have to put up with contempt from other physicians, those same physicians often change their tune should they themselves end up in therapy (or, one might add, should their children end up in therapy). Lastly, psychiatrists also have a responsibility to educate others about what they do. Just like in therapy, we cannot change others, but we can change ourselves. If we are unsatisfied with how we are viewed as a speciality, then it is up to us to do what we can to change that perception. Part of that image comes from our role in taking care of patients – not just taking care of their mental health, but their health in general. And that often comes down to working with physicians from other fields.

References

1. Kaplan HI. History of psychosomatic medicine. In: Sadock BJ, Sadock VA (eds) *Kaplan and Sadock's Comprehensive Textbook of Psychiatry*, 8th edn. Philadelphia, VA: Lippincott Williams & Wilkins, 2005; pp. 2105–2112.

2. Robinson D. *Conducting Psychiatric Consultations Explained*. Port Huron, MI: Rapid Psychler Press, 2000.
3. Engel GL. The need for a new medical model: a challenge for biomedicine. *Science* 1977; **196**: 129–136.
4. Fava GA. The decline of pharmaceutical psychiatry and the increasing role of psychological medicine. *Psychother Psychosom* 2009; **78**: 220–227.
5. Green MR. How to maintain your basic medical skills. In: Foreman T, Dickstein LJ, Garakani A (eds) *A Resident's Guide to Surviving Psychiatric Training*, 2nd edn. Arlington: American Psychiatric Association, 2007; pp. 8–10.
6. Lloyd GG. A sense of proportion: the place of psychiatry in medicine. *J Roy Soc Med* 1996; **89**: 563–567.
7. Lipsitt DR. Psychiatry and the general hospital in an age of uncertainty. *World Psychiatry* 2003; **2**: 87–92.
8. Green MR. Psychiatrists are "real doctors" too: finding your place in the world of medicine. In: Foreman T, Dickstein LJ, Garakani A (eds) *A Resident's Guide to Surviving Psychiatric Training*, 2nd edn. Arlington: American Psychiatric Association, 2007; pp. 5–7.
9. Van De Feltz-Cornelis CM, Van Os TW, Van Marwijk HW *et al.* Effect of psychiatric consultation models in primary care. A systematic review and meta-analysis of randomized clinical trials. *J Psychosom Res* 2010; **68**: 521–533.
10. Rigatelli M, Ferrari S, Uguzzoni U *et al.* Teaching and training in the psychiatric-psychosomatic consultation-liaison setting. *Psychother Psychosom* 2000; **69**: 221–228.
11. Diefenbacher A, Strain JJ. Consultation-liaison psychiatry: stability and change over a 10-year-period. *Gen Hosp Psychiatry* 2002; **24**: 249–256.
12. Strain JJ, Strain JJ, Mustafa S *et al.* Consultation-liaison psychiatry literature database (2003 update). Part I: Consultation-liaison literature database: 2003 update and national lists. *Gen Hosp Psychiatry* 2003; **25**: 378–385.
13. Huyse FJ, Herzog T, Lobo A *et al.* European consultation-liaison services and their user populations: the European Consultation-Liaison Workgroup Collaborative Study. *Psychosomatics* 2000; **41**: 330–338.
14. Huyse FJ, Herzog T, Lobo A *et al.* European Consultation-Liaison Psychiatric Services: the ECLW Collaborative Study. *Acta Psychiatry Scand* 2000; **101**: 360–366.
15. Huyse FJ, Herzog T, Lobo A *et al.* Consultation-Liaison psychiatric service delivery: results from a European study. *Gen Hosp Psychiatry* 2001; **23**: 124–132.
16. Dimsdale JE, Dantzer R. A biological substrate for somatoform disorders: importance of pathophysiology. *Psychosom Med* 2007; **69**: 850–854.
17. Smith GC. From consultation-liaison psychiatry to integrated care for multiple and complex needs. *Aust NZ J Psychiatry* 2009; **43**: 1–12.
18. de Jonge P, Honig A, van Melle JP *et al.* Nonresponse to treatment for depression following myocardial infarction: association with subsequent cardiac events. *Am J Psychiatry* 2007; **164**: 1371–1378.

19. Bradfield JWB. A pathologist's perspective of the somatoform disorders. *J Psychosom Res* 2006; **60**: 327–330.
20. Strain JJ, Blumenfield M. Challenges for consultation-liaison psychiatry in the 21st century. *Psychosomatics* 2008; **49**: 93–96.
21. Kathol RG, Kunkel EJS, Weiner JS *et al*. Psychiatrists for medically complex patients: bringing value at the physical health and mental health/substance-use disorder interface. *Psychosomatics* 2009; **50**: 93–107.
22. Katon W, Unutzer J, Wells K *et al*. Collaborative depression care: history, evolution and ways to enhance dissemination and sustainability. *Gen Hosp Psychiatry* 2010; **32**: 456–464.
23. Kathol R, Stoudemire A. Strategic integration of inpatient and outpatient medical-psychiatry services. In: Wise MG, Rundell JR (eds) *Textbook of Consultation-Liaison Psychiatry*, 2nd edn. Washington, DC: American Psychiatric Publishing Inc., 2002; pp. 995–1014.
24. Leue C, Driessen G, Strik JJ *et al*. Managing complex patients on a medical psychiatric unit: an observational study of university hospital costs associated with medical service use, length of stay, and psychiatric intervention. *J Psychosom Res* 2010; **68**: 295–302.
25. Trzepacz PT. The Delirium Rating Scale. Its use in consultation-liaison research. *Psychosomatics* 1999; **40**: 193–204.
26. Inouye SK, Schlesinger MJ, Lydon TJ. Delirium: a symptom of how hospital care is failing older persons and a window to improve quality of hospital care. *Am J Med* 1999; **106**: 565–573.
27. Inouye SK, Rubin FH, Wierman HR *et al*. No shortcuts for delirium prevention. *J Am Geriatr Soc* 2010; **58**: 998–999.
28. Monteleone P, Martiadis V, Maj M. Management of schizophrenia with obesity, metabolic, and endocrinological disorders. *Psychiatr Clin N Am* 2009; **32**: 775–794.
29. Hafizi S, Favaron E. Interferon-induced depression: mechanisms and management. *Br J Hosp Med* 2007; **68**: 307–310.
30. Duddu V, Husain N, Dickens C. Medically unexplained presentations and quality of life: a study of a predominantly South Asian primary care population in England. *J Psychosom Res* 2008; **65**: 311–317.
31. Jackson JL, Kroenke K. Prevalence, impact, and prognosis of multisomatoform disorder in primary care: a 5-year follow-up study. *Psychosom Med* 2008; **70**: 430–434.
32. olde Hartman TC, Borghuis MS, Lucassen PLBJ *et al*. Medically unexplained symptoms, somatisation disorder and hypochondriasis: course and prognosis. A systematic review. *J Psychosom Res* 2009; **66**: 363–377.
33. olde Hartman TC, Hassink-Franke LJ, Lucassen PL *et al*. Explanation and relations. How do general practitioners deal with patients with persistent medically unexplained symptoms: a focus group study. *BMC Fam Pract* 2009; **10**: 68.
34. Kanaan RAA, Lepine JP, Wessely SC. The association or otherwise of the functional somatic syndromes. *Psychosom Med* 2007; **69**: 855–859.

35. Diefenbacher A. Psychiatry and psychosomatic medicine in Germany: lessons to be learned? *Aust NZ J Psychiatry* 2005; **39**: 782–794.

36. Stone J, Hewett R, Carson A *et al.* The 'disappearance' of hysteria: historical mystery or illusion? *J Roy Soc Med* 2008; **101**: 12–18.

37. Sumathipala A, Siribaddana S, Abeysingha MR *et al.* Cognitive-behavioural therapy v. structured care for medically unexplained symptoms: randomised controlled trial. *Br J Psychiatry* 2008; **193**: 51–59.

38. Morriss R, Gask L, Dowrick C *et al.* Randomized trial of reattribution on psychosocial talk between doctors and patients with medically unexplained symptoms. *Psychol Med* 2010; **40**: 325–333.

39. Caplan JP, Epstein LA, Stern TA. Consultants' conflicts: a case discussion of differences and their resolution. *Psychosomatics* 2008; **49**: 8–13.

40. Shem S. *The House of God*. New York: Bantam Dell, 2003.

41. Kanner L. *Child Psychiatry*, 3rd edn. Springfield: Thomas, 1957.

42. Kraemer S. "The menace of psychiatry": does it still ring a bell? *Arch Dis Child* 2009; **94**: 570–572.

43. Olson AL, Kemper KJ, Kelleher KJ *et al.* Primary care pediatricians' roles and perceived responsibilities in the identification and management of maternal depression. *Pediatrics* 2002; **110**: 1169–1176.

44. Burket R, Hodgin J. Pediatricians' perceptions of child psychiatry consultations. *Psychosomatics* 1993; **34**: 402–408.

45. Connor DF, McLaughlin TJ, Jeffers-Terry M *et al.* Targeted child psychiatric services: a new model of pediatric primary clinician-child psychiatry collaborative care. *Clin Pediatr* 2006; **45**: 423–434.

46. Heneghan A, Garner AS, StorferIsser A *et al.* Pediatricians' role in providing mental health care for children and adolescents: do pediatricians and child and adolescent psychiatrists agree? *J Dev Behav Pediatr* 2008; **29**: 262–269.

47. Ross W, Chan E, Harris S *et al.* Pediatric experience with psychiatric collaboration. *J Dev Behav Pediatr* 2004; **25**: 377–378.

48. Buchanan RW, Heinrichs DW. The neurological evaluation scale (NES): a structured instrument for the assessment of neurological signs in schizophrenia. *Psychiatr Res* 1988; **21**: 335–350.

49. Chen EYH, Shapleske J, Luque R *et al.* The Cambridge neurological inventory: A clinical instrument for assessment of soft neurological signs in psychiatric patients. *Psychiatr Res* 1995; **56**: 183–204.

50. Sanders RD, Keshaven MS. The neurologic examination in adult psychiatry: from soft signs to hard science. *J Neuropsych Clin N* 1998; **10**: 395–404.

51. Morihisa JM, Rosse RB, Cross CD. Laboratory and other diagnostic tests in psychiatry. In: Hales RE, Yudofsky SC (eds) *The American Psychiatric Press Synopsis of Psychiatry*. Arlington, VA: American Psychiatric Press, 1996; pp. 271–301.

52. Hollander E, Kaplan A, Schmeidler J *et al.* Neurological soft signs as predictors of treatment response to selective serotonin reuptake inhibitors in obsessive-compulsive disorder. *J Neuropsych Clin N* 2005; **17**: 472–477.

53. Gurvits TV, Gilbertson MW, Lasko NB *et al.* Neurological status of combat veterans and adult survivors of sexual abuse PTSD. *Ann NY Acad Sci* 1997; **21**: 468–71.
54. Moore DP, Jefferson J. *Handbook of Medical Psychiatry*. Boston: Mosby, 1996.
55. Jones KL. *Smith's Recognizable Patterns of Human Malformation*. Philadelphia: Elsevier, 2006.

CHAPTER 15

Where they need us... Opportunities for young psychiatrists to help in developing countries

Felipe Picon

Department of Psychiatry, Federal University of Rio Grande do Sul, Porto Alegre, RS, Brazil

Introduction

In recent years there has been a significant increase in awareness and concern about mental health problems affecting developing countries. In 2001, the World Health Organization Report *Mental Health: New Understanding, New Hope*[1] brought light to the difficulties and possible ways of dealing with this challenge. Unfortunately, mental health problems are a common burden in developing countries, with more than 25 % of people worldwide presenting with at least one psychiatric disorder at some point in their lives.[1] This report and others on psychiatric training[2,3] clearly show the efforts towards the development of mental health care worldwide.

According to the World Bank,[4] developing countries are those countries with middle and low rates of gross national income (GNI) per capita. This group encompasses the majority of the countries in the world, and comprises 5.5 billion people of the 6.7 billion people in the world today.[5] These countries present a wide variety of stages of economic development, sociocultural characteristics, historical and ethnic backgrounds, even though they all fall into the same category.

Just as these countries have economic and social needs, psychiatric care is also a field that requires attention. Considering the burden of

How to Succeed in Psychiatry: A Guide to Training and Practice, First Edition.
Edited by Andrea Fiorillo, Iris Tatjana Calliess and Henning Sass.
© 2012 John Wiley & Sons, Ltd. Published 2012 by John Wiley & Sons, Ltd.

psychiatric disorders, the improvement of mental health status is also a primary goal for overall development. Early career psychiatrists are among the key professionals charged with the development of psychiatry and mental health care in these countries. Opportunities arise despite the sometimes overwhelming difficulties these countries face.

The public image of psychiatry

Historically, in many developing countries mental health problems were either dealt with by traditional healers or as a problem to be segregated from the community in centralized asylums.[6] Knowledge and attitudes about mental disorders among the general population, and also among primary health-care workers, are generally rudimentary or inaccurate. This situation causes an important obstacle for the adequate provision of care for those in need.[7] In many countries, knowledge about how to treat mental disorders is undermined by prejudices and false beliefs, usually related to the supposed dangerousness of psychiatric patients or to the impossibility or difficulty of treating mental disorders. The way the general population perceives psychiatry and psychiatric patients has a crucial role in the delivery of psychiatric treatment and influences the status of mental health professionals, with a consequent detrimental effect on medical students' attitudes toward psychiatry.[8] It is imperative that comprehensive and innovative strategies are introduced for the general population and mental health care workers in order to improve their understanding of how psychiatric disorders can be recognized, managed and prevented.

In the last decades, progressive changes in the way psychiatry is seen by the general population enabled the development of governmental policies for better mental health assistance in many developing countries. Following the Italian movement from 1978,[9] when the mental health system was shifted from asylums to community-oriented services, psychiatric reforms happened in various countries,[10–12] thus creating a growing demand for trained professionals. The need arose not only for more psychiatrists, but also for nurses, social workers and psychologists with a focused training in the care of the mentally ill. Overall, more opportunities for early career psychiatrists can be created and more mental health facilities developed if the general public's knowledge about psychiatry and mental health issues is improved and if fears and prejudices about psychiatric patients are reduced.

Economic influences

Several studies link poverty and/or economic difficulties with a greater susceptibility to psychiatric disorders.[13–16] Lund *et al.*[16] showed that variables such as education, food insecurity, housing, social class, socio economic status and financial stress have a relatively consistent and strong association with common mental disorders (depression and anxiety) while others, such as income, employment and particularly consumption, were more equivocal. Pragmatic actions, such as supplying money directly to those in need, showed both positive and negative impacts on mental health, as reported by Plagerson et al.[17] This study explored the potential for a poverty alleviation programme to contribute to breaking the vicious cycle between poverty and common mental disorders. The influence of socioeconomic status in enhancing the risk for mental disorders is of particular importance for early career psychiatrists in developing countries, because their work will eventually have to face these economic aspects. A review of 11 community studies on the link between poverty and common mental disorders in six low- and middle-income countries (Brazil, Chile, Indonesia, Lesotho, Pakistan and Zimbabwe) showed an association between indicators of poverty and the risk of mental disorders, the most consistent being low levels of education. This study also showed the vicious circle of direct and indirect costs of mental illness and a worsening economic situation – as the severity and duration of mental illness increases, the less economically active that person becomes.[18]

Early career psychiatrists should be aware of these aspects and of the possible difficulties that might arise when working in these countries. Although early career psychiatrists usually may be able to find many different alternatives and solutions to clinical and organizational problems, in particular in difficult situations, they are not able to supply any economic aid for their patients. In order to create better mental health policies, the best way to help is to work in collaboration with local governments; early career psychiatrists can contribute by participating in research activities that will serve as basis for the inclusion of mental health on the agenda of development agencies and international non-governmental organizations.[18]

Where do they need us?

There is a shortage of psychiatrists to meet the needs of mental health care even in high-income countries.[19–21] In low- and middle-income countries, this lack of specialists is even more profound.[22] In some countries the lack of psychiatrists is also related to an very unequal distribution of professionals within the country. In Brazil, for example, there is a higher proportion of psychiatrists working in the states nearest to the coast, while the interior of the country has very few professionals in this field. In their study, Moraes et al.[23] focused only on the availability of child and adolescent psychiatrists, and a slightly better status for adult psychiatrists would be expected. Brazil is an example of a country with an appreciable number of psychiatric training institutions (68 residency programmes with a total of 967 residents per year)[24] and a considerable number of new psychiatrists per year (around 367), but it still faces a shortage. Opportunities for early career psychiatrists in Brazil are currently high as the country is experiencing a period of economic growth, social improvements and also approval of new psychiatry residency programmes,[25] with more jobs for trainees and for supervisors.

India, the second most populated country in the world, also has an insufficient number of psychiatrists. It is a multicultural society where people frequently seek help from religious and traditional healers for mental health problems, although in many parts of the country modern health services are available. During its 10-year duration, the Indian National Mental Health Programme increased significantly the budget for mental health care services, which led to improvement of training opportunities for the different mental health professionals. Moreover, there has recently been a major increase of private psychiatric institutions to cater to growing demand from increasingly affluent sectors of society.[26]

In Africa, many countries are following the World Health Organization statements for the development of community-based mental health services. This model of care seems difficult to adopt in these countries, mainly because of the acute shortage of trained professionals, the absence of social services and also the dominant role of traditional healers in dealing with mental disorders.[27] However, these challenging scenarios present many opportunities for early career psychiatrists. Alem *et al.* report that in Ethiopia there are only 18 psychiatrists for 77 million people, and that there is no clinical psychologist nor any trained social worker.[27] This situation is similar to that in other African countries, where the few available psychiatrists work in the main cities. The situation seems to be even more serious in countries like the Republic of Chad, Eritrea and Liberia, where there is only one psychiatrist per country, and in Rwanda and Togo, where only two psychiatrists are active.[28] South Africa is undergoing significant changes in the organization and delivery of mental health care. Even with the heritage of an under-resourced, fragmented, racially inequitable service, heavily reliant on chronic custodial treatment in large centralized institutions, the new policy has strengthened the importance of community-based, comprehensive and integrated mental health services.[29]

Egypt also has recently undergone important mental health policy changes. A six-year mental health reform programme (2002–2007; Egymen) was initiated through an Egyptian-Finnish project, which brought still ongoing improvements in the way health organizations are structured.[30] Kenya also implemented reforms in its health system in order to deal with mental health problems more equitably.[31] Vietnam, still characterized by unclear policy and a number of limitations, has initiated the mapping of its mental health situation as a first step towards a more comprehensive care of psychiatric patients.[32]

Countries undergoing severe social crisis, such as natural disasters, political conflicts and wars, are usually places where the population has severe need for medical and psychiatric help. A recently publicized example is Haiti, but there are many other examples worldwide. Physicians from many countries went to help in Haiti right after the earthquakes in 2010 and soon after a first phase of aid, mental health professionals were also requested.[33] Disaster psychiatry is a specific field within the specialty that has become increasingly necessary with the growing number of places where the population is struggling with a natural disaster, socio-political instability or armed conflict.[34] Another example is Indonesia, where the 2004 tsunami brought chaos to the country, which subsequently received psychiatric aid as well as many other types of medical and social assistance.[35] Sadly, situations like these are not likely to end. Early career psychiatrists will have opportunities to provide their help in these particularly difficult scenarios. Websites where readers can find relevant information on how to help in these situations are listed in Table 15.1.

The further development of structured mental health services in developing countries is another future challenge for early career

Table 15.1 Web-based references of opportunities for early career psychiatrists.

Airline Ambassadors International	http://www.airlineamb.org/
American Psychiatric Association Disaster Psychiatry Resources	http://www.psych.org/Resources/DisasterPsychiatry.aspx
AmeriCares	http://www.americares.org/
Association Medicale Haitienne	http://www.amhhaiti.org/
Haitian American Psychiatric Association	www.hapa84.com
Heart to Heart International	http://www.hearttoheart.org/
International Federation of Red Cross and Red Crescent Societies	http://www.ifrc.org
Medecins sans Frontières/Doctors without Borders	http://www.doctorswithoutborders.org
Operation USA	http://www.opusa.org/
Pan American Health Organization	http://new.paho.org/
The Salvation Army International	http://www.salvationarmy.org/
United Nations	http://www.un.org/
World Health Organization	http://www.who.int/

psychiatrists. Saxena *et al.* suggested five key areas for expansion to achieve general adult mental health care: (i) outpatient or ambulatory clinics; (ii) mobile community mental health teams for outreach services; (iii) acute inpatient care; (iv) long-term community-based residential care; and (v) rehabilitation, occupation and work.[28] However, it is important to say that the amount of work necessary to accomplish these tasks is overwhelming in most of the developing world. In Brazil, for example, the same wave of reforms as happened in other countries has been ongoing since 1986. The government is still investing in new Psychosocial Care Centers (CAPS – *centro de atenção psicossocial*) around the country. These facilities are designed to assist patients in their own community with a multi-professional approach that includes psychiatrists, neurologists, nurses, nutritionists, pharmacists, speech therapists, psychologists, social workers, music therapists, occupational therapists, physiotherapists, physical education teachers and nursery technicians.[36] Psychiatrists can also work as supervisors for other mental health professionals. The system being developed in Brazil accords with the proposal by Saxena *et al.*[28] and enhances the job opportunities for young psychiatrists as many of these centres are created.

Another major focus for early career psychiatrists is to advance scientific knowledge of mental health. Up to now most psychiatric scientific knowledge has come from developed countries. Since psychiatric disorders very often have socio-cultural influences, the use of findings from American or European studies might not fully apply to populations from the developing countries. In 2009, Kieling *et al.*[37] found 222 indexed publications; of these, 213 originated from high-income countries, only 9 (4 %) derived from middle-income countries and none was from a low-income country. With the help of the World Psychiatric Association, in two years four new journals were included in the databases: one from Brazil, two from South Africa and one from Turkey.[37] The aspirations of early career psychiatrists to change these figures will be of vital importance for enhancing the representation of clinicians and researchers from low- and middle-income countries in the international scientific community.

Apart from the purely scientific importance of this discrepancy, the development of research in developing countries may also contribute to changes in care delivery. As more and more well-conducted studies describe and analyse the many aspects of mental health in developing countries, more possibilities for funding will be created, because evidence from good research provides the knowledge needed for policy changes. Governments are more precisely guided when there is scientifically based knowledge of the problem to be dealt. Since each country has its own characteristics, ideally there should be country-specific scientific knowledge about what would be the optimal mental health situation for each individual country. Research from developing countries should become much more prominent in future, considering that the majority of psychiatric patients reside in these countries. This is a huge opportunity for contemporary early career psychiatrists.

Conclusions

Even though we cannot underestimate the burden that economic difficulties might place on a person or on a whole country, developing countries are full of opportunities for early career psychiatrists. However, young psychiatrists should be aware of the potential difficulties of delivering psychiatric treatment to an optimal standard, because of the socioeconomic restrictions that they and most of their patients will face. Also, young psychiatrists should be aware of the cultural difficulties that often surround mental health problems. One way of dealing with these difficulties is to be engaged in mental health policies and government programmes that aid and support the improvement of mental health assistance and the education of the population about mental health issues.

Overseas rotations are an important opportunity for early career psychiatrists from developing countries to improve their capacities and bring home wider knowledge and experience.[38] Also, applying as a mental health professional volunteer with one of the many non-governmental organizations worldwide is an important way to gain know-how in disaster psychiatry while making a great difference for the survivors. Helping people from other countries in extreme and difficult situations, like natural disasters or in refugee camps, can also be a great opportunity for personal as well as professional development.

Other opportunities for career improvements have been highlighted by the World Psychiatric Association, including fellowships in well-recognized universities and academic institutions.[39] As for implementing community mental health care for adults with mental illness, guidelines and lessons learned from worldwide implementation of these services can be found online.[40] Also, materials to help the better delivery of standard psychiatric treatments are increasingly available online.[41] Certainly, early career psychiatrists from all developing countries have a difficult but thrilling challenge ahead of them.

References

1. World Health Organization. *Mental Health: New Understanding, New Hope*. The World Health Report. Geneva: World Health Organization, 2001.
2. World Health Organization. *Atlas: Psychiatric Education and Training Across the World 2005*. Geneva: World Health Organization, 2005.

3. World Health Organization. *Atlas: Child and Adolescent Mental Health Resources: Global Concerns, Implications for the Future.* Geneva: World Health Organization, 2005.
4. World Bank. How we classify countries. Available at: http://data.worldbank. org/about/country-classifications.
5. World Bank. You think! Development. Available at: http://youthink. worldbank.org/issues/development.
6. Broadhead J, Piachaud J, Birley J. Helping to promote psychiatry in less developed countries. *Adv Psychiatr Treat* 1999; **5**: 213–220.
7. Ganasen KA, Parker S, Hugo CJ *et al.* Mental health literacy: focus on developing countries. *Afr J Psychiatry* 2008; **11**: 23–28.
8. Fazel S, Ebmeier KP. Specialty choice in UK junior doctors: is psychiatry the least popular specialty for UK and international medical graduates ? *BMC Med Educ* 2009; **9**: 77.
9. Burti L. Italian psychiatric reform 20 plus years after. *Acta Psychiatry Scand* 2001; **410**: 41–46.
10. Ablard JD. Authoritarianism, democracy and psychiatric reform in Argentina, 1943–83. *Hist Psychiatry* 2003; **14**: 361–376.
11. Hirdes A. The psychiatric reform in Brazil: a (re)view. *Ciencia y Saude Coletiva* 2009; **14**: 297–305.
12. Keller RC. Pinel in the Maghreb: liberation, confinement, and psychiatric reform in French North Africa. *Bull Hist Med* 2005; **79**: 459–499.
13. Flouri E, Tzavidis N, Kallis C. Adverse life events, area socioeconomic disadvantage, and psychopathology and resilience in young children: the importance of risk factors' accumulation and protective factors' specificity. *Eur Child Adolesc Psychiatry* 2010; **19**: 535–546.
14. Nikulina V, Widom CS, Czaja S. The role of childhood neglect and childhood poverty in predicting mental health, academic achievement and crime in adulthood. *Am J Commun Psychol* 2010 (epub ahead of print).
15. Cerdá M, Diez-Roux AV, Tchetgen ET *et al.* The relationship between neighborhood poverty and alcohol use: estimation by marginal structural models. *Epidemiology* 2010; **21**: 482–489.
16. Lund C, Breen A, Flisher AJ *et al.* Poverty and common mental disorders in low and middle income countries: A systematic review. *Soc Sci Med* 2010; **71**: 517–528.
17. Plagerson S, Patel V, Harpham T *et al.* Does money matter for mental health? Evidence from the Child Support Grants in Johannesburg, South Africa. *Global Public Health* 2010; **11**: 1–17.
18. Patel V, Kleinman A. Poverty and common mental disorders in developing countries. *Bull World Health Organ* 2003; **81**: 609–615.
19. Tijdink JK, Soethout MB, Koerselman GF *et al.* The interest shown by medical students and recently qualified doctors in a career in psychiatry. *Tijdschrift voor Psychiatrie* 2008; **50**: 9–17.
20. Gowans MC, Glazier L, Wright BJ *et al.* Choosing a career in psychiatry: factors associated with a career interest in psychiatry among Canadian students on entry to medical school. *Can J Psychiatry* 2009; **54**: 557–564.

21. Becker EA, King B, Shafer A *et al* Shortage of child and adolescent psychiatrists in Texas. *Texas Med* 2010; **1**: 106.
22. Kohn R, Saxena S, Levav I *et al*. The treatment gap in mental health care. *Bull World Health Organ* 2004; **82**: 858–866.
23. Moraes C, Abujadi C, Ciasca SM *et al*. Brazilian child and adolescent psychiatrists task force. *Rev Bras Psiquiatr* 2008; **30**: 294–295.
24. Ministério da Educação do Brasil. Residências em Saúde. Available at: http://portal.mec.gov.br/index.php?option=com_content&view=article& id=12263&Itemid=507.
25. Brasil.gov. Ministérios da Saúde e Educação vão criar novos programas de residência médica (www.brasil.gov.br/noticias/arquivos/2010/12/3/minis- terios-da-saude-e-educacao-vao-criar-novos-programas-de-residencia- medica).
26. Khandelwal SK, Jhingan HP, Ramesh S *et al*. India mental health country profile. *Int Rev Psychiatry* 2004; **16**: 126–141.
27. Alem A, Jacobsson L, Hanlon C. Community-based mental health care in Africa: mental health workers' views. *World Psychiatry* 2008; **7**: 54–57.
28. Saxena S, Thornicroft G, Knapp M *et al*. Resources for mental health: scarcity, inequity, and inefficiency. *Lancet* 2007; **370**: 878–889.
29. Lund C, Flisher AJ. South African Mental Health process indicators. *J Ment Health Policy* 2001; **4**: 9–16.
30. Jenkins R, Heshmat A, Loza N *et al* Mental health policy and development in Egypt – integrating mental health into health sector reforms 2001–9. *Int J Ment Health Syst* 2010; **24**: 17.
31. Kiima D, Jenkins R. Mental health policy in Kenya – an integrated approach to scaling up equitable care for poor populations. *Int J Ment Health Syst* 2010; **28**: 19.
32. Niemi M, Thanh HT, Tuan T *et al*. Mental health priorities in Vietnam: a mixed-methods analysis. *BMC Health Serv Res* 2010; **10**: 257.
33. Bailey RK, Bailey T, Akpudo H. On the ground in Haiti: a psychia- trist's evaluation of post earthquake Haiti. *J Health Care Poor U* 2010; **21**: 417–421.
34. López-Ibor JJ Disasters and mental health: new challenges for the psychiatric profession. *World J Biol Psychiatry* 2006; **7**: 171–182.
35. Bender E. Psychiatrist answers plea to help Tsunami victims. *Psychiatr News* 2005; **40**: 10.
36. Ministério da Saúde do Brasil. Saúde Mental no SUS. Available at: www.ccs. saude.gov.br/saude_mental/pdf/SM_Sus.pdf.
37. Kieling C, Herrman H, Patel V *et al*. A global perspective on the dissemination of mental health research. *Lancet* 2009; **374**: 1500.
38. Rege S. Psychiatry in the land of the Sphinx: is an overseas elective justified? *Australas Psychiatry* 2008; **16**: 277–280.
39. Fiorillo A, Lattova Z, Brahmbhatt P *et al*. The Action Plan 2010 of the WPA Early Career Psychiatrists Council. *World Psychiatry* 2010; **9**: 62–63.

40. Thornicroft G, Alem A, Antunes Dos Santos R *et al.* WPA guidance on steps, obstacles and mistakes to avoid in the implementation of community mental health care. *World Psychiatry* 2010; **9**: 67–77.
41. Patel V, Thornicroft G. Packages of care for mental, neurological, and substance use disorders in low- and middle-income countries: *PLoS Med* 2009; **6**: e1000160.

CHAPTER 16

Professional responsibility in mental health: what early career psychiatrists really need to know

Alexander Nawka[1] and Gregory Lydall[2]
[1]Department of Psychiatry, First Faculty of Medicine, Charles University, Prague, Czech Republic
[2]Castel Hospital, La Neuve Rue, Guernsey; University College London, London, UK

Professional responsibility

Medical practice takes place within a society that expects certain standards of care from its physicians.[1] As a profession, medicine is characterized by high moral standards, including a strong commitment to the well-being of others, mastery of a body of knowledge and skills, and a high level of autonomy.[2] Psychiatry, as an integral part of medical practice, shares those standards. However, its unique clinical and ethical tensions differ to some extent from other branches of medicine.[3]

Professional responsibility implies multiple commitments – to patients, to fellow professionals, and to institutions or systems within which health care is provided.[3] It is based on mutual trust between society and professional groups.[4] Psychiatrists are often expected to make high-risk decisions in complex clinical situations. Thus, occasionally the psychiatric profession may be exposed to greater public scrutiny and criticism than other medical disciplines.[5] Early career psychiatrists should understand the real-life application of the concepts essential to being a professional psychiatrist, and be prepared for some of the most important challenges facing our profession.

How to Succeed in Psychiatry: A Guide to Training and Practice, First Edition.
Edited by Andrea Fiorillo, Iris Tatjana Calliess and Henning Sass.
© 2012 John Wiley & Sons, Ltd. Published 2012 by John Wiley & Sons, Ltd.

Professional responsibility and humanism

Professional responsibility is the legal and moral duty of a professional to apply his or her knowledge in ways that benefit the patient and wider society, without causing harm to either. Medical professionalism as we understand it today demands placing the interests of patients above those of the physician; setting and maintaining standards of competence and integrity;[6] and providing expert advice to society on matters of health.[7]

Traditionally, professionalism contains moral commitments that include a diverse range of components like empathy, respect and compassion, as well as standards expected of a physician like appropriate dress, language and habits.[7] Humanism, on the other hand, comprises a set of deep-seated personal convictions about one's obligations to others, especially those in need. Humanism manifests itself in such personal attributes as altruism, duty, integrity, respect for others and compassion.[8] These characteristics are considered essential in medical professionals too. Physicians whose professionalism lacks a solid foundation in humanism are in danger of deviating from the ethical commitments of medicine. Cohen describes the link between the concepts as: *'Humanism provides the passion that animates authentic professionalism'*.[8] One might be humanistic without being professional, but it is almost impossible to be professional without having strong humanistic roots. Simply put, humanism is *what we are* and professionalism is *what we do*. Importantly, professionalism can be learned and internalized.[9]

Professional responsibility in psychiatry

The word 'professional' traditionally means a person who has obtained a degree or qualification in a given professional field. A professional is a member of a vocation founded upon specialized educational training. Historically, professions were complex social structures, which derived from the guild system of specialized competencies. The guild system was intended to organize specialized and complex bodies of knowledge in such a way as to address both individual and societal needs.[10]

Psychiatrists are physicians with specialized knowledge of mental illness and its treatment, whose core function is to care for mentally ill patients and their families.[11] Psychiatrists share the same ethical ideals as all physicians, and are committed to the principles of compassion, fidelity, beneficence, trustworthiness, fairness, integrity, scientific and clinical excellence, social responsibility and respect.[3] Whether they are diagnosticians, treating psychiatrists, teachers, scientists or consultants, all psychiatrists are expected to follow these principles.[3]

The daily work of psychiatrists poses distinct ethical challenges. Mental illnesses directly affect thoughts, feelings, intentions, behaviours, relationships and capacity – those attributes that help define people as individuals. The therapeutic alliance between psychiatrists and patients struggling with mental illness thus has a special ethical nature.[3]

Moreover, because of their unique clinical expertise, psychiatrists are entrusted with a heightened professional obligation, that prevent patients from causing harm to themselves or others. Psychiatrists may consequently at times be required to treat patients against their will or to breach the usual expectations of confidentiality.[3]

Psychiatrists may also be called upon to assume duties of importance to society, such as consultation on legal or organizational issues. These features of psychiatric practice may therefore create greater asymmetry in interpersonal power than in other professional relationships and introduce ethical issues of broad social relevance. For all these reasons, psychiatrists are encouraged to be especially attentive to the ethical aspects of their work and to act with great professional responsibility.[3]

Core professional responsibilities

Psychiatrists' ability to discharge their role as described above is predicated on the fulfilment of the ethical principles that ground the field.[12] The core responsibilities of medical professionalism are altruism, accountability, excellence, judgment, duty, honour and respect. These are defined in more detail in Table 16.1. These responsibilities and values serve as the foundation for public trust in psychiatry, and form the basis of psychiatrists' privileged position, allowing them to enter into the lives of patients in such a deeply personal and meaningful way.[16]

Threats to professional responsibility

There are many signs that medical professionalism is under threat in the twenty-first century. Recent medical history has seen public scandals within psychiatry related to ills such as greed, misrepresentation, abuse of position and power, breaches of confidentiality and sexual harassment. Commercialized health-care markets and intrusion of market forces in the practice of medicine might also undermine the ethical foundations of medical practice and dissolve the moral precepts that have historically defined the medical profession.[17] The profession must learn from these errors, and take steps to reduce their recurrence. Complacency, paternalism, arrogance, inability to self-regulate and poor leadership also have no place in our profession.[18]

Challenges for early career psychiatrists

The six vignettes that follow may stimulate the reader to ponder over the core responsibilities and their related dilemmas, which might be

Table 16.1 Concepts of the core responsibilities.

Concept	Description
Altruism	Altruism is based on a dedication to serving the best interests of the patient and contributes to the trust that is central to the psychiatrist-patient relationship.[13] Altruism necessitates that the psychiatrist treats patients compassionately and respectfully. Psychiatrists must advocate for improved care and strive to reduce health-care inequalities and discrimination, whether based on race, gender, socioeconomic status, ethnicity, religion, or any other social category[13]
Accountability	Accountability goes beyond respecting the law by upholding professional standards of responsibility, governance and liability. Psychiatrists make complex clinical decisions and take responsibility for the clinical consequences. Where the law counteracts the best interests of the patient, the psychiatrist should feel confident in challenging the law using legal means. Psychiatrists are expected to work collaboratively to maximize patient care, be respectful of one another, and participate in the processes of self-regulation, including remediation and discipline of members who have failed to meet accepted professional standards[13]
Excellence	During training, psychiatrists must learn the relative effectiveness and risks of treatments for different disorders. Psychiatrists have a life-long duty to continue to study, apply and advance scientific knowledge, as well as maintaining their professional competence. In addition, excellence implies a capacity to see the wider picture encompassing public health and prevention issues. Overlapping with altruism, psychiatrists should also advocate for social, economic, educational and political changes that ameliorate suffering and contribute to human well-being[14]
Judgment	The practice of psychiatry is distinguished by the need for judgment in the face of uncertainty. There are currently no definitive diagnostic tests for psychiatric illness, so judgment in the face of complex evidence is a unique psychiatric skill. Without judgment, professional practice is merely technical work. There might not be a 'right' answer, but the 'best' answer in the circumstances that can be justified by the reasoning behind the decision. Psychiatrists take responsibility for these judgments and their consequences (also see 'Accountability'). Up-to-date knowledge and skills provide the explicit scientific and experiential basis for such judgments[3]

(continued overleaf)

Table 16.1 (Continued)

Concept	Description
Duty	By the principle 'duty' we mean accepting inconvenience and risk to meet patients' needs. Being available and responsive when 'on call' and providing the best possible care regardless of the patient's ability to pay, failure to follow a treatment plan, or missing an appointment. Duty also means an ongoing commitment to the patient, using psychiatric expertise for the welfare of the community, and teaching and mentoring the next generation of psychiatrists[14]
Honour	Honouring confidentiality is essential to psychiatric treatment. The rule of doctor-patient confidentiality is based in part on the special nature of psychiatric therapy as well as on the traditional ethical relationship between psychiatrists and patients. Patients' willingness to make painful, stigmatizing or embarrassing disclosures depends on their trust in the psychiatrist-patient relationship and expectation of confidentiality.[15] Psychiatrists must ensure that patients are completely and honestly informed before the patient has consented to treatment and after treatment has occurred. Psychiatrists have an obligation to recognize, disclose to the general public, and deal with conflicts of interest that may arise in the course of their professional duties and activities.[13] Where necessary to protect the safety of patients or others, psychiatrists may be bound to break confidentiality
Respect	Psychiatrists must respect human life and the dignity of the individual; they must also have respect for patient autonomy and empower people to make informed decisions about their treatment. Where patients have capacity, their decisions about their care must be paramount, with the caveat that their decisions are in keeping with ethical practice and do not lead to demands for inappropriate care. Psychiatrists must respect patients, families, nurses, medical students and colleagues. Psychiatrists should therefore never exploit patients for any sexual advantage, personal financial gain or other private purposes

revealed when dealing with real-life events. Together with the scenarios, comments with the possible solutions on the issues are provided.

In Scenario 1, issues related to research in psychiatry and informed consent are presented; these include dilemmas concerning *altruism, judgment* and *respect*.

Scenario 1

I was asked by a senior researcher from my hospital whether I would like to participate in a study dealing with social rehabilitation of patients with schizophrenia. The senior researcher explained to me that informed consent is not needed in this study, as the patients will probably not understand it correctly. Part of the study involved a questionnaire on the history of sexual abuse in the family. The study did not consider how to offer patients a chance to discuss those sensitive topics after the interview. I expressed my concerns to the senior researcher; however, his response was uncaring and he did not communicate these concerns to the patients' treating clinicians. I was very disappointed and wanted to stop my involvement in this study.

Comments
Psychiatrists should strive to protect patients' best interests at all times, especially those lacking mental capacity to protect themselves. This should apply in both clinical and non-clinical (such as research) scenarios. Informed consent and best interest principles should form the basis of all interactions and interventions between psychiatrists and their patients.[15]

In Scenario 2 we present issues dealing with impaired colleagues and how to respond to the unethical conduct of colleagues. This scenario includes dilemmas concerning *accountability, duty* and *respect*.

Scenario 2

Early in my career as a psychiatric trainee I was sharing accommodation with a colleague, who soon became a friend. He was often withdrawn, untalkative, distracted and he looked sad. It took me more than a year to find out that he had been struggling with misuse of sedatives and hypnotics. Complaints were received from patients and staff about his emotionally distant approach and reluctance to engage, as well as lateness. I also recollected that whole packages of benzodiazepines had gone missing from the ward. I confronted him about his problem. He was then very angry and said that if I reported him I would be a traitor. On the one hand I didn't want to cause him more trouble, but on the other hand I knew that it might easily lead to neglect of his responsibilities and result in risk to patients. I didn't know what to do.

Comments

All physicians including psychiatrists must ensure that their health is robust enough to facilitate safe treatment of patients. However, physical and mental health issues, including substance misuse, can lead to ill-health amongst psychiatrists leaving them and, more importantly, their patients vulnerable. It is important that every psychiatrist recognizes the importance of maintaining their own good health in the delivery of high-quality patient care. Additionally, to protect the best interests of patients, all psychiatrists have a responsibility to raise any concerns about the health of their colleagues, initially directly with the colleague and if necessary with others, through appropriate channels.[15]

In Scenario 3 are issues that include dealing with sensitive information and the use of electronic media, which cover the concepts of *excellence, judgment* and *honour*.

Scenario 3

The board exam was imminent. A reporter from the local newspaper approached me via a social networking website after I had recently published an article on social phobia in a magazine. She liked the article and explained that she was also experiencing similar problems, which was why she was using electronic media instead of personal communication. It felt like I was chatting to both journalist and patient, which was confusing for me. After half an hour of an interesting chat, I accidentally found an identifiable detail about the patient I had described in the magazine. I felt dreadful. I asked the journalist not to name the patient under any circumstances, and she promised not to. After the chat I had thoughts that I had crossed the line. In the end the journalist kept her word and prepared a very interesting and educational article for her local newspaper without mentioning any patient details.

Comments

Patient confidentiality is a prime responsibility of all doctors, especially psychiatrists – given both the sensitive nature of the information often revealed in therapy sessions as well as the mental state of a patient, which might affect their capacity to protect their own information. Breaking confidentiality is a very serious decision and confidentiality should only be breached when a judgment is made that not breaching confidentiality would threaten the safety of the patient in a significant way. Any patient information should only be revealed to a third party with the explicit, specific and capacious consent of a patient. Accidental breaches of confidentiality should in most circumstances be discussed with the patient, but this also depends on the patient's mental state at the time (and their overall best interest) and local policies and national legislation governing such breaches. As depicted in this example, whilst it is important to engage with the media to raise the profile of mental illness and reduce the stigma related to it, this should never be a forum for breaching patient confidentiality, and any such discussions should be restricted to general information regarding mental health issues rather than specific information about an individual patient, unless the patient has consented to this and has mental capacity to give such a consent.[15]

In Scenario 4, issues about the just distribution of scarce resources and financial conflicts of interest in relations with the pharmaceutical industry are presented. These include dilemmas concerning the concepts of *altruism, honour* and *respect*.

Scenario 4

The hospital I joined had a longstanding relationship with the pharmaceutical industry, and had received significant funding from this relationship over the years. Patients in clinical trials for industry would often be prioritized for investigations and treatment to meet research deadlines. When a representative from a pharmaceutical company asked me to assist in a trial, I was almost honoured. Part of my contract with the hospital was to arrange a CT scan for all the patients with bipolar disorder enrolled in a study. On one occasion, a patient from neurology was sent for an urgent CT scan but was only scanned after three patients in an industry-sponsored trial in order to meet a study deadline. In this case, the delay in scanning resulted in late diagnosis of an intracranial bleed, with resultant morbidity for that patient. The indication for routine CT scans of our patients had never been questioned because of the 'tradition' of the hospital. However, after that incident I could no longer participate in such studies. I was ashamed of what my hospital had been doing for funding.

Comments
There are important overall gains for patients consequent on health-care professionals engaging in research in collaboration with the pharmaceutical industry. Additionally, such research can often provide important resources that would otherwise not be available to a significant number of patients. However, individual and collective patient care must never be compromised by any conflict of interests that might arise for psychiatrists or their health-care organizations because of such collaborations, and such collaborations should only be undertaken with the explicit understanding that evidence-based medicine, overall patient care and individual patient's best interests would always take precedence over any other interests or arrangements.[15]

In Scenario 5 we discuss seeking professional consultation and innovative clinical practice, which cover dilemmas concerning *accountability, excellence* and *judgment*.

Scenario 5

I have an elderly patient with recurrent depression since childhood. Despite our best treatment her condition deteriorated. I had followed the national and international guidelines, had searched the literature and followed my clinical experience. I had tried combinations of antidepressants, augmentation and lastly electroconvulsive therapy, but to no effect. Both she and I were becoming desperate. I presented the case to an older, more experienced colleague, who suggested I refer her for deep brain stimulation. I discussed at length the risks and benefits with the patient, observing that this was a relatively new treatment with a small body of evidence. It turned out to be the best thing I could do for the patient. Since the surgery, she has made a marked improvement, although with some residual symptoms. I still remember when she returned from the hospital and thanked me for finding the best solution in her case.

Comments
An important aspect of good psychiatric practice is for psychiatrists to realize the limitations of their own expertise. This could relate to individual patients or to particular diagnostic groups. This is particularly relevant for patients where the next steps of management are unclear due to their complex presentation or poor

response to treatment. Individual psychiatrists should develop their own pathways for seeking support from other members of the multidisciplinary team, their peers and their senior colleagues, both through formal and informal routes as this manner of external reflection is likely to improve patient outcomes and enhance a psychiatrist's own experiential learning.[15]

In Scenario 6 the issue of involuntary psychiatric treatment is presented, which encompasses dilemmas concerning *altruism, accountability* and *duty*.

Scenario 6

I was about to finish work on a Friday afternoon, and was looking forward to a pleasant weekend. On my way out of the clinic I encountered an ambulance, which had just brought in an agitated patient. My colleague on call was waiting and commented that this was his seventh admission. His telephone rang, and he was called to a ward emergency. I wished him good luck, but on my way to the car, I felt that this would be a situation in which I would appreciate help if I were in his shoes. I offered to see the agitated patient, who presented with a first episode of psychosis. He had already harmed himself and his father and required several hours to assess, admit involuntarily and start initial treatment. Because it was an involuntary admission, I had to deal sensitively with the patient, his family and receiving ward staff. I missed my weekend arrangements but felt satisfaction in helping a patient and a colleague. But it is never easy, and especially not on a Friday afternoon.

Comments

This vignette highlights two important principles, one of a sense of altruism and duty, and the other of enhancing patient autonomy, even under difficult circumstances. Firstly, understanding their overall duty to help other patients and their colleagues should be at the core of professionalism for all doctors, including psychiatrists. Additionally, especially in circumstances where patients are very ill and distressed, all efforts should be made to enhance patient autonomy, and involuntary admissions should only be used as a last resort. In circumstances where involuntary treatment is being considered, this should not be for the sake of expediency. In fact, more not less time should be spent initially trying to work collaboratively with the patient to support voluntary treatment and, if this is not possible, then resources should be expended in dealing sensitively with the patient and their carers with regards to involuntary treatment.[15]

Teaching professional responsibility in psychiatry

Imparting the theory and practice of professionalism to the next generation of doctors is clearly an essential part of continuing the strong traditions of professionalism in medicine. Similarly, teaching professional responsibility is arguably integral to raising awareness and professional standards in psychiatry. This has been recognized by a number of medical and psychiatric organizations around the world, including the American Medical Association[14] and the Royal College of Psychiatrists.[1]

In addition to a theoretical knowledge base, key skills that enhance professionalism must therefore be inculcated into the psychiatrist's character, from medical school through specialty training, and continued throughout specialist professional development – a process of 'personal professional and civic development underpinned by a strong ethical and moral framework'. The key to achieving this is learning the skills to apply knowledge and engage in reflective practice.[19] Creuss[20] recommends the use of experiential learning and role modelling in teaching professional responsibility, and notes that support from institutions is a requirement for this to succeed. Brainard and Brislen[12] recommend that administrators, medical educators, residents and students alike must show a personal commitment to the professionalism curriculum and address deficiencies in the learning environment and in individual and institutional professional behaviour. But, as Bhugra noted:[6] 'how these [skills] are learnt and taught needs further debate'.

Conclusions

Early career psychiatrists face many professional challenges and opportunities. Professional responsibility is particularly important in psychiatry because of the unique position and skills of the psychiatrist.

Medical professionalism is an essential part of being a psychiatrist.[21] We suggest that medical professionalism must form an essential part of undergraduate medical studies as well as psychiatric specialist training.[22] Courses in ethics, the humanities (literature, history, philosophy, religion and the arts) and human values sensitize clinicians by raising awareness and by developing critical reflection skills. In addition, appreciating the close link between theory and practice is essential, especially for those at the beginning of their careers.[12,20] Furthermore, we suggest that it becomes an important part of continuing professional development and appraisal systems for specialists. The unwillingness or inability of a trainee or specialist to fulfil all their core responsibilities as a psychiatrist should result in the profession recognizing these issues in a timely manner and making active attempts to remedy or address them. If these remediation steps are unsuccessful, patient interests should remain paramount, and an effective, self-regulating profession must consider exclusion of such individuals.[2]

Although direct evidence is lacking that more robust teaching of professionalism will lead to better health outcomes, patients certainly understand the meaning of poor professionalism and associate it with poor medical care. The public is well aware that an absence of professionalism is harmful to their interests.[3] Psychiatrists must therefore respect the rights of patients, colleagues and other health professionals. We must continue to study, apply and advance scientific knowledge, maintain a commitment to medical education, and make relevant information available to patients, colleagues and the public. Psychiatrists, across the specialties, have possibly the greatest appreciation of patients as individuals, and as people. As professionals, we have many skills, but most important amongst these is our role as empathic doctors,[23] who always have to adhere to the golden rule: 'treat others as you would like to be treated'.

Acknowledgement

The authors would like to thank Dr. Amit Malik MRCPsych, DGM for his unwavering support and editing of the chapter.

References

1. Bhugra D. Renewing psychiatry's contract with society. *The Psychiatrist* 2008; **32**: 281–283.
2. Williams Jr. The future of medical professionalism. *S Afr J Bioethics Law* 2009; **2**: 48–50.
3. Working Party of the Royal College of Physicians. Doctors in society. Medical professionalism in a changing word. *Clin Med* 2005; **5**: 5–40.
4. Sullivan WM. Medicine under threat: professionalism and professional identity. *Can Med Assoc J* **162**: 673–675.
5. Cruess RL, Cruess SR, Johnston SE. Professionalism and medicine's social contract. *J Bone Joint Surg* 2000; **82**: 1189.
6. Bhugra D. Professionalism and psychiatry: past, present, future. *Australas Psychiatry* 2009; 17: 357–359.
7. Goldberg JL. Humanism or professionalism? The white coat ceremony and medical education. *Acad Med* 2008; **83**: 715–722.
8. Cohen JJ. Viewpoint: linking professionalism to humanism: what it means, why it matters. *Acad Med* 2007; 82: 1029–1032.

9. Cruess RL, Cruess SR, Steinert Y. Teaching medical professionalism. New York: Cambridge University Press, 2009.

10. Barondess JA. Medicine and professionalism. *Arch Intern Med* 2003; **163**: 145–149.

11. Brown N, Bhugra D. 'New' professionalism or professionalism derailed? *The Psychiatrist* 2007; **31**: 281–283.

12. Brainard AH, Brislen HC. Viewpoint: learning professionalism: a view from the trenches. *Acad Med* 2007; **82**: 1010–1014.

13. ABIM Foundation, ACP–ASIM Foundation, and European Federation of Internal Medicine. Medical Professionalism in the New Millennium: A Physician Charter. *Ann Intern Med* 2002; **136**: 243–246.

14. American Medical Association. Declaration of professional responsibility medicine's social contract with humanity. Available at: http://www.ama-assn.org/ama/pub/physician-resources/medical-ethics/declaration-professional-responsibility.shtml [accessed 7 February 2011].

15. Principles of ethics and professionalism in psychiatry. Proposed changes to APA guidelines. Available at: http://www.stanford.edu/group/psylaw seminar/Ethics.htm [accessed 25 August 2010].

16. Roberts LW. Professionalism in psychiatry: a very special collection. *Acad Psychiatry* 2009; **33**: 429–430.

17. Relman AS. Medical professionalism in a commercialized health care market. *Cleveland Clin J Med* 2008; **75**: 33–36.

18. Page DW. Professionalism and team care in the clinical setting. *Clin Anat* 2006; **19**: 468–472.

19. Schon D. *Educating the Reflective Practitioner: Towards a New Design for Teaching and Learning in the Professions.* San Francisco: Jossey Bass, 1987.

20. Cruess RL. Teaching professionalism: theory, principles and practices. *Clin Orthop Relat Res* 2006; **449**: 177–185.

21. Chard D, Elsharkawy A, Newbery N. Medical professionalism: the trainees' views. *Clin Med* 2006; **6**: 68–71.

22. Bhugra D. Professionalism and psychiatry: the profession speaks. *Acta Psychiatr Scand* 2008; **118**: 327–329.

23. Malhi GS. Professionalizing psychiatry: from 'amateur' psychiatry to 'a mature' profession. *Acta Psychiatr Scand* 2008; **118**: 255–258.

CHAPTER 17

The role of ethics in psychiatric training and practice

Cecile Hanon,[1] Defne Eraslan,[2] Dominique Mathis,[3] Abigail L. Donovan[4] and Marianne Kastrup[5]

[1]EPS Erasme, Antony, France
[2]Department of Psychiatry, Faculty of Medicine, Acibadem University, Istanbul, Turkey
[3]Institut Paul Sivadon, Hôpital de l'Elan Retrouvé, Paris, France
[4]Harvard University, Massachusetts General Hospital, Boston, MA, USA
[5]Centre for Transcultural Psychiatry, Psychiatric Centre Copenhagen, Denmark

Introduction

Ethics is an object of knowledge; it is neither a science, nor an institutional system of rules, nor a know-how. Medicine has always been concerned by ethics, indeed, medical practice is characterized by ethical concerns: its object is another person, its motive is empathy for the suffering of others and its purpose is the promotion of health for others.

The origins of ethical theories date from antiquity and its philosophers; its foundations can be traced to thinkers such as Aristotle, Plato, Galileo, Descartes, Levi-Strauss, Kant, Nietzsche, Sartre and Levinas. It was after the Second World War that contemporary medical ethics was born with the Nuremberg Code, enacted in August 1947 and composed of ethical rules set by the International Military Tribunal that tried the doctors who worked at the Nazi extermination camps.

New technologies, new knowledge (e.g. intensive care, organ transplantation, medical imaging, medically assisted procreation, abortion, genetic prediction, psychosurgery and coercive measures), scientific research, market demands, nationalization of health services and demands of society with regard to medicine all can lead physicians into ethically

How to Succeed in Psychiatry: A Guide to Training and Practice, First Edition.
Edited by Andrea Fiorillo, Iris Tatjana Calliess and Henning Sass.
© 2012 John Wiley & Sons, Ltd. Published 2012 by John Wiley & Sons, Ltd.

confusing situations. Alongside these recent issues, more traditional but equally difficult ethical dilemmas related to medical situations can arise.

Psychiatrists must have the means to identify and analyse the values and conflicts in care situations, research and public health and then make balanced ethical decisions.

Ethical principles and the therapeutic relationship: from paternalism to autonomy?

Two models of doctor-patient relationship exist: the paternalistic and the autonomic models. According to the paternalistic model, based on the principle of asymmetrical charity, the doctor supports and protects the patient, discharges him or her from the responsibility of the decision, and maintains the patient in a state of partial ignorance. This model is no more satisfying now.

Public accountability restricts traditional paternalistic forms of practising psychiatry or conducting research. The influence of the market and industry introduces forms of rationality that have to be reconciled with the traditional scientific, therapeutic or altruistic goals of the profession and its quest for knowledge based on the empirical sciences.[1]

Efficiency and diversification of treatment, and the development of medical information and its accessibility (indeed, a less 'savant' medicine has less to say) challenge this asymmetrical relationship and bring increased patient autonomy.

The autonomic model, theorized by H.T. Engelhardt,[2] describes the medical relationship as one in which the patient, fully informed, is responsible for the decisions regarding his or her treatment. The doctor is just a care provider under the guise of a contractual negotiation.

Respect for autonomy entails the need to respect an individual's right to self-determination and the patient's right to make decisions regarding health and care, provided that he/she has the capacity to do so. That issue leads directly to the concept of consent.

With increasing multiculturalism, it is important for doctors to be aware that patients coming from a non-Western context may not be familiar with the autonomic model focusing upon the consent of the individual patient and may find it natural to include others – typically the family – in their decision-making.

In real-world practice there are times when paternalism must override patient autonomy. For example, when a patient is at risk of harming him/herself or others, the psychiatrist may choose to act paternalistically and hospitalize the patient involuntarily, in order to ensure his/her safety. In this case, such paternalism may be considered 'beneficent' paternalism.

Beneficence or non-maleficence?

Beneficence is the requirement to consider the potential benefits arising from a course of action and balancing these benefits against the potential risks. Clinicians should always act for the benefit of patients. Non-maleficence is the requirement not to cause harm, and refers to Hippocrates' maxim 'Primum non nocere'.[3]

Consent

Consent is the agreement of the patient with the treatment decision of the doctor. The decision, when subjected to the consent, brings a value of interpellation. The patient questions: 'I suffer, help me'. The doctor replies: 'Here is what I decide for you, do you agree?'

The term *informed* consent has evolved largely since the 1950s. The legal standard for information disclosure, for example, continues to evolve and still varies by jurisdiction. One can apply the 'professional standard', in which the amount and content of disclosure is determined by what most physicians would traditionally disclose.

Another standard, with an increasing emphasis on patient autonomy, is the 'reasonable person standard'. This standard requires that psychiatrists disclose what a reasonable person would want to know (an accurate description of the proposed treatment, the risks and benefits of that treatment; any relevant alternatives and their potential risks and benefits; and the risks and benefits of no treatment at all). Thus, withholding information about side effects, for example, in the hope of increasing compliance, is not acceptable.

The manner in which information is presented, the choice of facts that are included or omitted, and the selection of alternatives that are offered, all can have distinct effects on patient decisions. For example, regarding consent to medication, some authors have found that information about the risk of treatment was more abstract for patients when expressed as a percentage. It could be more informative to compare such risks to those of everyday life, like driving or playing sports, so that patients have a point of reference when making decisions.

Psychiatry has two basic characteristics: the uniqueness of the relationship with the person and the fact that mental disorders can affect the ability to understand and to integrate information related to the therapeutic decision, and can prevent the patient from discerning, expressing and enacting his/her specific authentic and enduring personal values.

The doctor's request for consent to treatment, and thus the acceptance of a potential rejection, is based on the principle of respect for patient autonomy. Autonomy comprises an individual's ability to function in cognitive, affective and volitional domains. What would be free (volitional and emotional function) and informed (cognitive function) consent of a patient suffering from a psychiatric disorder?

Furthermore, the experience of dependence, societal marginalization and insufficient access to clinical care, may create a situation of desperation that may interfere with voluntary decision-making. It is important to note that these vulnerabilities need not confer incapacity, but rather complicate voluntary decision-making. Nonetheless, these vulnerabilities should be explored in order to optimize a patient's decision-making. This is particularly important in psychiatry where, even if patients are decisionally capable, both internal and external factors (e.g. the patient's illness, stigma, lack of resources) can make them vulnerable to coercive influences.

Exceptions to informed consent

Genuine emergencies do not require informed consent. Emergency care occurs in the framework of implied or presumed consent. Care for children or incompetent patients requires consent from parents or legally recognized surrogates. Patients may also waive their right to informed consent. This exception, however, presumes competence to do so.

Because the concepts of autonomy and informed consent have a legal basis, they may cast the clinical situation in an adversarial light. This view is antithetical to ethical practice. Although the ultimate choice on consent is made by an individual patient, autonomous choice does not take place in a vacuum; it must be nurtured by continued dialogue.

Ultimately, the ideal understanding of informed consent is an important reminder of respect for the rights of patients and the need for transparent, collaborative and enduring alliances. Psychiatrists who strive to develop these relationships will easily exceed the requirements of ethics and law.[4]

How to make a therapeutic decision?

Decision-making can be divided into three phases:[5]

1. Before the decision. The concordance between medical knowledge and clinical reality leads to the diagnosis or treatment decision and recommendation. The psychiatrist's experience, theoretical orientation and personality also play a role.
2. The decision itself. There are differences between what a doctor explains, what the patient understands, and the memories of both participants of the experience. The decision is not only the automatic result of logical consideration of the issues and resources, it includes a commitment by the person, the doctor or the patient, who produces an act of will.

3. The implementation of the decision. The implementation of the treatment evolves over time and requires adjustments according to the response and reaction of the patient.

In the USA, a physician may make a clinical assessment about a patient's ability to make a rational and informed treatment decision. This assessment is called a capacity evaluation, and can only be made in real time for a specific treatment question. If a patient lacks more global capacity, the case is referred for judicial review and a judge will determine global competence for all medical decision-making. If a judge deems a patient to be incompetent, a third party may be appointed as a substitute to make decisions. When a third party is appointed, this individual has the obligation to make medical decisions based on 'substituted judgment', that is, based upon what they believe the patient would have chosen to do, rather than based upon their own ideals or values.

The capacity evaluation is based upon professional, not legal standards, and typically includes the four criteria outlined by Applebaum and Grisso: (i) the ability to express a stable and consistent treatment choice over time; (ii) the ability to understand the medical facts relevant to the specific illness, and the treatments offered, including risks and benefits; (iii) the ability to appreciate the relevance of these facts to the patient's life and their individual situation; and (iv) the ability to manipulate all of these data in a logical manner.[6] The level at which capacity standards are applied also depends upon a risk-benefit analysis of the specific case. Specifically, the consequences of the patient's decision must be weighed against the potential treatment outcome. In a scenario of high treatment benefit with low treatment risk, the standard for capacity to refuse this treatment option should be more stringent than a situation in which the treatment benefit is low but the risks are high. This consideration allows for optimal protection of both the patient's autonomy and their physical well-being.

Bioethics

The evolution of philosophical reflection, practical needs of regulation in practice and research, and public awareness of rights and duties have led to the development of a new form of applied ethics, known as *bioethics*. Presented as a form of *global ethics* concerned with the impact of science and technology on human affairs and the moral obligations of humankind to the environment, it has been expanded to cover issues related to equity of access to health care, autonomy of patients in decision-making, forms of beneficence that are not paternalistic, and analysis of harm and risk in research and therapy. It is not the content, however, but the style of reasoning and debate that more essentially characterizes modern medical bioethics.[7]

Ethics in psychiatric research

Psychiatric residency is a period during which many young doctors participate in research for the first time in their lives. In many European countries, carrying out at least one clinical or preclinical study is compulsory for completing residency. In the USA, conducting a research study is not a training requirement, but many psychiatric residents will choose to participate in research regardless. Therefore, it is important to learn about and to apply ethical principles of psychiatric research during residency training.

Ethical issues concerning psychiatric treatment and research have always been a concern for the public. Muroff et al.[8] showed that the public is more willing to allow research on patients with general medical illnesses than on those with psychiatric illnesses. The authors state that this finding might be related to the public's perception of severity of medical illnesses and the view that people with psychiatric disorders may be less capable of informed and voluntary decision-making. Furthermore, it was perceived that many psychiatric patients may undergo forensic measures or receive coercive treatment, which further complicate the issue of informed consent.

This finding may reflect stigmatization of psychiatric research, and trainees may be similarly hesitant to conduct psychiatric research. Research has shown that most of the patients involved in both clinical and non-clinical studies (including trials of medication and other biological therapies, such as ECT) found psychiatric research to be beneficial and did not experience subjective distress.[9,10]

Therefore, efforts should be made to overcome this stigmatization, which might preclude valuable research. In-depth knowledge and vigorous application of ethical principles in psychiatric research might help prevent this risk.

Designing psychiatric research trials

Ethical considerations for research trials should be taken into account starting from the planning phase of the trial. Psychiatric research projects should be designed according to general principles of research ethics.[11] These principles are summarized in the Nuremberg Code, which helped form the foundation for the field of research ethics. They include the following requirements:[11]

- the participant's voluntary informed consent;
- the likelihood that the study will produce fruitful results;
- the minimization of the physical and mental suffering and risk to the participant;

- the proportionality of the study's risk to the importance of the problem examined by the research;
- the requirement that scientifically qualified individuals conduct the research;
- the participant's freedom to terminate his or her involvement during the study;
- the investigator's willingness to terminate the study if he or she has reason to believe that continuation is likely to lead to great harm to the participant(s).

The Declaration of Helsinki, published by the World Medical Association, takes the same principles into consideration and expands them.[12]

As discussed before, different characteristics of mental illness cause unique ethical concerns while doing psychiatric research. There are potential effects of mental illness on decision-making. As a result, informed consent and patient privacy are even more important in designing psychiatric research.

Informed consent in psychiatric research

The process of obtaining informed consent is perhaps the most important safeguard for carrying out ethical research. There are three major aspects of informed consent: information, decisional capacity and voluntarism.[13]

The information provided should include: (i) design and purpose of the study; (ii) risks and benefits of participation; and (iii) alternatives to participating in the study. The decision-making capacity of patients with severe mental illness depends on the nature of the decision to be made. For example, a participant who is capable of making a treatment decision may lack the capacity to understand the information about participation in a research study.[14]

Individuals who lack decision-making capacity may still participate in psychiatric research, using methods such as surrogate decision-makers and advance directives. The surrogate decision-makers should either make the decision according to what the patient would have wanted for himself/herself or what would best benefit the patient. If the patient has used a valid advance directive that states his/her preference regarding participation in research, it should be used when he/she lacks decision-making capacity. However, other possible motivations of the patient such as altruism and financial incentives should always be examined.[15]

Protecting private information in research

Protecting confidentiality is a key issue in general medicine and research, but because of the stigma associated with mental illness, even more caution should be taken while conducting psychiatric research. Investigators should protect the confidentiality of personal information throughout the research process.[16] As data on family members and non-familial significant others are also collected in many protocols, measures protecting personal information on patients' family members should also be taken.[17]

Confidentiality

Professional secrecy in psychiatry is based on the need to protect information disclosed during interviews with patients. Confidentiality concerns everything that has been seen, heard, understood or confided to the psychiatrist during treatment, and in particular events or news that someone wants to keep private, that are not commonly known, and that form part of the intimate nature of the individual.

The obligation of secrecy is part of the Hippocratic Oath: 'I will respect the privacy of my patients, for their problems are not disclosed to me that the world may know.' Not only the psychiatrist, but also every member of staff contributing to the care of the patient, is bound by confidentiality. Confidentiality also applies to all psychiatric records. This psychiatric information can only be shared with other doctors or medical staff if they are participating in the care of the patient.

The exceptions to confidentiality are governed by precise rules of law and detailed very precisely in each country. In the USA, the exceptions to confidentiality, particularly regarding the psychiatric treatment of adolescents and their rights to make certain treatment decisions, vary on a state-to-state basis. These exceptions usually include:
• demand and interest from parents of a child under 18;
• request by the guardian in the interests of the patient;
• court testimony;
• in state of necessity if the behaviour, attitudes and words of the patient indicate that he/she could seriously endanger the health or life of others;
• to protect the patient when he/she is unable to protect him or herself (due to disability, mental disorder or age under 18);
• in the case of children, the elderly, people with disabilities or mental disorders, the defence of the dignity and quality of life is primary.

Violation of confidentiality is a serious medico-legal issue and exposes the psychiatrist to various disciplinary, penal and economic sanctions. To avoid those medico-legal issues, some practical advice for early career psychiatrists can be given:
• Keep in mind the confidentiality issue in day-to-day practice, particularly in certain high-risk circumstances like waiting rooms, telephone

and voicemail messages, fax and email (consider entering a legal notice concerning the confidential information).

- Use caution in recording medical information.
- Keep medical records and all written information concerning patients in a safe place.
- Avoid casual discussion about patients with family or friends even if they are colleagues.

Forensic psychiatry

Forensic psychiatry raises some specific ethical issues. As a physician, it is clear that the forensic psychiatrist who works for the correctional services and prison systems is primarily responsible for the treatment and well-being of his/her patients, and is not an agent of social control. As such, this psychiatrist is bound to the same ethical rules as general psychiatrists. Moreover, the specific condition (e.g. prison) necessitates that the therapeutic boundaries (e.g. dealing with medical confidentiality) have to be clear and transparent to the patients.

Concerning forensic consultation, however, the ethical issues are more complex and have been the focus of many debates. One of the reasons is that, in the specific circumstances of the consultation, the forensic psychiatrist's main commitment is with justice and not with the interests of examinees. Therefore, the psychiatric expert is not bound to the same degree of confidentiality expected in ordinary clinical psychiatric practice. But the expert's work should be kept confidential outside the written report. The expert needs also to explain to the examinee the nature of the work at the beginning of the interview.[18]

When writing the report, adequate care must be taken to produce a balanced report. On the one hand, examinees should not be exposed unnecessarily (refer to the American Psychological Association recommendations in relation to fitness-for-duty evaluations, so that sensitive personal information may be omitted or summarized in the report provided that it does not compromise the efficiency of the document) but, on the other hand, vital information should not be omitted so that the work done is not compromised.[19]

The notion of 'fair care for the examinee' is fundamental in forensic practice and has been recently enhanced in literature. It is all the more important since the examinee is already exposed to a condition of vulnerability. Therefore, the basic ethical principle of non-maleficence should be kept in mind, with the goal of preventing additional and unnecessary suffering to the examinees.[20] The work of forensic psychiatrists should be performed with generosity and humaneness.[21]

Anticipated directives and Ulysses' contract

A. Kardiner, in his book *My Analysis with Freud*,[22] discusses the ethical question of psychiatric care: a psychoanalyst treats a patient engaged in the difficult business of contract killing. The psychiatrist learns that the patient has for years conscientiously performed his contracts for clients, but for some time he has presented with inhibition and can no longer operate. After a few sessions, the patient stops coming. The author's conclusion is: 'I never knew if I helped him recover from his ability or inability to kill.' This example shows the difficulty of fixing the limits of free will. Has the psychiatrist the right to ignore the social consequences of the patient's actions and focus only on his or her well-being?

In some cases, where the patient is liable to predictable relapses, such as manic episodes, the psychiatrist can utilize 'Ulysses' contract'. This refers to the Greek hero who, unable to resist the sound of the formidable but fearful mermaids' song, gets himself tied to the mast of his ship and commands his sailors not to remove him, even if he begs or orders them.[23] This contract represents an agreement between the patient and the doctor for care, even without consent, during crises. It demands a medical relationship that is stable and based on mutual trust; it pertains only to certain psychiatric disorders and only after the patient has already had two episodes with complete remission. The validity of the contract is defined, limited and signed in the presence of a third person. In the USA, such a contract may not be legally binding, but may be nonetheless useful in treatment.

Boundary violations

There are several ethical issues that more frequently arise in psychiatry compared to other medical specialties. These include boundary violations, of both a sexual and non-sexual nature.

The practice of psychiatry is, by its very nature, filled with intense emotion, and consists of regular, frequent and private contact with patients. These circumstances create a vulnerability for boundary crossings and violations. Boundary crossings are considered harmless deviations from the therapeutic frame, such as taking a patient's arm if he or she stumbles. Boundary violations are deviations from clinical practice that are potentially harmful and exploit the patient's emotional, physical or financial needs.

Boundary violations can be of either a non-sexual or sexual nature, and both have the potential for serious harm to the patient. Non-sexual boundary violations include engaging in a business relationship with a patient, or engaging in a social relationship outside of therapy. Financial boundary crossings and violations, which may arise particularly in private practice, for example, include lowering a fee beyond what is reasonable. Accepting a gift from a patient could also be considered a boundary crossing or violation, depending on the circumstance of the giving, the type and size of gift, and the expectations of the patient.

Sexual boundary violations include any intimate physical contact between the doctor and the patient. Some medical specialties condone intimate relationships between doctors and former patients when a certain time limit after the end of treatment has elapsed. However, most psychiatrists would subscribe to the principle 'once a patient, always a patient', meaning that sexual relationships with former patients, regardless of the time since treatment ended, are unethical.

It is critically important that early career psychiatrists are taught that all doctors are at risk for boundary violations. Denying this vulnerability prevents thoughtful analysis of motives and introspective examination. Early career psychiatrists should be educated about early warning signs, including idealizing the patient, and thus considering them as deserving special treatment, holding sessions 'after hours' or making house calls (when not part of one's standard practice), or allowing sessions to run longer than the standard time.[24] Another example would be writing statements that are not strictly based on evidence regarding the patient's condition in order to obtain certain social benefits. But the most important warning sign may be a reluctance to discuss the case with colleagues or supervisors. The early career psychiatrists should be immediately prompted by any of these warning signs to seek objective consultation to examine the case in depth.[25]

Conclusions

Of the branches of medicine, psychiatry is probably the one whose biological foundations are least clear, but at the same time is the most sensitive to developments in the fundamental sciences. As psychiatry involves both applied neuroscience and philosophical reflection, most ethical debates within its boundaries acquire a particular character, one that makes them more difficult to articulate or to handle.

In the light of that, the psychiatric profession has developed its own set of ethical guidelines governing the profession. In 1977 the World Psychiatric Association (WPA) formulated the Hawaii Declaration, which in 1996 was replaced by the WPA Declaration of Madrid,[26] outlining both general principles as well as specific guidelines. The existence of ethical codes is a necessary but not a sufficient step to prevent human rights violations. The founding father of the WPA Madrid Declaration, Ahmed Okasha,[27] has emphasized that guidelines, declarations, and so on do not by themselves prevent ethical breaches. Whether the individual psychiatrist behaves ethically is ultimately based on his/her personal sense of responsibility towards the patient and his/her judgment in determining what is a correct and appropriate conduct.

As such, education and training in medical ethics are especially relevant to psychiatry, and professionalism should be an integral part of the initial training offered to trainees and early career psychiatrists (see also Chapter 16). It should have several objectives:[28]

- To gain knowledge about fundamental medical ethical principles, as many may breach ethical codes simply because they are unaware of them.
- To identify and manage ethical dilemmas that commonly arise in clinical and research settings and populations (including treatment of children, adolescents, the elderly, involuntary patients, non-decisional patients, patients with substance abuse, patients seen for psychotherapy, patients involved in research protocols, boundary violations).
- To communicate truthfully, respectfully and effectively with patients, their families and clinical colleagues.
- To demonstrate a commitment to competence, confidentiality and appropriate relationships with patients, their families and clinical colleagues.
- To work diligently to decrease the stigma associated with mental illness.

This ethical approach should not be simply reduced to the norms of social conformity, but must be specific to the individual patient, to his/her human's status: the emergence of ethics may be there.

References

1. Lolas F. Bioethics and psychiatry: a challenging future. *World Psychiatry* 2002; **1**: 123–124.
2. Engelhardt HT. *The Foundation of Bioethics*, New York: Oxford University Press, 1986.
3. Katona C, Chiu E, Adelman S *et al*. World Psychiatric Association section of old age psychiatry consensus statement on ethics and capacity in older people with mental disorders. *Int J Geriatr Psychiatry* 2009; **24**: 1319–1324.
4. Kress JJ. Information, depressive illness and suicide risk: reflexive approach. *Ann Med-Psychol* 1999; **4**: 57.
5. Kress JJ. Ethics in psychiatry: information-consent-decision. In: *Where does Medicine go?* Presse Universitaire de Strasbourg, 2003, 25–30.
6. Appelbaum PS, Grisso T. Assessing patients' capacities to consent for treatment. *N Eng J Med* 1988; **319**: 1462–1467.
7. Hottois G, Parizeau MH. The words of Bioethics. *Encyclopaedic vocabulary*. Brussels: De Boeck University, 1993.
8. Muroff JR, Hoerauf SL, Kim SY. Is psychiatric research stigmatized? An experimental survey of the public. *Schizophr Bull* 2006; **32**: 129–136.

9. Jorm AF, Kelly CM, Morgan AJ. Participant distress in psychiatric research: a systematic review. *Psychol Med* 2007; **37**: 917–926.

10. Rosen C, Grossman LS, Sharma RP *et al.* Subjective ratings of research participation by persons with mental illness. *J Nerv Ment Dis* 2007; **195**: 430–435.

11. Barry LK. Ethical issues in psychiatric research. *Psychiatr Clin N Am* 2009; **32**: 381–394.

12. World Medical Association Ethics Unit. *Declaration of Helsinki*. WMA, 2010. Available at: http://www.wma.net/en/30publications/10policies/b3/index.html.

13. National Commission for the Protection of Human Subjects of Biomedical and Behavioral Research. *The Belmont Report: Ethical Principles and Guidelines for the Protection of Human Subjects of Research.* Washington, DC: U.S. Government Printing Office, 1979.

14. Roberts LW. Informed consent and the capacity for voluntarism. *Am J Psychiatry* 2002; **159**: 705–712.

15. Lieberman JA, Stroup S, Laska E *et al.* Issues in clinical research design: principles, practices, and controversies. In: Pincus HA, Lieberman JA, Ferris S (eds) *Ethics in Psychiatric Research.* Washington, DC: American Psychiatric Association, 1999; pp. 23–60.

16. American Psychiatric Association's Task Force on Research Ethics. Ethical principles and practices for research involving human participants with mental illness. *Psychiatr Serv* 2006; **57**: 552–557.

17. Lounsbury DW, Reynolds TC, Rapkin BD *et al.* Protecting the privacy of third-party information: recommendations for social and behavioural health researchers. *Soc Sci Med* 2007; **64**: 213–222.

18. Bush SS. Independent and court-ordered forensic neuropsychological examinations: official statement of the National Academy of Neuropsychology. *Arch Clin Neuropsychol* 2005; **20**: 997–1007.

19. Anfang SA, Wall BW. Psychiatric fitness-for-duty evaluations. *Psychiatr Clin N Am* 2006; **29**: 675–693.

20. Taborda J, Abdalla-Filho E, Garrafa V. Ethics in forensic psychiatry. *Curr Opin Psychiatry* 2007; **20**: 507–510.

21. Griffith EEH. Personal narrative and an African-American perspective on medical ethics. *J Am Acad Psychiatry* 2005; **33**, 371–381.

22. Kardiner A. *My Analysis with Freud.* Paris: Belfond, 1978.

23. Palazollo J, Julerot JM, Lachaux B. From ethics in psychiatry to the psychiatrist facing ethics. *L'Encéphale* 1999; **XXV**: 674–680.

24. Norris DM, Gutheil TG, Strasburger LH. This couldn't happen to me: boundary problems and sexual misconduct in the psychotherapy relationship. *Psychiatr Serv* 2003; **54**: 517–522.

25. Donovan AL, Messner E, Stern TA. Coping with the rigors of psychiatric practice. In: Stern TA, Fricchione GL, Cassem NH, Jellinek MS, Rosenbaum JF (eds) *The MGH Handbook of General Hospital Psychiatry*, 6th edn. Philadelphia: Saunders/Elsevier, 2010; pp. 659–666.

26. World Psychiatric Association. Madrid declaration on ethical standards for psychiatric practice. Available at: http://www.wpanet.org/detail.php?section _id=5&category_id=9&content_id=48.

27. Okasha A. The new ethical context of psychiatry. In: Sartorius N *et al.* (eds) *Psychiatry in Society.* London: Wiley, 2002, 134–137.

28. Ping Tsao CI, Guedet PJ. Ethics and professionalism preparation for psychiatrists-in-training: a curricular proposal. *Int Rev Psychiatry* 2010; **22**: 301–305.

CHAPTER 18

Coercive measures and involuntary hospital admissions in psychiatry

Valeria Del Vecchio,[1] Andrea Fiorillo,[1] Corrado De Rosa[1] and Adriana Mihai[2]

[1]Department of Psychiatry, University of Naples SUN, Naples, Italy
[2]Department of Psychiatry, University of Medicine and Pharmacy, Tg Mures, Romania

Introduction

Involuntary hospital admissions and coercive measures towards patients with mental disorders are controversial but sometimes necessary medical procedures. A recent review[1] showed that involuntary placement of mentally ill people is not associated with a higher risk of negative outcome; however, it may have a strong impact on specific outcome domains, such as satisfaction with treatments and quality of life.

Available epidemiological data show that rates of involuntary hospital admissions are significantly different across European states, ranging from 12.4/100 000 inhabitants in Italy to 232.5/100 000 in Finland, and also within the same countries.[2,3] The maximum duration of involuntary placement (Table 18.1), as well as the clinical conditions requiring an involuntary hospital admission are also very different in the various European contexts;[4] they include severe psychotic or affective disorders; suicide risk; marked cognitive impairment; behavioural disorders with aggression and agitation; severe danger for a patient's own life or for that of others; and an urgent need for a patient's psychiatric treatment.[5,6]

However, only limited data are available on procedures for involuntary hospital admission of mentally ill patients,[1] although several attempts have been made to standardize rules and instruments,[7-10] such as the publication of *Mental Health Legislation and Human Rights* by the World

How to Succeed in Psychiatry: A Guide to Training and Practice, First Edition.
Edited by Andrea Fiorillo, Iris Tatjana Calliess and Henning Sass.
© 2012 John Wiley & Sons, Ltd. Published 2012 by John Wiley & Sons, Ltd.

Table 18.1 Maximum duration of involuntary placement in selected countries.

Country	Maximum duration of placement	Reapproval after
Italy	7 days	After 1 week
Israel	7 days (head of the ward – next 7 days); minors – 30 days	After 3 and 6 months Minors – every 3 months (juvenile court)
Sweden	4 weeks	After 4 weeks, 4 and 6 months
Germany	Preliminary: 6 weeks Regularly 1 to 2 years	Preliminary: 3 weeks Regularly: after 6 months (only 1 land)
UK	Diagnostic purposes: 28 days Treatment: 6 months	After 28 days, after 6 months
Greece	6 months	After 3 months
Bulgaria	1 year	After 1 year
Czech Rep.	1 year	After 3 months
Romania	15 days	After 15 days
Slovakia	1 year	After 1 year
Spain	Not defined	Report every 6 months
Lithuania	Not defined	Not defined
Poland	Not defined	Not defined

Health Organization in 2003,[11] in which the issue of compulsory hospital admissions was specifically addressed from a legal and a technical perspective rather than from a clinical one.

Family associations and political bodies recently asked for the development of European guidelines and/or for the dissemination of good clinical practice recommendations on involuntary hospital admission and on the use of coercive measures, thus emphasizing the urgent need to find an international consensus.[12] Such consensus would be in line with one of the general goals of the European Union, namely the harmonization of health-care opportunities for EU citizens.[13,14] Within the EU, it is the Council of Europe that is charged especially with monitoring respect for EU citizens' human rights.

In this chapter we will provide an overview of the most frequently adopted coercive measures in psychiatry, and we will give some practical suggestions on how to improve the practice of involuntary hospital placements.

Coercive measures

The use of coercive measures in daily psychiatric practice is quite common,[15–17] although it has been recently criticized,[15] as it would represent a failure in psychiatric care.[18] Coercive measures include: (i) forced admission to a psychiatric hospital; (ii) involuntary detention after a voluntary admission; (iii) seclusion/isolation in a room that the patient is not allowed to leave; (iv) restraint/fixation by holding and/or mechanical devices; (v) forced medications, among which the most frequently used are haloperidol, zuclopenthixol and diazepam.[15] Data from a recent study carried out in 10 European countries and funded by the European Commission indicate that the most frequent reasons for the use of coercive measures are aggression against others, threats to patients' health, autoaggression, aggression against property, prevention of escape and inability to care for oneself. Among forced medications, the most frequently used drugs are first-generation antipsychotics and benzodiazepines. Interestingly, the use of coercive measures in psychiatric wards is not influenced by technical characteristics, such as rate of beds in the catchment area, number of staff per treatment place or number of beds per room.[15]

Some general advices may be particularly helpful for early career psychiatrists when dealing with patients who have aggressive or disturbing behaviours. The use of coercive measures must comply with existing legislation, national standards, and relevant ethical norms and policies. A justifying state of emergency and/or a court's decision that legitimizes the use of this measure must exist. Coercive measures should be applied only when other interventions or de-escalation strategies have been ineffective or are inappropriate, and they should never be used as a punishment or for reasons other than strictly therapeutic ones. The least restrictive effective method should be used, and it should be discontinued as soon as the emergency situation has ended; finally, patients' dignity, privacy and safety should be preserved at all times during the application of coercive measures.

Over the past decade, several programmes aimed at minimizing the use of coercive measures during psychiatric treatments have been proposed;[19–23] knowledge of these may be particularly helpful for early career psychiatrists. The key elements of these programmes include: (i) change in policy or leadership; (ii) external review or debriefing; (iii) data use; (iv) training of mental health professionals; (v) consumer and family involvement; (vi) increase in staff-patient ratio or use of crisis response teams; and (vii) changes in programme structure.[24]

Involuntary hospital admissions

Clinical conditions and legal prerequisites

An involuntary hospital admission should be performed only if the following clinical prerequisites are simultaneously present:

1. the patient is suffering from a serious mental disturbance;
2. the patient needs urgent therapeutic hospital-based interventions;
3. the patient does not agree to such care, so that the care cannot be given with his or her consent.

Involuntary hospital admissions should be ordered and performed according to the current national mental health laws, other relevant laws and regulations relating to mental health care. The herein defined basic criteria of mental health conditions, as well as additional criteria (e.g. dangerousness) legitimizing involuntary admission, must be fulfilled. In the following paragraphs suggestions on how to perform involuntary hospital admissions are reported, according to the EUNOMIA collaborating study, recently carried out in 12 countries.[25]

Professionals involved in the procedures of involuntary hospital admissions

Community mental health team

The physician, on first visiting the patient, should collect all potentially useful information regarding the patient's situation from all available sources, such as relatives, friends, colleagues, social workers, police officers and other professionals.

The first clinical examination should take place in a safe and quiet place, preferably in a four-eyes-situation or in the presence of very few persons (such as a nurse or a person whom the patient trusts). The physician should then issue a certificate, in which the mental disturbances and other relevant elements causing the need for hospitalization should be clearly reported, including a statement that the necessary prerequisites are fulfilled. After this preliminary clinical examination, the physician can involve the paramedical professionals, defining clear tasks for each of them. The patient can be moved to a first-aid station if there is a need for a general medical check, or for ascertaining the presence of alcohol/drug intoxication, which may have contributed to the development of psychiatric symptoms. Information on a patient's socio-demographic and clinical characteristics must be transferred to the hospital team before the patient's arrival.

Hospital mental health team

Upon a patient's arrival at the hospital, a full mental status examination should be performed by the ward psychiatrist. After having carefully examined the patient, the psychiatrist is responsible for the final decision about the patient's involuntary hospital admission. Information about a patient's hospital admission must be provided by the psychiatrist to the relevant authorities as soon as possible.

Nurses and other paramedical professionals: (i) must prepare the room and the bed before the patient's arrival. If the ward psychiatrist agrees, they: (ii) can take part in the clinical evaluation; (iii) must check the patient's personal belongings; (iv) must guarantee direct daily contact with him/her while maintaining calm, active and supportive behaviour; (v) must inform the patient about the ward's rules and report on his/her physical monitoring in the appropriate records.

Police

The physician can ask for police involvement in a patient's examination and/or when taking the patient to the hospital only when all alternatives have been considered, and only upon a written documented request.

The aim of police involvement is to avoid patients' aggressive and disruptive behaviour to doctors, other mental health professionals, and other involved persons (i.e. relatives), and not to protect the patients against illegal and humiliating treatment by psychiatrists. Police officers should explain to patients their role and the reasons for their intervention, and should inform them about their rights, avoiding aggressive physical and verbal behaviour.

All applied coercive measures should be reported in the patient's clinical record, including reasons for their application, and a clear description of how they have been performed. The record should always be at the judge's disposal.

Judiciary

The judge, before formulating any decision about a patient's admission, must collect information from patients, relatives and community mental health professionals, enquiring about the patient's actual clinical situation directly from the ward psychiatrist. In cases where orders that led to an involuntary hospitalization were not carried out within 48 hours, the circumstances under which the orders were issued should be re-examined.

If a hearing is required under national legislation (e.g. in the Czech Republic, Lithuania, Slovakia, Spain and Germany), this should take place in a comfortable and safe room, possibly located within the ward. During the hearing, the judge should involve the ward psychiatrist in order to integrate the available information with clinical details. The judge's decision should be made only after all persons participating in the involuntary admission procedure have been heard.

Relationship with the patient

Before being admitted to the hospital, patients should receive the relevant information about their admission as well as about diagnostic and therapeutic measures that have to be undertaken.

Patients are allowed to bring to the hospital documents and personal belongings, and they should be granted the possibility of staying in contact with their relatives and with the relevant authorities. Moreover, patients can receive visits and use the telephone. If the patient's mental status is significantly influenced by delusions or hallucinations, or by threats to others, the use of the telephone should be anyway allowed, but only in the presence of a mental health professional. Contacts by the patient with people outside the ward cannot be limited by anyone; in particular, letters written by the patient cannot be censored.

If necessary, cultural brokers can support the patient to overcome possible linguistic and cultural differences, which can influence the duration of hospitalization and the needs for care.

Relationship with the relatives

Unless expressly prohibited by the patient, relatives can be involved in the procedures of involuntary hospital admission (e.g. in order to get valid information about the clinical manifestations of the disorder before the admission) and should receive relevant information about the current admission, its presumed length and prescribed treatments, by phone or face to face, from the physicians involved. If the patient agrees, close relatives can be involved in the initial clinical assessment; during hospitalization, the patient should be granted the possibility of daily contact with his/her relatives.

Ethical aspects

All interventions provided during an involuntary hospital admission must follow the principle of the 'least restrictive alternative'. During the procedure, the following issues should always be considered:
1. It is necessary to reach a quick and clear decision about hospitalization, in the patient's interest.
2. The patient can ask to be taken to the hospital with his/her relatives, and he/she should ideally be admitted to the closest hospital.
3. The entire procedure should have a limited time frame – overly long waits should always be avoided.
4. Nobody can be involuntarily hospitalized without being assessed by a psychiatrist.

5. This assessment should be carried out in the most comfortable conditions while ensuring the necessary level of safety for both the examining physician and for the patient.

If at all possible, the admitted patient should be firstly located in a single room, in order to guarantee him/her a safe and calm environment. He/she should have regular contacts with mental health professionals, which should be held with reciprocal respect and understanding.

Communication must be adequate for the clinical state of the patient, and information should be clearly given during each step of the procedure: patients should be clearly informed about their rights, diagnosis, prognosis and treatment. If the patient does not provide his/her informed consent, it is forbidden to convey information on his/her clinical conditions to others.

The involuntarily admitted patient must have the opportunity to use his/her right of lodging an appeal with the relevant court and consult a trustworthy lawyer.

Coercive measures should always be considered as a last resort, and only when all other possible specific strategies for aggression management have failed. They are allowed only in the framework of existing legislation, national standards, and relevant ethical norms and policies. Applied coercive measures must be recorded in the patient's clinical file by the physician; in this file, information about persons ordering coercive measures and those executing them, the duration of coercive measures, and a patient's physical and mental condition should be reported. A more detailed description of ethics in psychiatry is provided in Chapter 17.

Therapeutic plan

The community mental health team, ward professionals and social workers should always develop a 'shared' therapeutic plan for the patient even when he/she has been involuntarily hospitalized. This plan should be devised after a careful evaluation of the patient's socio-demographic and clinical characteristics, care options, personal strengths and weaknesses, as well as his/her life expectations. The therapeutic plan should be agreed with the patient, if his/her mental status is such as to provide informed consent. If the patient is not able to provide it, the therapeutic plan should be agreed with his/her key relatives or with significant others; however, during the hospitalization process the physicians should continually try to obtain the patient's informed consent.

Proposals to improve patients' health care

Community and hospital-based mental health teams should organize periodical meetings, seminars and focus-groups with users' involvement on the main aspects of major mental disorders and of involuntary admissions. Moreover, training courses for the different professionals should be regularly planned, taking into account management strategies for aggressive or disturbing behaviours, diagnosis and treatment of the most frequent mental disorders, legal and administrative aspects of involuntary admissions, as well as specific communication skills and problem-solving strategies.

Conclusions

The avoidance of all coercive measures in psychiatric practice is an unrealistic goal, and early career psychiatrists should be aware of the need to use involuntary treatments. However, these should be practised according to national legislations and guidelines, if available, and always with a therapeutic focus. There is the need to:

1. Develop good clinical practice recommendations or guidelines on involuntary hospital admission and on the use of coercive measures.
2. Improve mental health care during psychiatric hospitalizations.
3. Guarantee patients' rights during involuntary hospital admission.
4. Increase patients' satisfaction with this procedure.
5. Promote collaboration among the different professionals involved in the hospital admissions.
6. Improve knowledge about current laws and appropriate procedures, with meetings and seminars for all involved parties and professionals.

References

1. Kallert TW, Glöckner M, Schützwohl M. Involuntary vs. voluntary hospital admission – a systematic review on outcome diversity. *Eur Arch Psy Clin N* 2008; **258**: 195–209.
2. Dressing H, Salize HJ. Compulsory admission of mentally ill patients in European Union Member States. *Soc Psych Psych Epid* 2004; **39**: 797–803.
3. Zinkler M, Priebe S. Detention of the mentally ill in Europe – a review. *Acta Psychiatr Scand* 2002; **106**: 3–8.
4. Laffont I, Priest RG. A comparison of French and British mental health legislation. *Psychol Med* 1992; **22**: 843–850.
5. Baca-Garcia E, Diaz-Sastre C, García Resa E et al. Suicide attempts and impulsivity. *Eur Arch Psy Clin N* 2005; **255**: 152–156.
6. Quirk A, Lelliott P, Seale C. Service users' strategies for managing risk in the volatile environment of an acute psychiatric ward. *Soc Sci Med* 2004; **59**: 2573–2583.
7. Priebe S, Badesconyi A, Fioritti A et al. Reinstitutionalisation in mental health care: comparison of data on service provision from six European countries. *Brit Med J* 2005; **330**: 123–126.

8. Abas MA, Vanderpyl J, Robinson E *et al*. Socio-economic deprivation and duration of hospital stay in severe mental disorder. *Br J Psychiat* 2006; **188**: 581–582.

9. Abas M, Vanderpyl J, Robinson E *et al*. More deprived areas need greater resources for mental health. *Aus NZ J Psychiat* 2003; **37**: 437–444.

10. Abas M, Vanderpyl J, Le Prou T *et al*. Psychiatric hospitalization: reasons for admission and alternatives to admission in South Auckland, New Zealand. *Aus NZ J Psychiat* 2003; **37**: 620–625.

11. World Health Organization. *Mental Health Legislation & Human Rights (Mental health policy and service guidance package)*. Geneva: World Health Organization, 2003.

12. Kallert TW, Rymaszewska J, Torres-González F. Differences of legal regulations concerning involuntary psychiatric hospitalization in twelve European countries: implications for clinical practice. *Int J Forensic Ment Hlth* 2007; **6**: 197–207.

13. Kallert TW. Coercion in psychiatry. *Curr Opin Psychiat* 2008; **21**: 485–489.

14. Kallert TW, Glöckner M, Onchev G *et al*. The EUNOMIA project on coercion in psychiatry: study design and preliminary data. *World Psychiatry* 2005; **4**: 168–172.

15. Raboch J, Kalisová L, Nawka A *et al*. Use of coercive measures during involuntary hospitalization: findings from ten European countries. *Psychiatr Serv* 2010; **61**: 1012–1017.

16. Steinert T, Lepping P, Bernhardsgrütter R *et al*. Incidence of seclusion and restraint in psychiatric hospitals: a literature review and survey of international trends. *Soc Psych Psych Epidemiol* 2010; **45**: 889–897.

17. Lay B, Nordt C, Rössler W. Variation in use of coercive measures in psychiatric hospitals. *Eur Psychiat* 2011; **26**: 244–251.

18. Bernstein R. Commentary on the "choice" between seclusion and forced medication. *Psychiat Serv* 2008; **59**: 212.

19. Smith G, Davis RF, Bixler E *et al*. Pennsylvania state hospital system's seclusion and restraint reduction program. *Psychiat Serv* 2005; **56**: 1115–1122.

20. Hellerstein DJ, Staub AB, Levesque E. Decreasing the use of restraint and seclusion among psychiatric inpatients. *J Psychiat Pract* 2007; **13**: 308–317.

21. Martin A, Krieg H, Esposito F *et al*. Reduction of restraint and seclusion through collaborative problem solving: a five-year prospective inpatient study. *Psychiat Serv* 2008; **59**: 1406–1412.

22. Mihai A, Allen MH, Beezhold J *et al*. Are female psychiatry residents better to propose in emergency a voluntary hospitalization? *Psychiat Quart* 2009; **80**: 233–239.

23. Damsa C, Ikelheimer D, Adam E *et al*. Heisenberg in the ER: observation appears to reduce involuntary intramuscular injections in a psychiatric emergency service. *Gen Hosp Psychiat* 2006; **28**: 431–433.

24. Scanlan JN. Interventions to reduce the use of seclusion and restraint in inpatient psychiatric settings: what we know so far: a review of the literature. *Int J Soc Psychiat* 2010; **56**: 412–423.
25. Fiorillo A, De Rosa C, Del Vecchio V *et al*. How to improve clinical practice on involuntary hospital admissions of psychiatric patients: Suggestions from the EUNOMIA study. *Eur Psychiat* 2011; **26**: 201–207.

CHAPTER 19

Mental health problems of early career psychiatrists: from diagnosis to treatment strategies

Nikolina Jovanović,[1] Julian Beezhold,[2] Adriana Mihai,[3] Olivier Andlauer,[4] Sarah Johnson[5] and Marianne Kastrup[6]

[1]Department of Psychiatry, University Hospital Centre and Zagreb School of Medicine, Croatia
[2]Norfolk and Waveney Mental Health NHS Foundation Trust, United Kingdom University of East Anglia, Norwich, UK
[3]Psychiatric Department, University of Medicine and Pharmacy, Tg Mures, Romania
[4]Department of Psychyatry, University Hospital, Besançon, France
[5]Department of Psychiatry, University of Louisville, KY, USA
[6]Centre for Transcultural Psychiatry, Psychiatric Centre Copenhagen, Denmark

Introduction

Mental health has been recognized as an integral part of human health, which may be conceptualized as a state of complete well-being, and not merely the absence of psychiatric disorder.[1] A large body of evidence suggests that those who choose medicine for their profession are at increased risk for developing mental health problems, mostly depression, substance abuse and suicide.[2-7] Working as a physician inevitably includes high levels of stress, similar to the stress that fire-fighters, policemen, managers, war reporters or pilots face in their professional assignments. Psychiatry is no exception, even more since today's psychiatrists are expected to be experts in a wide range of issues (from prevention, diagnostics and biopsychosocial treatments of mental disorders to administrative work and health management), and these demands are very likely to have harmful consequences on the mental health of both residents and specialists. Since it is impossible to completely eliminate stress from everyday clinical work, the only way to increase resilience is to undertake an effective strategy

How to Succeed in Psychiatry: A Guide to Training and Practice, First Edition.
Edited by Andrea Fiorillo, Iris Tatjana Calliess and Henning Sass.
© 2012 John Wiley & Sons, Ltd. Published 2012 by John Wiley & Sons, Ltd.

that will preserve and improve the well-being of psychiatrists. However, a somewhat different strategy is needed to help those who already have developed significant mental health problems (discussed in detail later in the text). The very first step is to increase awareness in medical communities worldwide that these problems are not rare. In fact, it quite often happens that a colleague is visibly depressed or dysfunctional at work for months (or even for years), and their community tolerates or ignores these signs. Physicians (psychiatrists included), although notorious at avoiding getting psychiatric help, do get ill and need to be treated immediately and efficiently.

Early career psychiatrists: a high-risk group for developing mental health problems

A common belief (or prejudice?) is that psychiatrists choose psychiatry as a profession to resolve their own mental health difficulties, such as a traumatic childhood, family conflicts or abuse. Undoubtedly, some psychiatrists are genetically predisposed to develop mental illness because of similar cases in their families, but more important is that the majority of psychiatrists have personality traits, such as perfectionism and proneness to undue guilt and self-recriminations, that are extremely unfavourable in this context.[8] Alternatively, choosing a 'helping profession' might be a sign of higher levels of empathy, but also proneness to so-called 'secondary traumatization' through clinical work with psychiatric patients. In both cases, the problem might occur when these traits interact with professional stressful events, thus increasing the risk for the development of mental illness.

Residency training and the early years after becoming a licensed psychiatrist are an extremely stressful period due to long working hours, many night and emergency shifts, sleep interruptions and often a marked imbalance between professional experience and responsibility. Early career psychiatrists often face incompatible demands, such as expectations to provide the highest quality of care in situations with an excessive patient load. Moreover, since medicine is still a strongly hierarchical profession, it is not uncommon that residents experience harassment by teachers, higher level residents or nurses. This period of life (usually late 20s or early 30s) is also characterized by many private life stressors, such as marriage, parenthood, frequent shifts in the workplace and estrangement from supportive networks.[9] Co-occurrence of these stressful professional and private events might cause the development of mental health difficulties, particularly depression, in early career psychiatrists and also be a contributing factor to suicidal ideation.

Depression has been documented to affect around 10–15 % of medical students and residents.[10] However, because of stigma, it is very likely that self-reporting underestimates the true prevalence of this disorder in both populations. Not only is depression itself often extremely difficult to handle and treat, but also depressed physicians may turn to social isolation and use of alcohol, anxiolytics and sedatives, rather than making an appointment with a psychiatrist. Although data are limited, it is estimated that approximately 2 % of physicians currently have an active substance abuse problem and another 8–18 % will be affected at some point in their lives.[11,12] The question is: why do early career psychiatrists become depressed? Although a history of depression and the role of personality, especially self-criticism and neuroticism, can never be underemphasized or ruled out, it has been shown that one extremely important risk factor is related to stress at workplace, the so-called 'burnout syndrome'.

Burnout syndrome

This term was coined in 1974 by Herbert Freudenberger in his paper 'Staff burnout', in which the author discussed job dissatisfaction precipitated by work-related stress.[13] Today research indicates that burnout syndrome is a distinct syndrome with very serious consequences. It refers to an inadequate response to prolonged occupational stress, and conceptually is characterized by a triad of: (i) emotional overextension and exhaustion; (ii) negative, cynical and detached responses to others; and (iii) feelings of inefficacy and reduced personal accomplishment.[14] Different studies report widely different burnout rates among medical residents, ranging from 18 to 82 %.[15] The rate is approximately 40 % in psychiatric residents.[15] The syndrome itself poses a significant challenge during early training years, with levels tending to decrease in the second half of training.[16] Risk factors can be characterized as either occupational or individual ones. As regards *occupational risk factors*, some work characteristics, such as time demands, lack of control and work planning, and poor work organization seem to be strongly related to burnout. For example, no special consultation rooms, one room shared between many trainees, lack of intimacy and confidentiality could be related to perceptions of high stress at the workplace. Differences between the expectations of patients, their relatives and older colleagues, together with often unclear professional goals and an undeveloped professional self, could increase inner conflicts and the perception of workplace stress. Interestingly, time constraints that eventually contribute to work-life imbalance cause significant feelings of dissatisfaction.[17] Under or overloading of work could be quantitative, including the volume of work in time units, or qualitative, related to task difficulties. Both are correlated with a reduced professional satisfaction.

Quantitative overload is common when departments are understaffed. The stress from this situation, coupled with the desire of the individual to treat every patient adequately, may result in physical and emotional fatigue. An increased number of patients may result in less time available for each patient, leading to inadequate treatments and failure to meet goals. The inability of individuals to fully use their training could be defined as 'qualitative underload', and may occur in normal workload situations as well, because of limitations applied by other professions or organizations.[18]

As regards the *individual risk factors*, the cross-sectional design of the majority of the studies carried out so far prevent us from understanding whether burnout is a consequence or a cause of dissatisfaction in social and family relationships. Most probably avoidant, dependent, antisocial and passive-aggressive personality traits correlate with higher levels of emotional exhaustion.[17] The perception of losing control, time pressure, lack of respect and social support, as well as the perception of a mismatch between the individual and the workplace, may be relevant factors for developing the burnout syndrome.[19] The degree of perception of danger in the workplace could also predispose the individual to burnout. We should keep in mind that only a small proportion of aggressive acts against health personnel comes to light, and numerous unreported violent incidents go unrecorded.[20] Furthermore, brief and superficial contacts with patients may lead to feelings of emptiness, lack of personal accomplishment and negative feelings towards patients. Gender differences with respect to perceptions of stress by medical doctors have been well documented. Thus, female physicians have been found to have twice the risk of being daily stressed compared to their male colleagues, even when controlled for stressors in relation to daily life, working life and health.[21]

Suicide

The stigma attached to suicide seems to be greater in the medical community than in the general population.[8] As a consequence, it is not rare that the suicide of a physician is covered up in order to preserve their medical reputation. The preponderance of suicides among physicians compared to other professions has been shown consistently. The data indicate that the risk of completed suicide is up to 2.4 times higher in physicians than in the general population.[2] The profile of a physician at high risk for suicide is given in Table 19.1.[6] Psychiatrists with a dual diagnosis of mood disorder and substance use, together with the knowledge and easy access

Table 19.1 The profile of a physician at high risk for suicide.

Gender	Women > men
Age	≥45 years for women
	≥50 years for men
Marital status	Single, divorced or in dysfunctional relationship
Family status	Recent loss
Health status	Depression, anxiety, alcohol or other drug misuse (or addiction), workaholic, gambler, risk taker, thrill seeker, physical symptoms of chronic pain or chronic debilitating illness
Work	Change in (or threat to) status – autonomy, security, financial stability, increased work demands
Knowledge and access to means	Access to lethal medications; access to firearms

Adapted from Silverman (2000).[6]

to lethal means, are at very high risk of suicide. This scenario seems to be even more cogent for early career physicians, and more often women. On average, the USA loses the equivalent of at least one entire medical school class each year due to suicide (approximately 400 physicians).[22] All this indicates the necessity of educating young students, residents and early career psychiatrists about suicide and prevention strategies.

Global perspective on early career psychiatrists' mental health problems

European perspective

A small number of studies have explored the mental health status of early career psychiatrists in Europe. Being aware of this problem and its impact on service provision, an important initiative came from European residents and early career psychiatrists to comprehensively study this problem and offer possible solutions. The International Psychiatry Residents/Trainees Burnout Syndrome Study (BoSS) was designed with the aim to search for risk factors that may endanger and/or protect the mental health status of psychiatric trainees. The study started in 2008 in 35 countries from all over the world. Preliminary findings are available from six countries (Croatia, France, Romania, Italy, Hungary and the UK) in where the study has been completed.[23] The 1722 interviewed residents, who have a mean age of 31.92 years (±5.44), are female in 52.3 % of cases, ($N = 807$), married or engaged in a stable relationship ($N = 1090$, 70.3 %), suffer from moderate levels of burnout (Table 19.2). Looking at other facets of mental health, results from the BoSS indicate that approximately 5 % of the sample met criteria for major depression

Table 19.2 Three dimensions of burnout syndrome in psychiatry residents ($N = 1722$). Preliminary data from the International Psychiatry Residents/Trainees Burnout Syndrome Study (BoSS). Values obtained using the Maslach Burnout Inventory-General Survey (MBI GS).[14]

	Range of experienced burnout syndrome (normative values)	BoSS sample (mean ± SD)	Interpretation – level of burnout
Exhaustion	≤2 (low) 2.01–3.19 (moderate) ≥3.20 (high)	2.81 ± 1.47	Moderate
Cynicism	≤1 (low) 1.01–2.19 (moderate) ≥2.20 (high)	2.16 ± 1.46	Moderate
Efficacy	≥5.00 (low) 4.01–4.99 (moderate) ≤4.00 (high)	4.38 ± 1.07	Moderate

Table 19.3 Depression in psychiatry residents ($N = 1722$). Preliminary data from the International Psychiatry Residents/Trainees Burnout Syndrome Study (BoSS). Assessments based on the Patient Health Questionnaire (PHQ-9).[36]

PHQ-9	BoSS sample (*N*, %)
No depression	836 (48.5 %)
Minor depressive disorder	163 (9.5 %)
Major depressive disorder	112 (6.5 %)

Table 19.4 Suicide ideation and behaviour in psychiatry residents ($N = 1722$). Preliminary data from the International Psychiatry Residents/Trainees Burnout Syndrome Study (BoSS). Assessments based on the Suicide Ideation and Behaviour Questionnaire (SIBQ).[37]

SIBQ	BoSS sample (*N*, %)
Passive suicide ideation	371 (21.5 %)
Active suicide ideation	294 (17.0 %)
Suicide attempt	25 (1.45 %)

(Table 19.3), and 1 % attempted suicide. However, it must be noted that in some countries the numbers with serious suicidal ideation is up to 20 % (Table 19.4). The main goal of this study is to feed these data back to each country and try to create country specific interventions that may improve the mental health of psychiatric residents.

US perspective

The mental health of medical residents has received a great deal of attention in recent years in the USA. In July 2003, the Accreditation Council for Graduate Medical Education implemented work hour restrictions limiting the number of hours that residents could work. This is one step that has been taken to promote well-being in the USA. However, there are few data available to quantify the impact that these measures are having on the trainees' experience.[24] The 2008 North American Resident Wellness Survey suggested that psychiatric trainees in the USA may also be at risk for mental distress. In a sample of 893 respondents, 8 % indicated that they felt 'very stressed' and 47 % indicated that they felt 'stressed', compared with 28 % reporting feeling 'neutral' and 6 % feeling 'relaxed'. Fourteen percent indicated that they were dissatisfied with their mental health state.[25] A follow-up study was completed in 2009 showing high levels of reported stress that were consistent with the earlier study. Factors contributing to burnout and stress were investigated, and data are currently being analysed.[26] The BoSS study will soon be implemented in the USA and enable comparison with European nations.

Prevention and treatment

Barriers to appropriate care seeking

One of the reasons why physicians are at higher risk of developing mental health problems in comparison with the general population is that the list of barriers to appropriate care seeking seems to be significantly longer and more complex. The list of barriers includes:[27]

1. Inadequate education about the causes, about the effects on service provision, and about the possible treatments.
2. Unwillingness to take time off from work to be dedicated to protection and/or improvement of one's own health.
3. Concerns about confidentiality, stigma, discrimination in medical licensing, hospital privileges, and career progress.

Furthermore, physicians who decide to reach out for help may face limited understanding by their colleagues, who might not take the problems seriously enough, consequently leading to inadequate diagnosis and treatments. Unfortunately, medical training rarely addresses the issue of specialized training for a physicians' physician.[22] The American Foundation for Suicide Prevention invited 15 experts to evaluate the knowledge about physician depression and suicide, and about barriers to treatment. In 2003, a consensus statement was published in which transformation of professional attitudes and institutional policies to encourage physicians to seek help were strongly recommended.[28] The statement suggests that physicians create services for those suffering from mental health problems, such as drug abuse and suicide risk, learn how to recognize depression in themselves, teach these skills to students and residents, and learn about laws that might protect confidentiality and professional work in case of mental health problems.

Prevention strategies

Prevention strategies should focus on identified occupational and individual risk factors. This might lead to specific workplace interventions such as regular supervision or obligatory daily and weekly rest (primary prevention), together with the identification of at-risk colleagues who might be offered psychiatric consultations (secondary prevention), or psychiatric treatment and a more suitable workplace (tertiary prevention). An interesting approach, called 'Engagement' and described by Maslach and Goldberg in 1998,[29] is defined in terms of the same three dimensions as burnout, but with a focus on the positive aspects of those dimensions, rather than on the negative ones. Thus, engagement consists of a state of high energy (rather than exhaustion), strong involvement (rather than depersonalization), and a sense of efficacy (rather than a reduced sense of accomplishment). The concept of a burnout-to-engagement continuum enhances our perspective on how the organizational context of work can affect workers' well-being.[29] This multi-dimensional approach might be closer to the complex interactions between individual and environmental factors, similar to the psychiatric biopsychosocial perspective.

An extremely powerful tool in prevention and/or early recognition of depression and other mental health problems is a comprehensive education about risk factors and treatment options, starting with first-year medical students. In Japan, a 2-hour suicide intervention programme for medical residents has been developed, which consists of a 1-hour lecture and a 1-hour role-play session.[30] Participants' confidence and attitudes significantly improved after the intervention programme, but the effectiveness was limited after 6 months, which might indicate that education and intervention programmes should take place continually throughout the professional career.

Table 19.5 Mental health of early career psychiatrists – prevention strategies.

Primary prevention	Workplace interventions: increasing staff awareness, ensuring regular supervisions and peer support, ensuring reasonable workload, team building, regular rest and vacation
	Education throughout entire professional career: how to protect one's mental health and how to create a defined boundary between work and home
	Development of stress-reduction and wellness programmes including meditation, physical exercise, etc.
Secondary and tertiary prevention	Identification of at-risk colleagues and those who might be offered psychiatric consultations, or given a more suitable workplace or specialty

Creating a defined boundary between work and home has also been strongly suggested. Maslach summarized effective working through burnout by stating: 'If all of the knowledge and advice about how to beat burnout could be summed up in one word, that word would be balance – balance between giving and getting, balance between stress and calm, balance between work and home.'[31] It is important to support early career psychiatrists to identify and practise the individual activities and techniques. Prevention strategies are listed in Table 19.5.

Treatment

Treatment of depression and substance abuse in early career psychiatrists includes all validated procedures that are used in the general population. The only difference is that an approach to a colleague (now a patient) with mental health problems needs to address all the aforementioned obstacles, such as the fear of compromised confidentiality and reputation, and poor insight. To our knowledge, there is no consensus on a biological approach to treat burnout and no clinical trial on pharmacotherapy has been published yet. Most psychological interventions are group interventions: workshops on how to improve communication skills, conflict resolution, stress management, etc. Medical education can also be useful to reduce stress and improve self-efficiency: for example, peer-support groups on difficult cases, attendance at lectures or conferences, and involvement in professional organizations. Supervision might be of great use in helping residents: among other interventions, receiving a positive feedback from supervisors may foster the sense of self-efficacy.[32]

Table 19.6 Burnout syndrome – prevention and recovery strategies.

Plan life, not time	Evaluate all your activities, even the most trivial, to determine whether they add to your life. If they don't, get rid of them
Slow down	When rushed, ask yourself if you really need to be. What's the worst that can happen if you slow down? Tell yourself at least once a day that failure seldom results from doing a job slowly or too well
Learn to say no	Decide what things you can do, what things you must do, and what things you want to do, and delegate the rest to someone else either permanently or until you complete some of your priority tasks. Before you take on a new responsibility, finish or drop an old one
Schedule time for yourself	Find time each day for quiet thinking, reading, exercising or activities that you enjoy
Learn to meditate	Meditation is an effective way for stress management. It generally focuses on deep breathing, allowing tension to leave the body with each exhalation. Anyone can learn to meditate!
Go for a massage regularly	Massage is an excellent means of relaxation and self-care. Massage boosts the immune system, relieves stress and enhances general well-being
Maintain a social network	Friends are vital to our mental health. Connecting with friends who are positive and enthusiastic renews optimism and hope. Friends can also help us to be accountable when we strive to make changes
Develop a hearty laugh	Laughter boosts our immune system. Learn to differentiate between what is serious and what is not. Spend time with people who are funny and make you laugh. Laugh big deep belly laughs
Seek professional help	If you are concerned about your stress level or are experiencing burnout find a therapist who can work with you to improve your emotional and physical well-being

Adapted from MacDonald.[38]

Well-being may be very useful: relaxation, meditation and physical activities can help to reduce stress. The 'ROM' (Respiratory One Method), in which the subject focuses on the word 'one' with each exhalation, seems to be the simplest intervention and may be easily used by physicians.[33] We must underline that most of these strategies have shown some effect on intermediate variables rather than burnout itself, more specifically on only one of its dimensions, emotional exhaustion.[34] Burnout prevention and recovery strategies are listed in Table 19.6.

Conclusions

Early career psychiatrists are at increased risk of developing burnout syndrome, which may lead to depression (although the latter can also occur independently from burnout syndrome), substance misuse and suicide. These problems may have a negative influence on physicians' clinical performance and on patients' care. Furthermore, burnout can significantly reduce learning capacity and academic performance of sufferers. The role of education in prevention and recovery from mental illness cannot be overemphasized. It needs to be comprehensive and continual, starting with first-year medical students and lasting throughout the entire professional career. The ongoing education of medical students and physicians is the only way to overcome stigma within the medical profession regarding seeking psychiatric care.[35] Furthermore, mental health services need to be easily available to everyone in need. Physicians must have the opportunity to seek confidential mental health treatment at their earliest signs of distress in order to maximize their optimal functioning in an effort to prevent impairment.[35] As stated by Michael Myers:[8]

> We need to keep fighting the culture of medicine that rewards punishing work, harassment in our medical centers, inappropriate self-sacrifice, neglect of our families, and eschewing of our responsibility to each other as brothers and sisters in medicine. We need to laud physicians who "come out of the closet" and tell their personal stories of living with psychiatric illness. We need to listen to the stories of husbands, wives, and children of doctors. We need to fight stigma, in word and deed, until it is completely eradicated from our society.

Although the burnout syndrome has been well documented in the last 10 years, it still requires further in-depth studies because prevention and treatment strategies are poorly developed and/or validated. Our initiative to explore different facets of the mental health of psychiatry residents worldwide may serve as a starting point for the development of country-specific interventions.

References

1. De Rivero T, David A. Alma-Ata revisited. *Persp Health* 2003; **8**: 2–7.
2. Schernhammer ES, Graham AC. Suicide rates among physicians: A quantitative and gender assessment (meta-analysis). *Am J Psychiatry* 2004; **161**: 2295–2302.
3. Hawton K, Clements A, Sakarovitch C *et al.* Suicide in doctors: a study of risk according to gender, seniority and specialty in medical practitioners in England and Wales, 1979–1995. *J Epidemiol Commun Health* 2001; **55**: 296–300.
4. Ramirez AJ, Graham J, Richards MA *et al.* Mental health of hospital consultants: the effects of stress and satisfaction at work. *Lancet* 1996; **16**: 724–728.
5. Rosta J. Hazardous alcohol use among hospital doctors in Germany. *Alcohol* 2008; **43**: 198–203.
6. Silverman M. Physicians and suicide. In: Goldman LS, Myers M, Dickstein LJ (eds) *The Handbook of Physician Health: Essential Guide to Understanding the Health Care Needs of Physicians.* Chicago: American Medical Association, 2000; pp. 102–117.
7. Welner A, Marten S, Wochnick E *et al.* Psychiatric disorders among professional women. *Arch Gen Psychiatry* 1979; **36**; 169–173.
8. Myers M, Fine C. Suicide in physicians: toward prevention. *Medscape Gen Med* 2003; **21**: 11.
9. Tyssen R, Vlagum P. Mental health problems among young doctors: An updated review of prospective studies. *Harvard Rev Psychiatry* 2002; **10**: 154–165.
10. Goebert D, Thompson D, Takeshita J *et al.* Depressive symptoms in medical students and residents: a multischool study. *Acad Med* 2009; **84**: 236–241.
11. McBeth B, Ankel F. Don't ask, don't tell: substance use by resident physicians. *Acad Emerg Med* 2006; **13**: 1–3.
12. Boisaubin E, Levine R. Identifying and assisting the impaired physician. *Am J Med Sci* 2001; **322**: 31–36.
13. Freudenberger HJ. Staff burnout. *J Soc Issues* 1974; **30**: 159–165.
14. Maslach C, Jackson SE, Leiter MP. *Maslach Burnout Inventory Manual*, 3rd edn. Palo Alto: Consulting Psychologists Press, Inc., 1996.
15. Prins JT, Gazendam-Donofrio SM, Tubben BJ *et al.* Burnout in medical residents: a review. *Med Educ* 2007; **41**: 788–800.
16. Tzischinsky O. Daily and yearly burnout symptoms in Israeli shift work residents. *J Hum Ergology* 2001; **30**: 357–362.
17. Thomas NK. Resident burnout. *JAMA* 2004; **292**: 2880–2889.
18. Wolfe GA. Burnout of therapists inevitable or preventable ? *Phys Ther* 1981; **7**: 1046–1050.
19. Stoica M. *Stress, Personality and Performances in Management Efficiency.* Cluj-Napoca: Ed Risoprint, 2007.
20. Miret C, Larrea AM. The professional in emergency care: aggressiveness and burnout. *Ann Sist Sanit Navar* 2010; **33**: 193–201.

21. Hargreaves M, Petersson B, Kastrup M. Kønsforskelle og stress hos læger [Gender differences and stress among medical doctors]. Ugeskr Læg 2007; **169**: 2418–2422.

22. Andrew LB. Physician suicide. *Medscape Ref*. Available at: http://emedicine. medscape.com/article/806779-overview.

23. Jovanovic N, Beezhold J, Podlesek A. Mental health and well-being among early career psychiatrists. In: Fiorillo A, De Rosa C (eds) *Lo psichiatra del nuovo millennio: bisogni formativi, competenze cliniche e rischi professionali*. Milan: Sintesi InfoMedica, 2010; p. 59.

24. Fletcher K, Underwood W, Davis S *et al.* Effects of work hour reduction on resident's lives: a systematic review. *JAMA* 2005; **294**: 1088–1100.

25. Johnson S, O'Leary P. The 2009 North American resident wellness survey. Presented at the Association for American Directors of Psychiatric Residency Training Programs, Annual Meeting, Tucson, Arizona, 2009.

26. Johnson S, O'Leary P, Tamas R. Burnout in US psychiatry residents. Presented at the Association for Academic Psychiatry, Annual Meeting, Washington, DC, 2009.

27. Reynolds CF 3rd, Clayton PJ. Commentary: Out of the silence: confronting depression in medical students and residents. *Acad Med* 2009; **84**: 159–160.

28. Center C, Davis M, Detre T *et al.* Confronting depression and suicide in physicians: a consensus statement. *JAMA* 2003; **289**: 3161–3166.

29. Maslach C, Goldberg J. Prevention of burnout: new perspectives. *Appl Prevent Psychol* 1998; **7**: 63–74.

30. Kato TA, Suzuki Y, Sato R *et al.* Development of 2-hour suicide intervention program among medical residents: first pilot trial. *Psychiatry Clin Neurosci* 2010; **64**: 531–540.

31. IsHak WW, Lederer S, Mandili C *et al.* Burnout during residency training: a literature review. *J Grad Med Educ* 2009; **1**: 236–242.

32. Dory V, Beaulieu MD, Pestiaux D *et al.* The development of self-efficacy beliefs during general practice vocational training: an exploratory study. *Med Teacher* 2009; **31**: 39–44.

33. Ospina-Kammerer V, Figley CR. An evaluation of the respiratory one method (ROM) in reducing emotional exhaustion among family physician residents. *Int J Emerg Ment H* 2003; **5**: 29–32.

34. McCray LW, Cronholm PF, Bogner HR *et al.* Resident physician burnout: is there hope? *Fam Med* 2008; **40**: 626–632.

35. Worley LLM. Our fallen peers: a mandate for change. *Acad Psychiatry* 2008; **32**: 8–12.

36. Kroenke K, Spitzer RL, Williams JB. The PHQ-9: validity of a brief depression severity measure. *J Gen Int Med* 2001; **16**: 606–613.

37. Marušič A, Roškar S, Zorko M. Questionnaire on Suicide Ideation and Behaviour. In: Amresh KS (ed.) *Suicide Prevention in Developing Countries*. London: Gaskell, 2007; pp. 201–209.

38. MacDonald L. Burnout prevention and treatment strategies. 2000. Available at: www.lucymacdonald.com.

CHAPTER 20

Leadership, management and administrative issues for early career psychiatrists

Julian Beezhold,[1] Kate Manley,[2] Emma Brandon,[3] Victor Buwalda,[4] and Marianne Kastrup[5]

[1]Norfolk and Waveney Mental Health Care NHS Foundation Trust, United Kingdom
University of East Anglia, Norwich, UK
[2]Norfolk and Waveney Mental Health Care NHS Foundation Trust, Norwich, UK
[3]Norfolk and Waveney Mental Health NHS Foundation Trust, Norwich, UK
[4]Altrecht ggz, Utrecht/Den Dolder and Department of Psychiatry, Free University of Amsterdam, The Netherlands
[5]Centre for Transcultural Psychiatry, Psychiatric Centre Copenhagen, Denmark

> The future of psychiatry depends greatly upon its leaders, especially its academic leaders. Their beliefs and commitments will, to a considerable extent, determine the future of specialty.
>
> Samuel Berry Guze, 1992[1]

Introduction

Broadly speaking, the structure of many organizations has undergone a process of gradual evolution from the traditional hierarchical, bureaucratic arrangements of the past,[2] into a more horizontal, flexible style, where goals and objectives are the responsibility of smaller teams as opposed to large, formally constituted departments.[3]

Whilst the structure and organization of mental health services may be undergoing change, the need for leadership and the requirements for successful management remain constant. In order to maintain the core values of mental health service providers, it is necessary for some clinicians to take on leadership roles.[2]

How to Succeed in Psychiatry: A Guide to Training and Practice, First Edition.
Edited by Andrea Fiorillo, Iris Tatjana Calliess and Henning Sass.
© 2012 John Wiley & Sons, Ltd. Published 2012 by John Wiley & Sons, Ltd.

There appears to be widespread consensus that specialist training in most, if not all, specialties fails adequately to prepare residents for life as fully qualified specialists. In particular, early career psychiatrists rarely obtain adequate training in leadership and management skills to enable them adequately to meet the particular demands of their role.

The key competencies required for successful leadership by examining mainstream theory, as well as issues that are specific to the tasks and challenges confronted by mental health organizations, are too often neglected.

Leadership vs management

'Leadership' and 'management' are terms that are frequently used synonymously. In practice, many leaders may often simultaneously take on managerial roles – indeed, to be a successful leader requires managerial competence.[4] Conceptually, however, leadership and management are somewhat different. In broad terms, leadership is concerned with the pursuit of major, transformational change, whereas management is concerned in dealing with complexity.[5]

In the book *Leading Change*, Kotter makes the distinction as follows: 'Managing is a set of processes that can keep a complicated system of people and technology running smoothly. . . . The most important aspects of management include planning, budgeting, organizing, staffing, controlling, and problem solving . . . Leadership is a set of processes that creates organizations in the first place or adapts them to significantly changing circumstances . . . . Leadership defines what the future should look like, aligns people with that vision, and inspires them to make it happen despite the obstacles.'[5]

For an organization to be successful, it is required to adapt to a constantly shifting environment. Change is therefore vital for survival in the current era of competition for funding, resources and increasing pressure on organizations to meet targets for improved patient outcomes. The initiation and management of this organizational change is a fundamental principle of leadership.

Leaders are firstly required to define and communicate their vision of change for the future to others, and subsequently work alongside key members of the organization to provide a guiding alliance to lead the transformation.[2] To achieve the level of change necessary for the perpetuation of an organization, a combination of both effective leadership and appropriate management is required: 'Successful [organizational change] transformation is 70 to 90 percent leadership and only 10 to 30 percent management'.[5]

In order to fully understand the role of a leader, it is also necessary to examine the specific concepts of clinical and professional leadership in addition to the general terms leadership and management.

There is no agreed definition of clinical leadership; however, Edmonstone[6] has postulated that clinical leadership is 'leadership by clinicians of clinicians...all those who retained some clinical role but at the same time took on a significant part in matters of strategic direction, operational resource management and collaborative working with colleagues in their own and other clinical professions'. In this sense, clinical leadership relates more specifically to effecting those local changes in service improvement that result in improved patient care. Strategic vision is one of the most important tools at the disposal of the successful clinical leader – where, alongside colleagues, established clinical practice must be reviewed, and appropriate changes devised and implemented to provide improved service delivery. The role of clinical leadership is very much centred on evidence-based changes to patient care at a local level.[7]

As with clinical leadership, there is no solid definition of professional leadership. It involves the development of a professional identity (a shared set of attributes and values adopted within a profession), and advancing the contribution of the profession towards maintaining the values and achieving the objectives of the organization.[8]

On a general note, a psychiatrist's approach to acting as a spokesperson for mental health should also be considered here. Attitudes of other professionals and clinicians towards psychiatry may often be based on misunderstanding and stigma, and there is sometimes conflict between psychiatrists and the competing demands of other medical disciplines. However, it could be argued that psychiatrists are failing in their roles as professional leaders and representatives of their profession – that they must 'take a large measure of responsibility' for these problems, as a result of a 'long-standing collusion...and tolerance of unacceptable behaviour'.[9]

Organizational values and the concept of morality in leadership

Levin *et al.*[2] outline the concepts of managerial alliance and psychological contracts within organizations, which leaders should be aware of and consider as tools to aid them in successful leadership.

Managerial alliance refers to the key values of the organization, which are reflected by the leaders when carrying out their role, and the identification of these values by the other members of the organization. These values generally relate to the overall objectives or mission of the organization, helping to unify members and concentrate efforts towards a common goal.[10] From a mental health perspective, the key values will likely include a commitment to excellence in patient care and service delivery.

Psychological contracts, which are 'powerful cultural agreements that reflect nature of the work to be performed and organisational values ... a set of mutual expectations between leadership and subordinates',[2] relate to the unwritten rules or codes of conduct that both leaders and organization members expect of one another.

In their roles as both leaders and clinical providers, clinicians are often faced with conflict as they may encounter conflicting responsibilities.[11] However, if leaders are not successful in upholding the key values of the organization, or if either side violates their psychological contract, the result is a breakdown of organizational structure – a loss of trust, and an inability to function adequately as a team. It is therefore important for psychiatrists to consider these concepts when embarking on a new role that requires them to act as leaders.

In addition to upholding the core values of the organization, a moral perspective on leadership can also be adopted; Chervenak[4] suggests that managerial knowledge and skills can be used to both worthy and unworthy ends and therefore require a moral foundation. It is argued that 'the concept of the physician as the moral fiduciary of the patient should be the moral foundation of management decisions by physician-leaders', suggesting that physician leaders must apply professional virtues (namely self-effacement, self-sacrifice, compassion and integrity) in order to create a 'moral culture of professionalism' within the organizations in which they work.[4]

The need for leadership, management and administrative skills

Early career psychiatrists as a group tend to share a number of common needs and concerns, ranging from training deficits, problems coping with role change and workload, through to developing the skills required for surviving and thriving in their new roles.

A study of early career psychiatrists in the USA showed that moderate to severe anxiety was experienced by 78 % of early career psychiatrists, with 58 % experiencing depression.[12]

Researchers in different medical specialties have examined these issues. Their work highlights common themes and gives us some direction in how to approach these issues, for example internal medicine,[13] accident and emergency medicine,[14] geriatric medicine,[15] orthopaedics[16] and also hospital doctors.[13,17]

The UK London Deanery, responsible for cross-specialty postgraduate training in London, analysed early career specialist training events over several years. Delegates described the change from resident to early career specialist status as 'main challenge...was surviving', 'dramatic' and 'a host of unanticipated responsibilities that required skills [that they] didn't have'.[17] These early career specialists identified several needs for management skills, including business planning, negotiation, dealing with the problems of residents and other colleagues, conducting interviews, responsibility for decision-making, learning to say 'no' (where appropriate) in a constructive manner, prioritization skills for workload and administrative pressures, managing difficult relationships, all aspects of role change (such as how and where to obtain help when they are actually the person in charge), and the need for more information regarding the structure and organization of their broader and immediate work setting.

Robinowitz[18] describes two critical periods of time for psychiatrists who are newly appointed in leadership positions, which are pivotal for determining the course of their leadership: (i) the initial negotiations with the institution, and (ii) the 2–6-month period at the beginning of the post. Both of these critical periods occur early on, and they provide an opportunity for a new leader to identify what is required of them, elucidate goals, establish priorities and build a supportive infrastructure. It follows that psychiatrists who are inexperienced or ill-prepared for the demands of leadership are at a considerable disadvantage in this initial period.

Psychiatrists as leaders

Leadership is best characterized by vision and mission, and the courage, character, and ability to put the precepts of this vision and mission into sustainable action. Leaders combine their ideas and values with the necessary energy and effectiveness to implement them.

C. Robinowitz[18]

It has been postulated that psychiatrists are 'natural born leaders',[19] as they possess attributes that ensure they are well suited to leadership as a result of their professional training: 'Management is just psychiatry by other means'.[20] Psychiatrists may benefit in their role as leaders from their understanding of human interaction – from individual and group dynamics to their knowledge of the concepts of transference, projection and narcissism. They are also able to utilize well-honed communication skills to facilitate them in their role.[18] Alternatively, it could be argued that some attributes possessed by psychiatrists may hamper them in their efforts to act as a successful leader. Passivity, for example, which could be viewed as a useful technique employed when listening to patients and being empathetically responsive, is clearly a drawback for a leader, who may often be called upon to take decisive actions.[2]

Whether or not psychiatrists are well suited to leadership, patients and colleagues may well have expectations of them, often automatically looking to them as leaders. Despite leadership being a key component of an early career psychiatrist's role, it is well documented that training is lacking in this area.[21,22] There are even concerns that the whole profession of psychiatry faces a leadership crisis.[23] In contrast, the perspective of the corporate world is altogether different, and management training contributes a significant part of a career pathway.[24]

Within the health service, early career psychiatrists may find themselves working alongside policy-makers and administrators who have all undergone management training in order to fulfil their roles, compared with the limited exposure of psychiatrists to such training.[22] But this lack of training in leadership and management is not exclusive to psychiatry; it is evident in other medical disciplines: in a large survey of early career internists, the striking difference was noted between the 20–25 % of time commitment to managerial duties required in their posts and the 5 % of training devoted to preparation for this.[13]

As the notion of leadership is poorly addressed in training courses for psychiatrists, it is rare for them to consider leadership roles early in their original career plans. Further, there is a tradition of prioritizing research over leadership and thereby not paying sufficient attention to the acquisition of leadership competencies. Indeed, clinicians may end up in leadership roles rather 'by accident'.[25] This lack of focus on leadership may further allow other professions, such as nurses, to take over managerial roles as they may have better understood the need to focus on leadership.

In many cases, the lack of preparation for such a role coupled with the competing commitments of clinical work, research and home, results in few incentives for clinicians to adopt managerial or leadership roles. This is notable in the case of clinical leadership, where a survey of NHS Medical Directors[26] discovered that 80 % believed that the role of clinical leader was not an attractive career option for doctors, 90 % felt that there was no proper career structure to encourage medical staff to become clinical leaders, and 43 % did not even have a personal development plan.[25]

Leadership and management competencies

If you want to be a leader in psychiatry, you must be present

Norman Sartorius, speaking at the European Congress of Psychiatry, 2009

What constitutes a successful leader? The majority of the literature devoted to answering this question pertains to business and profit-making industries, and there is little writing specific to the subject of leadership in psychiatry. Whilst many useful parallels can be made with the corporate world, it is at the same time important to consider leadership in the context of the particular values, roles and challenges found within the mental health services.

The ingredients for effective leadership and management in psychiatry can be broadly summarized into a series of seven desirable 'core competencies'.[22,27] This list is by no means exhaustive, but is intended to provide an overview of the main areas in which successful leaders should have abilities.

1. *Organizational knowledge, tolerance for systems process.* Although the structure and processes of the management environment may be drastically different from the experience of clinical work, an ability to adapt and function in this area is obviously beneficial.

2. *Sound financial stewardship.* A knowledge of some of the important terminology involved in basic accounting, the costs required to achieve goals, and the available budget are all desirable. Additional qualifications or experience in finance are obviously beneficial, but are by no means a prerequisite as the majority of leaders in psychiatry will rely on advice from individuals with greater financial expertise.

3. *Strategy development.* In order to maximize competitive edge, the leader of an organization must be able to perform an assessment of the competition in order to select appropriate means of adaptation. Whilst this is crucial in the corporate business sector, the importance of this may seem less apparent when considering the provision of mental health services. However, health-care provision organizations can still be subject to competitive factors. Porter[28] describes the two questions that a leader should consider when assessing the potential for strategy development: '1) What is the structure of the industry in which you are functioning?, and 2) What is your own organisation's relative position in the industry?'

4. *Communication skills.* Communication skills are a vital component of effective leadership, and need to be utilized both within the team and beyond. Due to their overlapping knowledge, clinical leaders may also adopt a parallel role as interpreters: 'Making sense of the managerial agenda for clinicians and making sense of the clinicians' agenda for managers'.[25] A good leader must be able to negotiate effectively and possess well-developed conflict resolution skills. For many leaders in psychiatry, contact with the media often comprises part of the job – but

whilst formal media training can be an extremely useful asset, it is something to which residents are rarely exposed.

5. *Understanding of basic legal issues relevant to the position.* In addition to those issues that are relevant to their clinical practice, leaders should also be familiar with legal issues that may be specific to their leadership role – employment legislation regarding equal opportunities, or contractual negotiation, for example.

6. *Understanding of the basic principles of quality management.* Quality management can be viewed as the approach employed by an organization to achieve and sustain high-quality output. The principles of quality management were originally derived from industry, but quality management theory has been increasingly adapted and utilized by health-care provision organizations.[29]

7. *Broad knowledge base of medicine/psychiatry.* Leaders should of course have sound clinical acumen; in addition to this, however, it is the responsibility of the leader to continue to drive their professional development – learning new skills, meeting new clinical challenges and keeping up with the latest developments.

In addition to the core competencies listed above, consideration must also be given to time management and the prioritization of tasks – the 'final common pathway' of successful leadership.[2] The responsibilities of leadership and management can place immense demands on the time available to fulfil other commitments. Greiner[27] raises the important point that leaders must be willing to make sacrifices and commit themselves to undertaking their leadership roles and responsibilities: 'One basic litmus test is to determine if you will be able to attend 80 % of the new meetings and be an active contributor to the discussions. If you cannot make that commitment, then leadership is probably not a reasonable choice.'

Team-working and team-building

Finally, skills in team-working and team-building are of vital importance to good leadership, with efficient team-working having benefits for clinical care and patient outcomes.[30] The act of leadership itself has become less of an individual role and more a team-pursuit: studies in Canada have provided evidence for the success of leadership teams over individuals.[31] In Table 20.1 the necessary characteristics of an effective team leader are reported.

In addition to the key strategies described in Table 20.1, an effective leader must also be prepared to provide regular feedback regarding performance in order to ensure the continued smooth running of the

Table 20.1 Characteristics of an effective team leader.

- Being inspiring and bringing out the best in others
- Setting objectives and goals with clear and achievable outcomes
- Participating in recruitment of colleagues
- Facilitating the development of the next generation of leaders
- Delegating authority
- Arranging regular and effective team meetings
- Motivating the team to develop, through the promotion of training
- Organizing mentoring for colleagues
- Rewarding success

team and to maintain morale. 'Performance appraisal … reflects genuine interest in subordinate's work and is an opportunity to connect the individual with the organisation and reinforce organisational values'.[2]

A lack of feedback (positive or negative) can leave team members dissatisfied and disempowered – feeling as though 'no one cares' about their work. Psychiatrists as a group should already be aware of the impact of reward and reinforcement on behaviour and motivation, and the importance of giving positive feedback.[18]

Dealing with poor performance can be a very challenging part of a leadership role – it is important to remember to offer to help improve the situation when identifying areas for improvement and giving negative feedback.

In addition to providing feedback to the team, receiving feedback is an incredibly useful tool employed by effective leaders. Successful leadership can be evaluated in various ways – meeting targets or achieving goals are obvious measures of outcome, but 360-degree evaluations from colleagues can provide valuable information on leadership strengths and weaknesses to improve and develop future performance.

Targets for improvement

A study carried out by Cray and Lawrance[32] specifically included 'recommendations for best practice in relation to setting up newly appointed (early career specialists) for success'. The authors identified environmental factors, engagement with early career specialists, and a supporting and enabling management approach as being the three key areas for organizations to focus on when dealing with new specialists.

Environmental factors ranged from establishing and promoting mentoring and early career networks, through using appropriate feedback, acknowledgement and praise, to monitoring for bullying and adequate secretarial, office space and computer support.

The report recommended engaging early career specialists by using a formal welcome and induction process after planning for the new arrival. It went on to suggest using a constant process of feedback and review to examine barriers to engagement, career planning and also performance of both the employer and employee.

Methods for supporting and enabling early career specialists included planning and allocating time for specific training, using existing staff to welcome and support, for example with a 'buddy' system, reviews with senior medical managers from the outset, and setting up an early career specialists' network.

Regarding clinical leadership specifically, a study that focused on successful clinician – management relationships concluded that such productive alliances were marked by the following: '1) Open participative and inclusive modes of communication; 2) collaborative leadership styles (both clinical and managerial); 3) greater clinical input into managerial decision-making at all levels; 4) a shared focus on the centrality of managing the means of production; 5) ensuring continuity over time; 6) appropriate investment in organization development.'[33]

How the needs can be addressed

A study that compared leadership approaches between companies[34] found that in the most successful companies, leaders had adapted their approach to the needs of the company rather than adopting a leadership style that was reflective of their individual personality. It is a popular misconception that leadership is a quality that cannot be taught (i.e. it is either present or absent). The reality is that good leadership is present in degrees,[27] and can be enhanced with appropriate training.

Improvements to specialist training curricula worldwide are constantly being made, with a major shift in the direction of competency-based training. Some training organizations are now very aware of the concerns regarding the transition to early career psychiatrist posts and, for example, put significantly more emphasis on management training than in the past.[22,35]

Early career specialists who had been able to gain training that included actual responsibility during their training years reported that this had been extremely helpful.[17] However, there is an argument for beginning such training much earlier in a resident's career, and that by the end of training it might be too late to foster the good practices of effective leadership and management. The Royal College of Surgeons of Edinburgh responded to this need with the Adamson executive report regarding the training needs of early career surgeons. This led to the introduction of an increasingly popular two-day course focusing on the changing roles, responsibilities and unmet personal development needs of early career surgeons.[36]

Ham[37] examined the means by which clinicians are encouraged to take on clinical leadership roles. He argued that successful reform needs to focus on organizational development, not merely on leadership development, to create 'organizations in which professionals are willing to follow their peers who take on leadership roles'. Furthermore, it is suggested that research is required on the subject of leadership, specifically in healthcare organizations in order to positively influence leadership training and organizational structure and development.[37]

Mentoring relationships have received a lot of attention recently, for example in Canada, Pakistan and the UK.[9,38,39] There is also a growing evidence base that highlights the benefits of mentoring to individuals and companies,[40] and psychiatrists at any stage in their careers may benefit from mentoring.

The European Psychiatric Association has run a mentoring programme for the past few years whereby promising young psychiatrists are given the opportunity to be mentored by world-leading experts in their chosen field.[41] In the UK, the Department of Health and the Royal College of Psychiatrists have jointly and robustly recommended that 'new job descriptions [should] not be approved without a mentor being identified'.[42]

The mentoring relationship should not involve a mentor with line-management responsibility for the early career psychiatrist, and should be informal and supportive.[43] In the case of newly appointed consultants, meetings should be arranged regularly (at least once a month), with an agreed structure and agenda. The period of the mentoring relationship varies in length, but typical periods may be up to 2 years.[44]

Roberts et al.[45] outlined some of the aims and purposes of the mentoring relationship in a scheme that was established for new consultant psychiatrists in the UK, which can be applied to other mentoring relationships (Table 20.2).

Interestingly, early career specialists who had joined units with 'flat structured cooperative environments where everybody is involved in decision making' reported some of the most satisfactory experiences of transition.[17] This is a critical point for organizations as it has far wider implications than simply meeting the needs of early career specialists. Early career specialist groups and networks have spontaneously or deliberately been set up across the world, as reflected, for example nationally, in the structures of the American Psychiatric Association and the Italian Association of Psychiatrists. Many local level initiatives have sought to address exactly the same needs.

Table 20.2 Aims and purposes of the mentoring relationship.

- An opportunity for 'mature reflection'
- Confidential advice
- Exploration of professional coping mechanisms
- A sounding board – someone to listen
- Realignment to professional realities, e.g. fallibility and uncertainty
- Setting priorities and managing time
- Induction into the consultant role
- Exploration of organizational culture
- Exploration of guiding values
- Sharing of experience

From Roberts et al., 2002.[45]

Conclusions

Whilst psychiatry residents may possess several professional competences acquired through their training to aid them, they are mostly ill-prepared for the administrative, management and leadership challenges they will meet as their careers develop. Research has highlighted a number of key issues that are of particular concern to early career psychiatrists, and identified the measures that can be undertaken to ensure a smooth transition from resident to early career specialist. Some training programmes have responded to concerns by increasing the amount of management education provided to psychiatrists during their training years; however, there are arguments for initiating this much earlier in a resident's career.

For psychiatrists in various stages of their career, the mentoring relationship can be extremely useful – in particular, however, early career psychiatrists as a group may benefit from participation in mentoring schemes in order to make the adjustment to new leadership roles as smooth and efficient as possible.

When successful, leadership can be incredibly rewarding. Key qualities required for good management and leadership include: appropriate strategy development, organizational knowledge, communication skills and the ability to inspire and motivate others in the team. Efficient and effective leadership is desirable in that it has beneficial consequences for clinical care and patient outcomes. We have earlier noted that other professions have not hesitated to take advantage of any gap in leadership. In the light of this it is important to increase the awareness among early career psychiatrists of the critical role of leadership. Obtaining formal training, experience and qualifications in leadership can only strengthen our ability as psychiatrists to continue to lead the way in mental health.

References

1. Guze SB. *Why Psychiatry is a Branch of Medicine*. New York: Oxford University Press, 1992.
2. Levin BL, Henson A, Kuppin S. Leadership and training in mental health. In: Reid WH, Silver SB (eds) *Handbook of Mental Health Administration and Management*. Hove: Brunner-Routledge, 2003; pp. 22–40.
3. Bartlett C, Ghoshal S. Changing the role of top management: beyond systems to people. *Harvard Bus Rev* 1995; **73**: 132–142.
4. Chervenak F. The moral foundation of medical leadership: the professional virtues of the physician as fiduciary of the patient. *Am J Obstet Gynecol* 2001; **184**: 875–879.
5. Kotter J. *Leading Change*. Cambridge, MA: Harvard Business School Press, 1996; p. 25.
6. Edmonstone J. What is clinical leadership development? In: Edmonstone J (ed.) *Clinical Leadership: A Book of Readings*. Chichester: Kingsham Press: 2005; pp. 16–19.
7. Millward L, Bryan K. Clinical leadership: a position statement. *Leadership in Health Services* 2005; **18**: xiii–xxv.
8. Department of Health. *Medical Leadership Competency Framework*, 33rd edn. London: Department of Health, 2010.
9. Beezhold, J. The needs of new consultants. *Adv Psychiatry Treat* 2008; **14**: 321–325.
10. Levinson H. *Organisational Diagnosis*. Cambridge, MA: Harvard University Press, 1962.
11. Fitzgerald L. (2006) in Edmonstone J. Clinical leadership: the elephant in the room. *Int J Health Plann and Managem* 2009; **24**: 290–305.
12. Looney JG, Harding RK, Blocky MJ, Barnhart FD. Psychiatrists' transition from training to career: stress and mastery. *Am J Psychiatry* 1980; **137**: 32–36.
13. Mooney, A. *Royal College of Physicians New Consultant Survey*. London: Royal College of Physicians, 2003.
14. Beckett M, Hulbert D, Brown R. The new consultant survey 2005. *Emerg Med J* 2006; **23**: 461–463.
15. Sandler M. Training experience and views of recently appointed consultants in geriatric medicine. *J Roy Coll Phys* 1992; **26**: 44–46.
16. McKinstry B, Macnicol M, Elliot K *et al*. The transition from learner to provider/teacher: the learning needs of new orthopaedic consultants. *BMC Med Educ* 2005; **5**: 17.
17. Houghton A, Peters T, Bolton J. What do new consultants have to say ? *BMJ Career Focus* 2002; **325**: S145.
18. Robinowitz C. Psychiatrists as leaders in academic medicine. *Acad Psychiatry* 2006; **30**: 273–278.

19. Bickel J. Turning intellectual capital into leadership capital: why and how psychiatrists can take the lead. *Acad Psychiatry* 2007; **31**: 1–4.
20. Wilson D. The seven deadly sins of academic chairs. *Acad Psychiatry* 2006; **30**: 304–308.
21. Yu-Chin R. Teaching administration and management within psychiatric residency training. *Acad Psychiatry* 2002; **26**: 245–252.
22. Buckley P. Leadership development: more than on-the-job training. *The Psychiatrist* 2009; **33**: 401–403.
23. Licinio J. A leadership crisis in American psychiatry. *Mol Psychiat* 2004; 9: 1.
24. Hill S. How do you manage a flexible firm? The Total Quality Model. *Work Employ Soc* 1991; **5**: 397–415.
25. Edmonstone J. Clinical leadership: the elephant in the room. *Int J Health Planning Management* 2009; **24**: 290–305.
26. Nolan A. Clinical leadership. Structural instability. *Health Serv J* 2006; **116**: 25.
27. Greiner C. Leadership for psychiatrists. *Acad Psychiatry* 2006; **30**: 283–288.
28. Porter M. (1991) In Levin BL, Hanson A, Kuppin S. Leadership and training in mental health. In: Reid WH, Silver SB (eds) *Handbook of Mental Health Administration and Management.* Hove, UK: Brunner-Routledge, 2003; pp. 22–40.
29. Laffel G, Blumenthal D. The case for using industrial quality management science in health care organizations. *JAMA* 1989; **262**: 2869–2873.
30. Haynes AB, Weiser TG, Berry WR *et al.* A surgical safety checklist to reduce morbidity and mortality in a global population. *N Engl J Med* 2009; **360**: 491–499.
31. Denis J, Lamothe L, Langley A. The dynamics of collective leadership and strategic change in pluralistic organisations. *Acad Manage J* 2001; **44**: 809–837.
32. Cray S, Lawrance C. *Good Practice Guide to Consultant Recruitment and Retention.* Salomons, 2006.
33. Edmonstone J. *Building on the Best: An Introduction to Appreciative Inquiry in Health Care.* Chichester, UK: Kingsham Press, 2006.
34. Farkas C, Wetlaufer S. The ways chief executive officers lead. *Harvard Bus Rev* 1996; **74**: 110–122.
35. Bhugra D, Bell S, Burns A (eds). *Management for Psychiatrists,* 3rd edn. London: RCPsych Publications, 2007.
36. Bonner J. Preparing to consult. *BMJ Careers* 2005; **22**: 182–183.
37. Ham C. Improving the performance of health services: the role of clinical leadership. *Lancet* 2003; **361**: 1978–1980.
38. Puddester D. The early career psychiatrist: perspectives on academic and personal development. *Bull Can Psychiatr Assoc* 2003; Dec, 11–14.
39. Gadit A. Mentorship Program in Mental Health: Time to develop a new academic relationship. *J Pakistan Med Assoc* 2007; **57**: 527–528.
40. Oxley J. *Mentoring for Doctors: Signposts to Current Practice for Career Grade Doctors. Guidance from the Doctors' Forum.* London: Department of Health, 2004.

41. Fiorillo A, Volpe U, Calliess I, *et al*. Young psychiatrists' committee of the European Psychiatric Association: an essential tool for the future. *Eur Psychiatry* 2010; free communication pages.
42. Department of Health and Royal College of Psychiatrists. *Recommendations to Increase the Recruitment of and the Overall Numbers of Consultant Psychiatrists and to Improve their Retention*. London: Department of Health, 2004.
43. Dean A. Mentors for newly appointed consultants. *Adv Psychiatr Treat* 2003; **9**: 164–165.
44. Royal College of Psychiatrists. *Mentoring and Coaching* [OP 66]. London: Royal College of Psychiatrists, 2008.
45. Roberts G, Moore B, Coles C. Mentoring for newly-appointed psychiatrists. *Psychiatr Bull* 2002; **26**: 106–109.

CHAPTER 21

Why should I pay for it? The importance of being members of psychiatric associations

Andrea Fiorillo,[1] Iris Tatjana Calliess[2] and Domenico Giacco[1]
[1]Department of Psychiatry, University of Naples SUN, Naples, Italy
[2]Department of Psychiatry, Social Psychiatry and Psychotherapy, Institute for Standardized and Applied Hospital Management, Hannover School of Medicine, Germany

Introduction

Scientific associations have important implications for the professional development of medical doctors. It is extremely relevant to be part of a scientific community, whose members can share professional difficulties and problems and receive medical education and updated information on the most recent scientific advances in the field.[1] Usually, scientific associations reach their goals through three main tools: a congress, a website and a journal (with differences among the different associations, of course). While a website can rapidly and efficiently provide information concerning the life of the association and of its members, the main role of the congress is community building, by facilitating physical meetings and leading to establishment of networks, which are useful to reduce professional isolation; moreover, during congresses updated knowledge on scientific advances is provided. Finally, a journal and a bulletin play an important role in transferring information about the activities and scientific publications produced by a given association; moreover, they publish papers within the field of interest of the association.

Joining scientific associations may be particularly inspiring for junior doctors, who have the chance to improve their training curricula, update their professional knowledge and find a way to solve their job difficulties.

How to Succeed in Psychiatry: A Guide to Training and Practice, First Edition.
Edited by Andrea Fiorillo, Iris Tatjana Calliess and Henning Sass.
© 2012 John Wiley & Sons, Ltd. Published 2012 by John Wiley & Sons, Ltd.

The transition from residency to specialistic work nowadays represents an important challenge for early career doctors, mainly due to the greater relevance given to medical professional responsibility (in many countries, residents have tutors during their clinical activities, but not when they start their career), demanding workloads (which can, in turn, lead to professional isolation and burnout, described in detail in Chapter 19 of this book), and to working with patients who are, in most cases, simply different from those seen during residency years (unlike in other medical specialties, early career psychiatrists usually take care of the most difficult patients).[2]

Professional associations may play an important role in addressing at least some of the difficulties faced by early career psychiatrists. These associations bring peer groups together, thereby counteracting any feelings of loneliness, and influencing decisions about training and practice. Meeting periodically with other early career psychiatrists from one's own or other countries, comparing training programmes, becoming informed about common challenges in clinical practice and providing useful advice – all may contribute to improved training and daily clinical work.[3]

Several associations for early career psychiatrists are active in this respect worldwide. The first group of young colleagues aiming to start an association was the European Federation of Psychiatric Trainees, whose first Forum dates back to 1993. At the World Congress of Psychiatry in 1999, which took place in Hamburg, the first World Psychiatric Association (WPA) young psychiatrists' network was created, including all fellows to that Congress. Finally, the European Psychiatric Association started its own programme for young psychiatrists in 2004 during the Geneva Congress. Since then, the road has been long and fruitful.

In this chapter we will focus on scientific associations dedicated to trainees or to psychiatrists at their early career stages. Of course, this will not be an exhaustive review of all existing national and international psychiatric associations. Our aim is to provide useful information about the programmes for early career psychiatrists of the WPA and of the European Psychiatric Association. Room will also be given to the European Federation of Psychiatric Trainees, the first independent federation of postgraduate medical trainees. Finally, some examples of national associations will be provided.

World Psychiatric Association (WPA) – Early Career Psychiatrists Council (ECPC)

The WPA is the largest psychiatric association, representing more than 200 000 psychiatrists all over the world. In recent years it has developed several initiatives for early career psychiatrists (ECPs).

During the 1999 World Congress of Psychiatry, which took place in Hamburg, a list of young psychiatrists was invited to attend the congress and to establish the first WPA Congress Fellows Network. Currently, more than 350 ECPs from all over the world are included in this network and have periodical access to the activities of the WPA.

In 2003 the WPA Executive Committee established the Young Psychiatrists Council (WPA-YPC), including all trainees and ECPs registered to their national psychiatric associations. In 2009, the WPA-YPC was completely restructured and changed its name to the WPA Early Career Psychiatrists Council (WPA-ECPC), with one representative being nominated by each WPA Member Society for a 3-year mandate. The WPA-ECPC has been subdivided into five geographical areas, each with one coordinator: (i) Europe I, which includes Northern, Southern and Western Europe; (ii) Europe II, which includes Central and Eastern Europe; (iii) Asia/Australasia; (iv) Africa and the Middle East; (v) the Americas.

Aims

The WPA-ECPC aims to:
1. upgrade communication concerning ECPs between WPA Member Societies and WPA bodies;
2. identify and address problems concerning ECPs;
3. promote the participation of ECPs in the activities of the different sections of the WPA;
4. contribute to activities aimed to promote the professional development of early career psychiatrists.

Activities

The WPA-ECPC participates in several WPA activities:
1. The translation into several languages, and their adaptation to various national contexts, of three sets of slides of the WPA Programme on Depression and Physical Diseases. In particular, the slides on depression and diabetes have been translated into 16 languages (Azeri, Bangla, Bosnian, Croatian, Czech, Estonian, French, German, Indonesian, Italian, Japanese, Portuguese, Romanian, Russian, Spanish and Swedish). These slides are available on the WPA website (www.wpanet.org).
2. The conduction of surveys on training and practice of psychotherapy in Europe and on career choices after training.
3. The development, in collaboration with the WPA headquarters, of a section of the WPA website dedicated to ECPs, including information on the activities of the Council as well as other materials (papers, documents, announcements of meetings or publications, reports about

personal professional experiences), which may be of interest to early career psychiatrists worldwide.

4. The organization of symposia and meetings at the major WPA congresses and conferences.

5. The publication of papers on different issues related to psychiatric training.[4,5]

Further information on the WPA-ECPC is available at www.wpanet. org/subIndex.php?section_id=22&category_id=59.

European Psychiatric Association – Early Career Psychiatrists Committee (ECPC)

At the initial invitation of the European Psychiatric Association (EPA), an informal network of European young psychiatrists designed a specific scientific programme during the annual EPA congresses. This group of individuals, named the 'Young Psychiatrists Program Organizing Committee', had past involvement in the activities of the European Federation of Psychiatric Trainees. However, the committee structure was fragile and was not a part of the official body of the EPA, and its only mission was to develop a specific congress track for young psychiatrists at the European Congresses of 2005 in Munich and 2006 in Nice. After years of commitment, the leaders of the European Psychiatric Association recognized the need to create an officially recognized body for young psychiatrists; therefore, in 2007 the 'Young Psychiatrists' Committee' was officially founded with full committee status within the EPA. In 2010 the Committee changed its name into 'Early Career Psychiatrists' Committee'.

Aims

The Early Career Psychiatrists' Committee of the EPA was established with the specific aims to: (i) harmonize psychiatric training standards in Europe; (ii) promote quality of training across Europe; (iii) evaluate psychiatric training in Europe; (iv) understand young psychiatrists' and trainees' opinions about training and the first years of their professional life; (v) communicate these opinions to relevant European and national bodies; and (vi) promote and develop national young psychiatrists' and trainees' associations.[1]

In 2011, the Committee approved an Action Plan, which includes activities in the following four areas: publications, meetings, educational activities and research activities. For each of these activities, a workgroup has been nominated, including one EPA mentor and up to five European distinguished early career psychiatrists.

Early Career Psychiatrists' Congress Programme

The Early Career Psychiatrists' Programme takes place during the annual EPA Congress and includes special symposia, workshops, meet-the-experts sessions, happy-hour meetings with European leaders, interactive Continuing Medical Education (CME) courses and social events.

One of the initial goals of the programme was to facilitate a smooth integration of young psychiatrists into the annual European Congress and to allow those rather conference-inexperienced young doctors to network and to meet leaders in the psychiatric field. Therefore, in each Congress a 'lounge' space is dedicated to all young psychiatrists attending the conference. This lounge, which offers a unique opportunity for young psychiatrists to meet informally, is usually a large space with technical equipment that facilitates networking and communication among young colleagues.

Since 2007 a scholarship programme has been initiated to promote clinical and scientific excellence among ECPs, allowing the participation of European ECPs in the EPA Congress by covering their travel and accommodation expenses. Since 2008, a mentoring scheme for alumni/scholars has been implemented, with the valuable collaboration of well-known EPA leaders. Furthermore, in order to encourage scientific contributions from ECPs, every year research awards are granted to ECPs who have published the best scientific papers in international journals indexed in Current Contexts. Further information on the EPA Early Career Psychiatrists Committee is available at http://www.europsy.net/what-we-do/early-career-psychiatrists/.

European Federation of Psychiatric Trainees

The European Federation of Psychiatric Trainees (EFPT) is an independent, nonprofit, international federation of national associations of psychiatric trainees in Europe. The EFPT was created in 1992 by the personal initiative of a small group of psychiatric trainees from nine European countries, and formally established in 1993. Since then, the Federation has constantly expanded, each year organizing a Forum of all European psychiatric trainees. The active support provided to the establishment of new psychiatric trainees' associations has significantly enlarged the number of European countries participating in the EFPT Forum, which currently are more than 30.[6]

The Forum usually takes place at the end of the spring in the country of the President. One of the major achievements of the EFPT, so far, is the close collaboration with the Section and Board of Psychiatry of the UEMS (European Union of Medical Specialists). This allows the views of psychiatric residents to be considered when implementing changes to the training programmes.[6,7]

Aims

The EFPT's main objectives are:

1. To explore differences in psychiatric training across Europe.
2. To further the development of national psychiatric trainees' organizations in European countries.
3. To promote and represent the views and needs of psychiatric trainees to relevant international bodies.
4. To improve training in psychiatry at local levels.
5. To create networks among European psychiatric trainees.

Organization and activities

The general governing body of the EFPT is the General Assembly, which meets annually during the EFPT Forum. The General Assembly is composed of two delegates from each member country (with one vote per country) and elects the seven officers of the EFPT Board of Directors (president, president elect, immediate past president, child and adolescent representative, general secretary, IT secretary, treasurer) who perform executive functions for the federation. In the course of the Forum a poster session is organized each year with a different theme related to psychiatric training, and national delegates present the 'country reports', outlining the current situation of psychiatric training in all the participating countries.

The activities of the EFPT, during the Forum and throughout the year, are carried out through several working groups addressing issues related to psychiatric training, such as competency-based training, psychotherapy training, research experience, relationships with the pharmaceutical industry, etc. On completion of their activities, the EFPT working groups produce: (i) consensus statements, which are used to circulate the opinions of psychiatric trainees to the relevant bodies (UEMS, senior professional and scientific associations, political bodies, etc.); and (ii) publications in scientific journals. Further information is available on the EFPT official website: www.efpt.eu.

In Table 21.1 the most important achievements of the EFPT, and the Forums at which they were formalized, are reported in order to give readers an example of the development of an independent professional association.

National associations

In the next paragraphs some national associations of early career psychiatrists will be described. Of course, many other associations exist in the various countries and regions of the world, and a comprehensive list of these associations is provided in Table 21.2.

Table 21.1 Main achievements of the European Federation of
Psychiatric Trainees (EFPT) Forums.

1993 – Utrecht	Official establishment of the EFPT
1994 – Cork	
1995 – Copenhagen	Participation of EFPT representatives in the meetings of the UEMS (Union Européenne des Médecins Spécialistes) Board of Psychiatry
1996 – Lisbon	
1997 – Athens	Inclusion of all EU countries and several Eastern European countries in EFPT
1998 – Ghent	Election of the first EFPT Board
1999 – Tampere	Permanent seat in the UEMS Board
2000 – Berlin	Enhancement of the collaboration with the UEMS
2001 – Naples	Creation of the EFPT website
2002 – Sinaia	
2003 – Paris	Conduction of a survey on satisfaction with training
2004 – Cambridge	Start registration process as a NGO
2005 – Istanbul	Collaboration with the European Psychiatric Association
2006 – Riga	
2007 – Athens	Collaboration with the UEMS in the formulation of a Competency Based Training
2008 – Göteborg	
2009 – Cambridge	
2010 – Dubrovnik	Registration as a NGO based in Brussels (Belgium) Approval of the EFPT Bylaws
2011 – Prague	
2012 – Sorrento	

Italy

The Italian Psychiatric Society (Società Italiana di Psichiatria, SIP) was one of the first scientific psychiatric societies to create, in 2000, a specific programme for ECPs. A special area of the society, dedicated to young members, was established in order to facilitate the full integration of Italian ECPs into the activities of the society. The early career psychiatrists' committee is composed of a president and 17 regional coordinators, who meet at least four times a year to undertake joint projects and share local experiences. The principal aim of the committee is to promote the professional development of ECPs. To achieve this goal, five areas of work have been identified: (i) organization of educational events and activities, on the basis of the ECPs' training needs; (ii) identification of relevant areas for the training of ECPs, such as ethics and forensic psychiatry, psychopathology, clinical psychiatry and psychotherapy; (iii) mentoring by more experienced members; (iv) collaboration with other national and international societies of young psychiatrists; and (v) conduction of research projects for ECPs and publication of their results. Further information can be found at www.giovanipsichiatrisip.wordpress.com.

Table 21.2 National early career psychiatrists' associations.

Country	Association	Website
Austria	Austrian Association of Psychiatry and Psychotherapy – Psychiatric Trainees' section	
Belarus	Young psychiatrists' section of the Belarusian Psychiatric Association	groups.google.com/group/belyoungpsy
Belgium (Flemish part)	Vlaamse Vereniging Assistenten Psychiatrie (VVAP) (Flemish Association of Psychiatry Trainees)	www.kuleuven.be/vvap
Brazil	Programa de Desenvolvimento Profissional para Psiquiatras em Formação da Associação Brasileira de Psiquiatria	www.abpbrasil.org.br/medicos/psiquiatra_formacao/
Bosnia-Herzegovina	Association for residents and young psychiatrists and neuropsychiatrists	Under construction
Canada	Member-in-Training (MIT) Section of the Canadian Psychiatric Association	www.cpa-apc.org/browse/documents/171
Colombia	Comité de Residentes de Psiquiatría de la Asociación Colombiana de Psiquiatría	http://www.psiquiatria.org.co/BancoConocimiento/R/residentes/residentes.asp
Croatia	Croatian Young Psychiatrists and Psychiatric Trainees Section	www.mladi.psihijatrija.hr/?lang=en
Czech Republic	The Section of Young Psychiatrists of the Czech Psychiatric Association	www.psychiatrie.cz/index.php?option=com_content&view=section&id=5&Itemid=16
Denmark	Foreningen af Yngre Psykiatere (FYP)	www.dpsnet.dk
Egypt	Early Career Psychiatrists Section, Egyptian Psychiatric Association	www.epaegypt.com/StaticPage.aspx?SPID=8

Finland (Adult Psychiatry)	The Trainees' section of the Finnish Psychiatric Association	www.psy.fi
Finland (Child and Adolescent Psychiatry)	Trainee Section of the Finnish Society for Child and Adolescent Psychiatry	www.lpsy.org
France	Association Française Fédérative des Etudiants en Psychiatrie	www.affep.net
Germany	Young Psychiatrists (Deutsche Gesellschaft für Psychiatrie, Psychotherapie und Nervenheilkunde)	www.dgppn.de
Greece	Hellenic Association of Psychiatric Trainees	
Ireland	Trainee Committee, College of Psychiatry of Ireland	http://www.irishpsychiatry.ie/Postgrad_Training.aspx
Israel	The Israeli forum for psychiatric trainees	
Italy	Early Career Psychiatrists' Committee of the Italian Society of Psychiatry	www.giovanipsichiatrisip.wordpress.com
Japan	Japan Young Psychiatrists Organization (JYPO)	http://jypo.umin.jp/eng_home/n_represent.html
The Netherlands	Netherlands psychiatric trainees association (Subvereniging Assistenten Psychiatrie, SAP)	www.nvvp.net
Poland	Division of Psychiatric Training, Polish Psychiatric Association	www.ptp.cm-uj.krakow.pl/sks/index.php
Portugal	Associação Portuguesa de Internos de Psiquiatria (APIP)	www.apipsiquiatria.pt
Romania	Asociatia Medicilor Rezidenti in Psihitrie Din Romania	www.amrpr.ro

(continued overleaf)

Table 21.2 (Continued)

Country	Association	Website
Serbia	Serbian Young Psychiatrists' Section (SYPS)	www.ups-spa.org/
Sweden	The Swedish association of psychiatric trainees (SLUP)	http://www.svenskpsykiatri.se/utbildning_st.html
Switzerland	Schweizerische Vereinigung psychiatrischer Assistenzärztinnen und Assistenzärzte (SVPA) (in German) or Association suisse des médecins assistantes et assistants en psychiatrie (ASMAP) (in French)	www.svpa-asmap.com
Turkey (Adult Psychiatry)	Trainees' committee under the Psychiatric Association of Turkey	www.psikiyatri.org.tr/
Turkey (Child and Adolescent Psychiatry)	Turkish Association for Child and Adolescent Psychiatry	www.cogepder.org.tr/
United Kingdom	Trainees' section of the Royal College of Psychiatrists	www.rcpsych.ac.uk/specialtytraining/trainees/ptc.aspx
United States of America	Assembly Committee on Early Career Psychiatrists of the American Psychiatric Association	www.psych.org/Resources/EarlyCareerPsychiatrists.aspx

United Kingdom

The Royal College of Psychiatrists (RCP) is the representative body for psychiatrists and psychiatric trainees in the UK. It is responsible for the definition of professional standards, communication and health policy for psychiatry, and relations with other representative bodies. In particular, the RCP directly defines the standards and procedures for postgraduate training in psychiatry. Within the RCP, there is a specific section for psychiatric trainees, the Psychiatric Trainees' Committee (PTC), which consists of 40 members, elected from the Divisions (i.e. regional subgroups of England), Wales, Scotland, Northern Ireland, the Republic of Ireland and the British Armed Forces. The 40 representatives of the PTC have essentially two fundamental responsibilities: the first is participation in the general management and supervision of the RCP's activities (the PTC has representatives on all the main committees of the RCP); the second is more specific and refers to the formulation and ratification of the main aspects of educational policy, the implementation of periodic reviews of the psychiatric training curriculum and the definition of its standards. The RCP organizes the Annual Medical Education and Training Residential Conference, during which residents attend workshops and lectures by prominent experts on the management and the treatment of major mental disorders. Postgraduate trainees are actively involved in the preparation of these events and can present the results of their own research projects in specific sessions. Furthermore, four years ago the RCP established the College Education and Training Centre (CETC), whose aims are to promote high-quality training for postgraduate psychiatric residents and, in general, for psychiatrists, to facilitate collaboration between specific sections of the RCP and individual universities, and to organize high-quality training events on specific topics, in all training centres. Further information can be found on the official website of the Royal College of Psychiatrists: www.rcpsych.ac.uk.

Republic of Ireland

In the Irish College of Psychiatry, the Psychiatric Trainees' Committee and Section are active. The Committee supervises the psychiatric trainees' section, but also promotes and ensures the participation of early career psychiatrists in the activities of the College. The Section has the objective of contributing to the improvement of postgraduate training standards in Ireland. The representatives of the Irish ECPs always participate in the meetings of the Council and of the Faculty of the College, thus ensuring that the views of postgraduate trainees are represented in all the decisions made by these bodies. The Psychiatric Trainees' Committee meets regularly (on average every 4–6 weeks) and has frequent meetings with representatives of trainees in other specialties. The Psychiatric

Trainees' Section organizes an annual educational event, which aims to address relevant training issues and contribute to the professional development of early career psychiatrists. Further information can be found on the official website of the College of Psychiatry of Ireland: http://irishpsychiatry.ie/Postgrad_Training.aspx.

France
The Association Française Fédérative des Etudiants en Psychiatrie (AFFEP) is an independent association of French psychiatric trainees, founded in 1998, with the following main objectives:
1. To improve psychiatric training standards in France.
2. To participate in the European network of psychiatric trainees.
3. To carry out psychiatric research in the areas of neuroscience, epidemiology, clinical research, human sciences and psychotherapy.

Since 2007, the AFFEP has represented all postgraduate psychiatric trainees in France, and is organized as a federation of regional trainees' associations. The AFFEP has launched various initiatives aimed at the evaluation and improvement of psychiatric training in France. Networking among members is ensured by a dynamic and highly informative website and a mailing list. The Association elects a representative to the National Council of postgraduate trainees (Inter Syndicat National des Internes des Hôpitaux, ISNIH), the official delegate to the annual Forum of the EFPT and an official representative to the National Association of Psychiatry (Fédération Française de Psychiatrie). Finally, the AFFEP organizes educational events specifically dedicated to postgraduate psychiatric trainees, including the 'Day of the trainee' (Journée de l'Interne, organized at the beginning of each academic year and open to all trainees of the first year), and various training events on psychiatric and humanistic issues (anthropology, sociology, philosophy, etc.). Further information is available on the official website of the Association Française Fédérative des Etudiants en Psychiatrie: www.affep.net/.

Germany
The Association of German Young Psychiatrists and Trainees was founded in 2001. It is initially formed as a committee within the national senior psychiatric association. However, from the outset the creation of a network of psychiatric residents and the collaboration with other national bodies met some important needs of German ECPs. At the same time, several initiatives were implemented to promote the involvement of young psychiatrists in the annual meetings of the senior association. Within a few years, the section was formally established and the structure of its Board defined. Currently, the Association of German Young Psychiatrists and Trainees is well recognized nationally and internationally. It

is represents about 3800 young German psychiatrists. Each year, at the Congress of the senior association, specially tailored Young Psychiatrists' Programme is organized; in addition, regional training events are regularly held throughout Germany. In accordance with the standards of the European Union of Medical Specialists (UEMS). A special mentoring programme was established to encourage young doctors and senior medical students to start a career in psychiatry. A website is active to facilitate the diffusion of information in general and on job vacancies for young psychiatrists. Further information is available on the website of the German Association for Psychiatry, Psychotherapy and Nervous Diseases (DGPPN): www.dgppn.de.

United States

During its congresses, the American Psychiatric Association (APA) organizes specific sessions dedicated to ECPs, i.e. young American psychiatrists currently in postgraduate training or who have completed their training no more than 7 years ago. Furthermore, the APA established a committee, the Assembly Committee on Early Career Psychiatrists, with the principal aim of promoting the professional development of psychiatrists during their early career stages. This committee provides bi-directional communication between the APA and its younger members in the early stages of their psychiatric careers, in order to enhance the experiences of ECPs within the APA and to promote their professional development. In particular, the main objectives of the Assembly are: (i) to help identify and represent the interests of early career psychiatrists locally, regionally and nationally; (ii) to facilitate participation of ECPs within the membership and leadership of the APA and its district branches; and (iii) to contribute to policy-making and educational endeavours of the APA as they relate to the professional development of ECPs. Further information is available on the website of the APA – Early Career Psychiatrists Program: http://www.psych.org/Resources/EarlyCareerPsychiatrists.aspx.

References

1. Fiorillo A, Calliess I, Volpe U et al. Young Psychiatrists' Committee of the European Psychiatric Association: an essential tool for the future. *Eur Psychiatry* 2010; available at: http://www.europsy.net/wordpress/wp-content/uploads/2011/07/fiorillo_ypc.pdf?rs_file_key=6322561824e2fe7022a 438610355618.
2. De Rosa C. I primi passi nei dipartimenti di salute mentale italiani. In: Fiorillo A, Bassi M, Siracusano A (eds) *Professione Psichiatra: a practical guide.* Roma: Il Pensiero Scientifico, 2009; pp. 1–14.
3. Martinez DB. Getting involved: participating in professional organizations. In: Foreman T, Dickstein LJ, Garakani A (eds) *A Resident's Guide To Surviving*

Psychiatric Training, 2nd edn. Arlington: American Psychiatric Association, 2003; pp. 56–58.
4. Fiorillo A, Lattova Z, Brambhatt P, El Kholy H, Picon F. The Action Plan 2010 of the WPA Early Career Psychiatrists Council. *World Psychiatry* 2010; **9**: 62–63.
5. Fiorillo A, Brambhatt P, El Kholy H, Lattova Z, Picon F. Activities of the WPA Early Career Psychiatrists Council: the Action Plan is in progress. *World Psychiatry* 2011; **10**: 159.
6. Nawka A, Rojnic Kuzman M, Giacco D, Malik A. Challenges of postgraduate psychiatric training in Europe: a trainee perspective. *Psychiatr Serv* 2010; **61**: 862–864.
7. Rojnic Kuzman M, Nawka A, Giacco D *et al*. European Federation of Psychiatric Trainees (EFPT): the journey and the future. *Eur Psychiatry* 2010; free communication pages.

Index

How to Succeed in Psychiatry: A Guide to Training and Practice, First Edition.
Edited by Andrea Fiorillo, Iris Tatjana Calliess and Henning Sass.
© 2012 John Wiley & Sons, Ltd. Published 2012 by John Wiley & Sons, Ltd.